W Britt
Tonawanda
1918

THE SOURCES AND MODES OF INFECTION

By

CHARLES V. CHAPIN, M.D., Sc. D.

SUPERINTENDENT OF HEALTH, PROVIDENCE, R. I.
AUTHOR OF "MUNICIPAL SANITATION IN THE UNITED STATES"

SECOND EDITION REVISED AND ENLARGED

SECOND THOUSAND

NEW YORK
JOHN WILEY & SONS, Inc.
London: CHAPMAN & HALL, Limited
1916

Stanhope Press
F. H. GILSON COMPANY
BOSTON, U.S.A.

PREFACE.

THIS volume is intended to indicate the principles which should guide sanitary practice, and to show how recent laboratory work and the epidemiological study of disease have modified these principles. When I began work as health officer in 1884 the filth theory was still in favor, and it was generally believed that the germs of disease commonly grew in decaying organic matter. Yet contagion was recognized as an important factor in the spread of disease, and the isolation of the sick was more and more insisted upon. Fifteen years ago probably most health officials believed that the contagious diseases could be completely stamped out if only all persons sick with them could be isolated. The air was thought to be the chief medium for their transmission, and fomites the mechanism for their passage from place to place. Sanitary practice was based on these premises.

My own views concerning these matters became greatly modified year by year, partly owing to the rapidly accumulating knowledge of bacteria and other disease-producing organisms, and partly owing to direct observations on the manner in which the infectious diseases are disseminated, and on the effect of preventive measures.

It now appears that the growth of disease germs outside of the body is not frequent enough to be an important factor in the causation of disease, but their growth in the body without causing sickness, their latency as it were, often for many months, is a factor of very great significance. We know now that direct contact with the sick, or with healthy carriers of disease germs, is an exceedingly frequent mode of transmission, and that infection by means of the air, or from infected articles, is not nearly as common as was formerly believed.

We are now better able than ever before to attribute to water and milk their proper share in the distribution of infection. The recent discovery of the transmission of disease by insects gives us entirely new and most effective means of combating disease. It is time that sanitary measures directed against the infectious diseases should be modified to correspond with existing knowledge. Present-day theories and present-day practice are maintained largely by tradition, and to facilitate the adaptation of practice to the facts as we now know them, is the purpose of this book. Some modifications of sanitary practice are suggested, but no attempt is made to discuss details; rather are general principles presented, which it is believed ought to guide administrators in their work.

While some of the following pages may seem rather radical to many, I believe that practically all laboratory workers will agree with the contents of the first chapter, and that a large number of bacteriologists and health officers are convinced of the great importance of "carriers" and mild unrecognized cases. The tendency among many, too, is to lay less emphasis on infection by fomites, though perhaps few are ready to give up routine terminal disinfection for the common infectious diseases. So also there are very many careful observers who are attributing more and more importance to what is generally called contact infection.

The public health administrator is placed at great disadvantage because he is obliged to base his acts on knowledge which is far from exact. The laboratory workers have accumulated a vast mass of quite exact data in regard to the causative relation of bacteria and protozoa to disease, and no one appreciates this more than the writer, but there are many problems which the laboratory men cannot solve, and many others which they have failed to solve. The epidemiologist must study in the field the way in which disease is caused. He must use the statistical method, and the application of statistical methods to epidemiology is more difficult and less attractive than laboratory experiment.

We need to measure more carefully the relative importance of different sources of disease and different modes of infection. It is not so important to know that typhoid bacilli live in water for weeks, as it is to know that 99 per cent die in one week. It is not enough to discover that diphtheria bacilli can be recovered from articles in the sick-room; we must learn how often they are found and how often disease is traced to such a source. We have for years been much alarmed because tubercle bacilli are found in milk, but since a serious effort has been made to measure the actual danger, the alarm has greatly diminished. Doubtless the house fly has been the cause of typhoid fever, but in what percentage of cases we are profoundly ignorant. Healthy carriers of diphtheria have certainly transmitted the disease to others, and we should earnestly try to determine the amount of diphtheria caused in this way. The attempt is made in the following pages to estimate roughly, with the very imperfect material now available, the relative importance of different factors in the extension of infectious diseases. The conclusions must to a large extent be merely tentative, and as indicating lines for further study.

I am under great obligations to my friends Dr. H. W. Hill and particularly Prof. F. P. Gorham for many suggestions and criticisms, but neither is to be considered at all responsible for any of the views presented.

The book is intended primarily for health officers and physicians, but it is hoped that many others will find some parts interesting and suggestive.

CHARLES V. CHAPIN.

PROVIDENCE, April, 1910.

PREFACE TO SECOND EDITION.

So much new material has accumulated since the appearance of the first edition that it has been thought best to rewrite several parts of the book. Thus, recent experiments and particularly the observation that bacteria fresh from the body are usually less resistant than are "cultured" germs, indicate that the life of bacteria outside the body is even shorter than was supposed. It is in regard to carriers that literature has been accumulating most rapidly and several comprehensive articles, as well as very numerous reports of carrier infection, leave no room for doubt that in many diseases, as diphtheria, cholera, typhoid fever and cerebro-spinal meningitis, the carrier is a very important, if not the most important, factor in the spread of the disease. Also recent work has shown that contact with carriers is quite likely to be the key to the epidemiology of poliomyelitis. New evidence has been presented concerning the carriage of infection by milk and also by water, but I cannot see that the reality of the Mills-Reincke phenomenon, which depends upon the influence of water on so many forms of disease, has yet been established. Much work during the past two years has been devoted to insects as carriers of infection and several additional diseases have been shown probably to be so transmitted. One of the most interesting of these is typhus fever, and, if recent work is substantiated, much light will be thrown on its epidemiology. While there is more evidence than there was that the fly is a factor in the spread of the fecal-borne diseases, there does not as yet seem to be much warrant for the rather sensational literature with which the public is deluged. Studies in hospitals and elsewhere have confirmed the belief that air is of minor importance in the spread of disease. The views presented in the first edition in regard to the inutility of isolation under many conditions, and in regard to the small importance of fomites, were somewhat novel and it was suspected that they might be subjected to considerable criticism, but such does not seem to have appeared, and I still believe that, while isolation and bedside disinfection will in the future continue to be, when scientifically applied, of the utmost importance, much of the routine practice of health officials needs to be profoundly modified.

CHARLES V. CHAPIN.

Providence, July, 1912.

CONTENTS.

CHAPTER I.

LIFE OF DISEASE GERMS OUTSIDE OF THE BODY.

PAGE

Review of evidence of growth of disease germs outside of the body, anthrax, black leg, tetanus. — Typhoid bacilli in soil, feces, water, ice, oysters, milk. — Epidemiological evidence relating to typhoid fever. — Evidence relating to cholera, Mediterranean fever, plague, dysentery, bacteria of suppuration, diphtheria and various other diseases. — Reasons for former belief in "filth theory" of disease. — Epidemiological evidence against soil infection. — Conclusions. — Relations of these views to public sanitation...... 1

CHAPTER II.

CARRIERS AND MISSED CASES.

Importance of the subject. — Evidence of the occurrence of carriers and missed cases, and reference to disease caused by them in typhoid fever, cholera, dysentery, cerebro-spinal meningitis, diphtheria, glanders, influenza, pneumonia, gonorrhea, tuberculosis, leprosy, suppuration, tetanus, scarlet fever, smallpox, measles, protozoan diseases such as cattle fever, malaria, sleeping sickness, nagana, syphilis, amebic dysentery, poliomyelitis and yellow fever. — Review of evidence. — Conclusions.... 33

CHAPTER III.

LIMITATIONS TO THE VALUE OF ISOLATION.

The number of carriers and missed cases. — Not realized by health officials. — Failure of isolation in Providence. — Hospitalization has not materially lessened infectious disease. — Less isolation followed by less diphtheria in Providence. — Failure of isolation in institutions. — Failures in the isolation of measles, of cerebro-spinal meningitis, of smallpox. — Failure due to carriers and missed cases. — Difficulties in the isolation of diphtheria. — Absolute isolation not possible. — Moderate isolation sufficient. — Infection not so easy as was believed. — Isolation effective at the beginning of an outbreak, rarely later. — The more carriers the less effective is isolation. — True value of isolation hospitals. — Details of home isolation. — Summary.................... 133

CHAPTER IV.

INFECTION BY CONTACT.

PAGE

Transmission of gonorrhea by indirect contact. — Of syphilis in the same way. — Typhoid fever spread by contact. — Reasons why contact infection has been disregarded. — Mode of contact infection in typhoid fever. — Contact infection in dysentery. — Cholera. — Anchylostomiasis. — Gonorrhea. — Transfer of nasal and oral secretions by contact. — Presence of germs in secretions and on various objects. — Diseases do not spread from family to family in tenements. — No cross infection in hospitals except by contact. — Contact infection in tuberculosis. — Protection from contact infection a personal matter. — Need for urging personal cleanliness. 164

CHAPTER V.

INFECTION BY FOMITES.

Definition. — Fomites and yellow fever. — Examples of alleged fomites infection. — Infection by clothing, rooms, rags, money. — Fomites infection in tetanus, anthrax, typhoid fever, diphtheria, plague. — No evidence that fomites are of much importance. — Reasons for belief in fomites. — Effect of drying on bacteria of different kinds. — The finding of bacteria on fomites. — Drying of vaccine and smallpox virus. — Summary of bacteriological evidence. — Experimental work with yellow fever, plague. — Results of abandoning disinfection after scarlet fever and diphtheria in Providence. — Disinfection in other diseases. — School disinfection. — Views of other writers. — Conclusions. 212

CHAPTER VI.

INFECTION BY AIR.

Alleged aerial transmission of smallpox, scarlet fever, diphtheria, typhoid fever, influenza, measles. — Hospital experiments in aerial transmission. — Transmission of typhus fever and plague. — History of surgical technique shows that air-borne infection is of little moment. — Air-borne anthrax. — Bacteria not given off from moist surfaces. — Bacteria carried in dust. — Dust and the germs of typhoid fever, diphtheria, plague. — Dust and tubercle bacilli. — Finding of tubercle bacilli in dust. — Other bacteria in dust. — Droplet infection. — Finding of bacteria in air. — Experimental work with tuberculosis, Mediterranean fever, anthrax, plague. — Conclusions. 259

CHAPTER VII.

INFECTION BY FOOD AND DRINK.

PAGE

The Broad Street well. — North Boston well. — Typhoid fever due to water. — Cholera, dysentery, diarrhea. — The Mills-Reincke phenomenon. — Malaria and yellow fever. — Purification of water. — Ice. — Milk, number of outbreaks. — Mode of infection of the milk. — Typhoid fever, scarlet fever, diphtheria. — Ice cream. — Butter. — Streptococcus sore throat and milk. — Tuberculosis and milk, evidence of infection. — Bacilli in market milk. — Amount of tuberculosis due to milk. — Mediterranean fever, anthrax, foot-and-mouth disease, rabies. — Diarrhea. — Infection by meat. — Infection by shellfish. — Crawfish. — Watercress. — Celery. 316

CHAPTER VIII.

INFECTION BY INSECTS.

Insects as biological and as mechanical carriers. — Pioneer work of Smith and Kilborne in cattle fever. — Malaria. — Modes of control: quinia, isolation, screening; mosquito reduction; practical results. — Yellow fever carried by mosquitoes, not by fomites. — Control of yellow fever; quarantine, isolation; mosquito control; practical results. — Filariasis, sleeping sickness, kala-azar, dengue, pellagra, opilacoa, pappataci fever, oriental sore, typhus fever, relapsing fever, Rocky Mountain fever. — Bubonic plague and fleas. — Anthrax. — Carriage of bacteria on the bodies of insects. — Cockroaches and other insects. — Flies, experimental work. — Bacteria found on flies. — Habits and species. — Transmission of disease, murrina, tuberculosis, cholera, dysentery, diarrhea. — Flies and typhoid fever, local and seasonal distribution. — Evidence against theory. — Epidemiological evidence in favor of causal relation. — Privies, flies and typhoid fever. — Conclusions.......... 380

THE SOURCES AND MODES OF INFECTION.

CHAPTER I.

LIFE OF DISEASE GERMS OUTSIDE OF THE BODY

Former Theories. — From time immemorial miasms, malarias, vapors and emanations, gaseous or otherwise, have been believed to be the frequent cause of disease. These miasms were thought to arise from stagnant marshes, decaying vegetation, putrid animal matter, and indeed filth of every kind. This belief in the extra-corporal origin of disease reached its widest acceptance about the middle of the nineteenth century. The rise of the germ theory greatly strengthened it. The discovery of bacteria and of their wide distribution and almost universal growth in dead organic substances, and the theory that these bacteria were the real cause of disease, led men to look for the source of disease outside of the body, and chiefly in dead animal and vegetable matter. With the passing of the germ theory as a theory, and with the demonstration of the parasitic nature of so many of our most important and dreaded diseases, the opportunity was afforded for studying in detail the bacteria and protozoa which are the specific causes of these diseases. Much has been done by laboratory workers to unravel the life history of these minute forms, and it is well for us to examine the knowledge thus gained, and also the newer epidemiological observations on the spread of the infectious diseases, and in the light of these data question the belief that these diseases have their origin in the outer world rather than in the bodies of men or animals. Let us consider some of these diseases in detail.

Anthrax is not common in the United States, but it is of much interest from a scientific standpoint. It was the first disease definitely proved to be caused by bacteria. It is of particular interest in this connection because a relation to the soil has been better established for this than for any other disease. Practically all writers are agreed that the soil may become infected with anthrax, and remain so for a long time, and that animals pastured upon such soil contract the disease by taking the bacteria in with the food, or inspired air, or through abrasions of the skin. That this soil infection is not the sole, or perhaps even the most common source of infection, and that danger from this source has perhaps been somewhat exaggerated, is probably true. Thus Delépine [1] from studying recent outbreaks in Great Britain is convinced that the disease is perpetuated by a more or less direct contact, chiefly with unrecognized or concealed cases, and that there is no necessity for supposing a long continued soil infection, and no direct evidence for it as the principal source of the disease. McFadyean [2] cannot trace anthrax in Britain to the soil, and thinks it improbable that it grows there, or it would be more common. Moreover it does not grow well under 60°. Legge [3] notes that animal anthrax does not increase in the summer as it would be likely to if it were due to growth in the soil. Moore [4] does not think the bacillus maintains a saprophytic existence. In Louisiana [5] the extensive outbreak in the latter years of the nineteenth century was believed to be due to some extent to food infection, and to a large extent to direct inoculation

[1] Delépine, Pub. Health, 1904–5, XVII, 491.

[2] McFadyean, J. Comp. Path. and Therap., Edinb. and Lond., 1903, XVI, 35.

[3] Legge, Lancet, Lond., 1905, I, 695.

[4] Rep. Comm. of Agric. N. Y., 1907.

[5] Louisiana Agricultural Experiment Sta., Bull. No. 60, 2d. s., 1900.

by a species of horsefly, *Tabanus lineola.* Outbreaks of anthrax have occurred every few years in Louisiana for over half a century, and persistent soil infection has been alleged as their source. Very likely it is so to a certain extent, but on the other hand there is no doubt that the interval between the outbreaks may well be bridged over by a more or less direct connection between sporadic and unrecognized cases occurring in the interval. That such cases really occur is shown by Delépine's investigations of similar conditions in England. Nevertheless almost all veterinary and medical writers are agreed as to the long continued soil infection of certain areas. Evidence of this is forthcoming from France, Germany, England [1] and the United States. In England such infective areas are said to be the most numerous where refuse from mills using foreign wools is used for manure. In this country anthrax is believed to have been traced to morocco factories on the Delaware River using large numbers of foreign skins.[2] Some of the infected Delaware farms had new tenants with new cattle each year, but infection recurred. All the evidence pointed to persistent infection of the soil. Similarly infected farms or fields are reported from New Jersey,[3] from the Genesee valley [4] and from Louisiana.[5] Law reports that 200 cases in cattle, and 3 in human beings resulted in the space of two weeks, from the soil infection of a limited area. Dr. Leonard Pearson wrote me that the evidence is conclusive that soil infection with anthrax has existed in a number of places in Pennsylvania. Two instances have recently been reported which seem to show pretty conclusively that anthrax bacilli do grow in small ponds under

[1] Poore, The Earth in Relation to the Preservation and Destruction of Contagia, Lond., 1902, 9–21.

[2] Delaware Agricultural Experiment Sta., Bull. No. 32, 1896, 6.

[3] Rep. St. Bd. Health, N. J., 1904, 5.

[4] Law, Text-Book of Veterinary Medicine, Ithaca, 1902, IV, 195.

[5] Louisiana Agricultural Experiment Sta., Bull. No. 60, 2d s., Insert opp. 345, and 357.

natural conditions. Dr. J. Sinclair Holden, health officer of Sudbury, Co. Suffolk, England, writes that in 1905 the waste water from a horsehair factory was discharged into a small pond. There was evidently some seepage from this pond to another about 20 feet distant. The second pond, in the following year, was found to be so abundantly filled with the bacilli of anthrax that it seemed that there must have been free reproduction. Hastings [1] also reports that he examined a pond which had received anthrax-infected tannery refuse, and that this was teeming with the vegetative forms of the bacillus.

While there is a good deal of evidence, apparently conclusive, that soil may remain infected with anthrax for years, there also is evidence that the infection after a time disappears. Pasteur records instances of the infection dying out after a lapse of some years,[2] and in Delaware infection did not persist on all the infected farms.[3] The fact that anthrax has appeared at so many isolated points in England and the United States, and though in the majority of cases soil inoculation must have taken place, nevertheless the fact that the disease has never become widespread or long persistent locally is sufficient reason for the conclusion that its virus does not, in these countries at least, find a suitable soil. If it increases at all in the soil it is only for a time, and the tendency is for it to die out. In other words, the history of this disease is best explained on the hypothesis that the soil is infected chiefly if not exclusively by the spores, which may retain their virulence for years, but which rarely germinate in the earth.

Charbon Symptomatique. — Another animal disease known as black-leg, or in Europe as *charbon symptomatique*, is

[1] Hastings, Paper read at meeting of Society of American Bacteriologists, 1908.

[2] Poore, The Earth in Relation to the Preservation and Destruction of Contagia, Lond., 1902, 13.

[3] Delaware Agricultural Experiment Sta., Bull. No. 32, 1896, 7.

quite prevalent among cattle in this country. Like anthrax it is caused by a bacillus that forms spores. Veterinarians are agreed that soil areas become infected with black-leg and may remain so for some time. Undoubtedly this infection may be explained, as is the infection by anthrax, as due simply to the resistance of the spores, and does not necessarily require the actual multiplication of the germs in the soil.

Tetanus or lockjaw, even before it was known to be due to a bacillus, was believed to occur with exceptional frequency in limited areas. It has been stated by numerous writers that there is a strip of land near Red Bank, New Jersey, where tetanus is decidedly endemic. The disease was also said to be formerly extremely common, especially among animals, on the eastern end of Long Island, but that it has now become quite rare in that locality. This alleged local prevalence on Long Island has been, in this country at least, one of the most frequently used arguments in support of soil infection, but Overton[1] has shown that the published statements cannot be verified, and that the disease has not been especially prevalent in that locality. I have corresponded with various officials in New Jersey, but have never been able to obtain any evidence of the alleged local infection at Red Bank. Tetanus is more common in the southern than in the northern parts of the United States, and is a very important cause of death in the West Indies. Before the organization of the present efficient health department in Havana there were often 200 deaths or more annually from infantile tetanus, due to infection of the navel. It has long been recognized that tetanus follows wounds in which dirt is forced deep into the tissues, and that garden earth is especially dangerous. Even well-established evidence of persistent local infection does not prove growth in the soil. It might be due to a great variety of causes.

Thus it has been explained that the bacilli of tetanus are very widely distributed because these bacteria are natural

[1] Overton, Long Island M. J., Brooklyn, 1907, I, 176.

inhabitants of the healthy intestines of domestic animals, particularly the horse. Hence they are found in profusion wherever the manure from these animals falls, and soiled skin and clothing are not likely to carry them. Theobold Smith,[1] however, says that there is no evidence that the tetanus bacilli are normal inhabitants of and multiply in the intestines of animals. He inclines to the view that their home is in the soil. Vincent[2] after introducing tetanus spores into the stomach of a rabbit could find no evidence of multiplication, and he, too, thinks a saprophytic existence probable. The tetanus bacillus forms spores which may retain their vitality for 16 years, so that it is not surprising that lands have been known to remain infected for several years.[3] These spores, or the bacilli, are said to have been found in gelatine,[4] in blank cartridges,[5] and on balls of lamp wick used in Havana for tying the umbilical cord.[6] While the soil, and dirt generally, contain tetanus bacilli or their spores, there is no direct evidence to show that they are propagated outside of the body. The fact that they do not grow in the presence of air would indicate that this is not the case, and the distribution of the disease and its comparative rarity would also lead to this conclusion. It is not, of course, to be denied that the tetanus bacillus may lead a saprophytic existence. It is very possible that it may do so, but it certainly can be affirmed that at present we have no proof that it does so, and all observed facts relating to the bacillus, or the disease caused by it, may be explained without assuming any such hypothesis.

It is suggestive that the pathogenic bacteria which are oftenest assumed to grow in the soil are the very ones the

[1] Theobold Smith, J. Am. Ass., Chicago, 1908, L, 929.

[2] Vincent, Compt. rend. Soc. de biol. Par., 1908, LXV, 12.

[3] Villar, J. Comp. Path. and Therap., Edinb. and Lond., 1897, XX.

[4] Tuck, J. Path. and Bacteriol. Edinb. and Lond., 1904, IX, 38.

[5] Dolley, J. Am. M. Ass., Chicago, 1905, XLIV, 466.

[6] Junta Superior de Sanidad de la Isla de Cuba, Suplemento y Noto Adicional, 1902–3, 4.

spores of which may retain their vitality for years. Is it not more likely that it is persistence of spores, rather than growth of the bacilli themselves, that in most instances maintains the soil infection ?

Typhoid Bacilli in Soil. — It has been amply demonstrated that water, milk, soil and various other materials are, when sterile, suitable media for the growth of the typhoid bacillus. But this fact is of little practical importance, as sterile materials are not ordinarily found in nature, but on the contrary almost everything which could possibly be considered a culture medium for typhoid and other disease germs is swarming with bacteria, mostly of entirely harmless varieties. There has been much painstaking work to determine whether typhoid bacilli actually do grow, or even retain their vitality, in or on a great variety of substances. The difficulties in this sort of experimentation are considerable, and not the least is that of picking out the typhoid bacillus from among other forms. Robertson[1] and Firth and Horrocks[2] seem to have made the most elaborate experiments in regard to its growth in soil, and to have worked under more natural conditions than most observers. Robertson found that by moistening soil from time to time with bouillon he could keep the bacillus alive for 11 months, and even cause it to grow. Firth and Horrocks did not find any evidence of increase in soil under a great variety of conditions. When conditions were favorable it could be recovered up to 74 days. In peat it could only be recovered after 13 days. More recently Mair[3] has been able to recover the bacillus from unsterilized soil in large numbers, for 20 days, and in small numbers, up to 70 or 80 days. He found no evidence of increase. Great care was taken not to introduce any nutritive medium with the bacilli. Unlike most observers, Mair found that in sterile soil the bacilli disappear more rapidly,

[1] Robertson, Brit. M. J., Lond., 1898, I, 69.
[2] Firth and Horrocks, Brit. M. J., Lond., 1902, II, 936.
[3] Mair, J. Hyg., Cambridge, 1908, VIII, 37.

in 11 days in fact. He believes that this is due to the chemical composition of the particular soil used. Smith[1] working with similar soil, unsterilized, could not recover the organism after 25 days, and the average duration in the soil was 15 days. Calvagno and Calderini[2] spread upon the soil some typhoid excreta. It was found that the bacilli could be recovered from the surface of the soil for 12 to 20 days and from the deeper portions, 20 centimeters, for 40 days. Most observers, as Koch,[3] Karlinski,[4] Uffelmann,[5] Martin,[6] Pfuhl[7] and others agree that it does not grow in soil, though it may retain its vitality at times for months. Savage[8] found that it died rapidly in tidal mud, though a few bacilli could be recovered after five weeks. Klein[9] could not find the organism in dead animals buried in earth, after 20 days, but Loesner[10] found it after 96 days.

Typhoid Bacilli on Vegetables. — Recently Creel[11] has investigated the chance of vegetables becoming infected with typhoid bacilli. He planted radishes and lettuce in soil which was watered two or three days later with a fecal emulsion mixed with a 24-hours-old agar culture of the typhoid bacillus. Some of the plants were grown indoors and some in the open air more or less exposed to sunshine. The leaves and stems were examined every 3

[1] Smith, Rep. on Occurrence of Typhoid Fever in Belfast, 1902, quoted by Mair.

[2] Calvagno and Calderini, Ztschr. f. Hyg. u. Infectionskrankh., Leipz., 1908, LXI, 188.

[3] Koch, Die Bekämpfung des Typhus, Berl., 1903, 14.

[4] Karlinski, Arch. f. Hyg., München u. Leipz., 1891, XIII, 302.

[5] Uffelmann, Centralbl. f. Bakteriol. [etc.], Jena, 1894, XV, 133.

[6] Martin, Rep. Med. Off. Local Gov. Bd., Lond., 1900–1901, XXX, 508.

[7] Pfuhl, Ztschr. f. Hyg. u. Infectionskrankh., Leipz., 1902, XL, 555.

[8] Savage, J. Hyg., Cambridge, 1905, V, 146.

[9] Klein, Rep. Med. Off. Local Gov. Bd., Lond., 1898–9, XXVIII, 363.

[10] Loesner, Arb. a. d. k. Gsndhtsamte, Berl., 1896, XII, 448.

[11] U. S. Pub. Health and Mar. Hosp. Serv., Pub. Health Rep., 1912, XXVII, 187.

days for the bacilli, and they were found, but not constantly, for periods varying from 10 to 31 days. The author considers that these experiments demonstrate the possibility of the transmission of typhoid fever by means of uncooked vegetables grown in infected soil, and so they do. Yet it often happens that the soil is manured a long time before the seed is planted, so that the bacilli have a chance to die out, and doubtless often the conditions are less favorable than in the experiments, owing to excessive rains, or prolonged drought, or very hot weather; and it is also true that the use of fresh night soil as a fertilizer in the more civilized countries is rapidly diminishing, so that it is not unlikely, after all, that raw vegetables are only occasionally a source of typhoid fever. If, too, as now seems probable, bacilli in feces are less resistant than those from cultures, the danger would be less than at first sight appears from these experiments. There can, however, be no doubt that this is a real source of danger, and that human excrement should not be used for fertilizing vegetables and low-growing fruits which are to be eaten raw. The futility of attempting to cleanse them by ordinary washing or rinsing is shown by Creel, who without success tried to cleanse a lettuce leaf by three washings with a pipette and by stirring in water.

Typhoid Bacilli in Feces.— According to Park,[1] typhoid bacilli soon die out in feces, usually in a few hours, but he has recovered them up to the tenth day. He suggested that this variation may depend on the constitution of the feces. On the other hand, Levy and Kayser [2] note the persistence of typhoid bacilli in a cemented privy vault up to 5 months, and Pfuhl [3] recovered them after 3 months from feces mixed with garden earth. Delépine [4] states that typhoid bacilli

[1] Park, J. Am. M. Ass., Chicago, 1907, XLIX, 852.

[2] Levy and Kayser, Centralbl. f. Bakteriol. [etc.], I Abt. Orig., Jena, 1902, XXXIII, 489.

[3] Pfuhl, Ztschr. f. Hyg. u. Infectionskrankh., Leipz., 1902, XL, 555.

[4] Delépine, Rep. Health of Manchester, 1907, 82.

will survive in a privy for a year. His investigation was made in 1898, 13 months after the use of the privy by a patient. Meanwhile the vault had been disinfected several times. Apparently, however, its use by a carrier was not excluded. Calvagno and Calderini recovered typhoid bacilli from a privy vault for 30 days and from a barrel for 25 days. Morgan and Harvey [1] could not recover typhoid bacilli from a privy vault later than 18 days. Semple and Greig [2] found that urine containing 60,000,000 bacilli per cubic centimeter kept at 80° F. was free from them in 72 hours, and that feces under similar circumstances lost them in 96 hours. Mosebach [3] sought for typhoid bacilli in privy vaults belonging to houses where carriers resided but where there had been no frank case of typhoid fever for years, and had no difficulty in recovering the germs. Johnstone [4] in studying the Janet Hill outbreak, which was probably due to carriers, could find no bacilli in 6 samples of soil from the yard of a house where there had been persistent typhoid fever. Rogers [5] found that the bacillus lived only a few days in filtered septic tank effluent.

Typhoid Bacilli in Water. — Jordan and Russell[6] imitated natural conditions by enclosing inoculated water in colloidal sacs to permit of osmosis, and these were placed in the Chicago River, a sewage-polluted stream. They could recover the bacilli for from 3 to 7 days only. Russell and Fuller [7] repeated these experiments with substantially the same results, though they kept the bacillus alive in lake

[1] Morgan and Harvey, J. Roy. Army Med. Corps, 1909, XII, 587.

[2] Semple and Greig, Sc. Memoirs, Med. and San. Dept., Gov. India, 1908, XXXII, 40.

[3] Mosebach, Centralbl. f. Bakteriol. [etc.], I Abt., Jena, 1909, LII, Orig., 170, 773.

[4] Johnstone, Rep. Med. Off. Local Gov. Bd., Lond., 1909–10, XXXIX, 166.

[5] Rogers, Brit. M. J., Lond., 1903, II, 639.

[6] Jordan and Russell, J. Infect. Dis., Chicago, 1904, I, 641.

[7] Russell and Fuller, J. Infect. Dis., Chicago, 1906 [Suppl. No. 2], 40.

water from 8 to 10 days. Houston[1] has made some careful quantitative studies of the life of the typhoid bacillus in raw London tap water. In eighteen series of tests the average reduction during the first week was 99.9 per cent, but a few could be recovered up to the eighth week.

More recently Houston[2] has compared the bacilli fresh from a carrier with the same strain after cultivation and he found that while the former usually lived over 5 weeks, the latter in 9 tests died in 1 week, in 3 tests in 2 weeks and in 1 test in 3 weeks. He also drank, without bad results, on 10 different days a half pint of water to each half pint of which had been added, from 23 to 28 days previously, fresh urine from the carrier containing 218,000,000 bacilli.

Morgan and Harvey[3] came to a similar conclusion as regards the comparative viability of typhoid bacilli from cultures and from excreta. They consider that cultures are worthless for practical tests of the viability of the bacillus. As most of the tests have been made with cultures, it seems highly probable that the persistence of the typhoid bacillus outside of the body is not as great as many of the experiments would indicate. Houston[2] has made careful search for typhoid bacilli in raw Thames and Lea waters which are more or less polluted with sewage. From 215 samples of water aggregating 116,900 cubic centimeters, 20,771 colonies were isolated for study, but only 2 proved to be typhoid bacilli. These examinations continued through the year.

Wilson and Dickson[4] report that they have developed a new method for isolating the typhoid bacillus from water by which they can recover a single bacillus from 100 c.c. of water. They claim that they can, by their method, show the presence of the bacillus when other methods fail to

[1] First Rep. on Research Work, Met. Water Bd., Lond.
[2] Seventh Rep. on Research Work, Met. Water Bd., Lond.
[3] Morgan and Harvey, J. Roy. Army Med. Corps, 1909, XII, 587.
[4] Wilson and Dickson, J. Roy San. Ins., Lond., 1911, XXXII, 9.

reveal it and that conclusions as to the rapid disappearance of the bacillus, based on other methods, are consequently erroneous. They found that the typhoid bacillus could be recovered from water up to the twenty-third day. But it may be that a single bacillus in 100 c.c. is so extremely unlikely to cause infection that somewhat coarser methods may yield results more indicative of the practical danger.

Field[1] found that typhoid bacilli would survive in sea-water for from 6 to 8 days, but that 50 per cent died in 24 hours. Herdman and Boyce[2] found no evidence of the multiplication of the typhoid bacillus in sea-water but, on the contrary, it entirely disappeared in about 3 weeks, the larger part of the reduction taking place during the first few days.

Recent careful observations have shown that in potable waters typhoid bacilli are able to survive much longer in winter than in summer. Ruediger[3] had noticed that the number of colon bacilli in the river supplying Grand Forks, N. D., was 4 or 5 times greater in winter than in summer. Believing that the excess in winter was due to the longer life of the bacilli at that season he tested the question by hanging in the river at different seasons celloidin sacs containing large numbers of typhoid bacilli. It was determined that in the winter, when the river was covered with about 30 inches of ice, the typhoid bacilli lived 5 or 6 times as long as in the summer. In summer he floated down the river two dialyses containing large numbers of bacilli and after 54 hours only 0.11 per cent was left in one and 0.013 in the other. Ruediger attributes the greater longevity in winter in part to the inter-relation of different organisms and in part to the cutting off of the sun's rays by the ice. Houston[4] placed typhoid bacilli in tanks at different temper-

1 Field, Rep. Dept. Health, City of New York, 1904, I, 451.
2 Herdman and Boyce, Rep. Thompson Yates Lab., 1898-9, I.
3 Ruediger, J. Am. Pub. Health Ass., 1911, I, 411.
4 Seventh Rep. on Research Work, Med. Water Bd., Lond.

atures and found that a reduction which took place in 2 weeks at 64.4° F. required 3 weeks at 50°, 4 weeks at 41° and 5 weeks at 32°.

Wheeler finds that in well water with considerable pollution, at room temperature, and with the exclusion of light, a considerable increase of typhoid organisms may take place. Konradi also claims that this bacillus can maintain a saprophytic existence in water, but his methods have been criticised, and, in some experiments at least a good deal of nutrient material was added to the water with the organisms. The report on typhoid fever in the District of Columbia[1] quotes from Kubler and Neufeld, and Stroezner and Tavel, instances of alleged longevity of the typhoid bacillus in well water or, in Tavel's case, in tap water, but secondary contact infection was not in any instance absolutely excluded. On the other hand, the infection in a reservoir in Scranton was proved to have died out within 8 weeks.[2]

Pfuhl[3] found bacilli in tap water after 28 days, but not after 31 days. In artificially inoculated seltzer water it lived for 27 days. Hill,[4] however, could not recover it from various carbonated " soft drinks " after 14 hours.

Typhoid Bacilli in Ice. — Various writers have studied the life of typhoid bacilli in ice, and Prudden,[5] Winslow,[6] Park,[7] Jordan, Russell and Zeit,[8] Clark,[9] Smith and Swingle[10] and Wheeler[11] have shown that they tend to disappear gradually,

[1] U. S. Pub. Health and Mar. Hosp. Serv., Hyg. Lab. Bull. No. 35, 178.
[2] N. York M. J. [etc.], 1907, LXXXV, 1025.
[3] Pfuhl, Ztschr. f. Hyg. u. Infectionskrankh., Leipz., 1902, XL, 55.
[4] Hill, Rep. Bd. of Health, Bost., 1904, 53.
[5] Prudden, Med. Rec., N. Y., 1887, XXXI, 341.
[6] Winslow, J. Mass. Ass. of Bds. Health, Bost., XI, 133.
[7] Park, J. Bost. Soc. M. Sc., 1899–1900, IV, 213.
[8] J. Infect. Dis., Chicago, 1904, I, 660.
[9] Clark, J. Mass. Ass. Bds. Health, Bost., XI, 124.
[10] Smith and Swingle, Science, N.Y., 1905, n. s. XXI, 481.
[11] Wheeler, J. Med. Research, Bost., 1906, XV, 269.

somewhat as they do in the water from which the ice is obtained. It must also be remembered, when considering the possible danger from ice, that the experiments of Sedgwick and Winslow and Clark show that when water freezes 90 per cent of the contained bacteria are excluded from the ice.

Typhoid and Oysters. — Herdman and Boyce [1] found that in oysters artificially infected typhoid bacilli could be recovered up to the tenth day. The bacilli did not increase in the oyster but probably perished in the intestine. In clean water the oysters freed themselves from typhoid bacilli in from 1 to 7 days.

Gorham [2] has made extensive studies of the contamination of oysters in Narragansett Bay which is considerably polluted by sewage. No attempt has been made to isolate the typhoid bacillus but attention has been devoted to *B. coli.* It has been found that while there is not much seasonal variation in the colon content of the water there is a very great variation in the colon content of the oysters which are quite free from these bacilli during winter weather. The same phenomenon has been noticed by Pease in New York and by Freeman in Virginia. Gorham believes that during the winter the oyster assumes a condition approaching hibernation and during this time the ciliary movement ceases, and with it the current of water over the gills, and feeding stops. No water is taken in from the outside and the bacteria in the oyster are gradually eliminated. Is it not safe to assume that the oyster is equally free from typhoid bacilli in the winter, at least in the northern United States?

Field [3] found that when typhoid bacilli were planted in living oysters they rapidly died and none could be recovered after the ninth day. When the oysters were dead

[1] Herdman and Boyce, Rep. Thompson Yates Lab. 1898-9, I.
[2] Gorham. Am. J. Pub. Health, 1912, II, 24.
[3] Field, Med. News, N. Y., 1904, LXXXV, 571.

or dying, there was a very considerable increase. Klein [1] found that in oysters kept in sea water typhoid bacilli would live from 6 to 7 days, but if kept out of the water, for 11 days. In other shellfish their life was longer.

Typhoid and Milk. — Sterile milk serves as an excellent culture medium for the typhoid bacillus, but ordinary market milk is not favorable for its growth, owing to the rapid production of lactic acid. Bassenge [2] says that when milk has soured to the extent of 0.3°–0.4° Soxhlet, and has continued in this condition for 24 hours, the bacilli are destroyed. Neufeld [3] states that they usually disappear from ordinary milk in from 2 to 3 days. Pfuhl [4] found the bacillus persisting in the milk for 13 days. Rosenau and McCoy have studied this question and reviewed the literature.[5] They find that raw milk, when first drawn, has a feeble antiseptic action, and typhoid and dysentery bacilli, when added to it, decrease slightly at times, but within 48 hours their numbers increase enormously. Eyre [6] also states that the typhoid bacillus may increase in milk to enormous numbers, but as the milk he experimented with was drawn under careful aseptic precautions, it is quite likely that his findings would not obtain in ordinary milk, owing to the hostile influence of lactic-acid and other bacteria.

If typhoid bacilli increase in number in ordinary market milk, extensive outbreaks ought to be expected in our large American cities, where the milk is handled by large dealers drawing their supply from many producers situated at long distances, so that the milk is from 48 to 72 hours old before

[1] Klein, Tr. Path. Soc. Lond., 1905, LVI, 23; Med. Press & Circ., 1905, LXXIX, 264.

[2] Bassenge, Deutsche med. Wchnschr., 1903, XXIX, 675, 697.

[3] Neufeld, Kolle u. Wassermann, Handbuch [etc.] Jena, 1903, II, 213.

[4] Pfuhl, Ztschr. f. Hyg. u. Infectionskrankh., Leipz., 1902, XL, 555.

[5] U. S. Pub. Health and Mar. Hosp. Serv. Hyg. Lab. Bull. No. 41, 449.

[6] Eyre, J. State M. Lond., 1904, XII, 728.

it reaches the consumer. Any dilution ought to be more than balanced by the alleged increase in the bacteria. But nearly all of the American milk outbreaks reported in Bulletin 41 of the Hygienic Laboratory were on small routes where the interval between infection and delivery was short. No outbreaks due to railroad milk were reported from Boston, New York, Philadelphia, Chicago, Buffalo, Baltimore, or St. Louis, and of one hundred and twenty-nine outbreaks in American cities only two instances were reported, namely in Washington, D. C., in which typhoid infection was brought in over a railroad.

Boers,[1] Bruck[2] and Pfuhl[3] have demonstrated the persistence of typhoid bacilli in butter up to 27 days, but few if any outbreaks have been traced to this article of food.

Mayer[4] states that paratyphoid bacilli will retain their vitality in dried human feces for a year and a half.

No bacteria can grow except in the presence of moisture, so an increase of typhoid bacilli on clothing, furniture, woodwork, etc., is not to be looked for. The duration of life under such conditions is sometimes shorter and sometimes longer than it is in the presence of moisture. This will be discussed further in another connection.

It must be confessed that the experimental evidence relating to the growth and vitality of typhoid bacilli outside the body is by no means conclusive. The evidence seems to be, however, that they rarely if ever increase in numbers, and in most instances they tend to die off, and that quite rapidly, often in a few days, or even hours.

Epidemiological Evidence. Soil. — There is not much epidemiological evidence that typhoid bacilli retain their vitality outside of the body for more than a few weeks or

[1] Boers, cited in U. S. Pub. Health and Mar. Hosp. Serv. Hyg. Lab. Bull. No. 41, 24.

[2] Bruck, Deutsche med. Wchnschr., 1903, XXIX, 460.

[3] Pfuhl, Ztschr. f. Hyg. u. Infectionskrankh., Leipz., 1902, XL, 555.

[4] Mayer, Münch. med. Wchnschr., 1908, LV, 2218.

perhaps occasionally for a few months, and there seems to be no such evidence of their increase, except sometimes in milk. Westcott[1] reports an instance where a well continued infected for 20 months. It was claimed that the conditions were such that continuous infection could not have taken place, but this does not appear to have been the fact. The numerous instances given in the Report on Typhoid Fever in the Spanish War[2] as showing the growth of typhoid bacilli in the soil, are by no means conclusive. Infected soil was supposed to have caused outbreaks in various army corps, but other sources could not be in any case excluded, and the chances of other modes of infection in an army are very great. The infection was supposed to have remained many months, and it is possible that it may have in some instances done so. As a matter of fact 90 per cent of the volunteer regiments in the Spanish War sooner or later became infected whether encamped on a polluted site or not. Koch[3] believed from epidemiological as well as from bacteriological evidence that it is very rare for an outbreak to be due to long continued soil pollution, and that the possibility of the growth of the bacillus outside the body may be neglected. In 1902, Koch undertook the investigation of the typhoid fever which had prevailed for some time in several villages in Trier. As a result of his labors, every typhoid case and typhoid carrier in four of the villages was isolated, and the outbreak ceased, showing that it was due entirely to contact infection and not to soil infection.

Epidemiological Evidence. Water. — Numberless outbreaks of typhoid fever have been traced to infected waters. In some instances the pollution of rivers is continuous, and the cities supplied from them suffer from a uniformly high

[1] Westcott, J. State M. Lond., 1899, VII, 104.

[2] Abstr. of Rep. on the Origin and Spread of Typhoid Fever in U. S. Military Camps during the Spanish War of 1898, Wash., 1900, 206–209.

[3] Koch, Die Bekämpfung des Typhus, Berl., 1903, 14, 19.

death rate from this disease. In most instances water outbreaks are of an explosive character, the onset is sudden and they often end suddenly, though sometimes the decline is gradual owing to the development of a certain number of secondary cases due to contact infection. A few days' or sometimes a single day's pollution is sufficient to account for the whole outbreak. Three outbreaks of this kind have occurred in Providence, and in one instance it was clearly traced to the throwing upon the banks of the river of the excreta from an infected family. The Providence watershed covers about ninety-six square miles, and had upon it in 1900 a population of some 35,000, a large part in villages along the banks, but some scattered in hamlets and farms over the whole area. The death rate from typhoid fever in Rhode Island is not less than 20 per 100,000 in the country districts, which means seven deaths per annum on the watershed. As the fatality is not over 10 per cent, there must be seventy cases, and if we add the " carriers," the number of persons each year distributing typhoid bacilli on the watershed must be at least one hundred, and perhaps very much greater. It is also certain that disinfection of excreta is practiced to such a slight extent as to accomplish very little. The fact that for years the city has had no outbreak of disease, and no excess due to the water, as is shown by the typhoid death rate which for several years has varied from seven to twenty-six per one hundred thousand, indicates that the typhoid bacilli, which are being continually deposited on the watershed, fail to multiply. Exactly similar conditions prevail on the watersheds of Pawtucket, Newport, Woonsocket, Hartford and New Haven, only to mention those cities in my neighborhood with which I am personally familiar. And the general testimony of all epidemiologists is that municipal water supplies are never continuously infected unless comparatively fresh excreta from typhoid-infected persons pass directly and continuously into them. Nevertheless it is certain that typhoid bacilli must be continually discharged onto the soil, and we are justified in considering the freedom from infection of the surface waters coming from such areas a strong evidence that the growth of the typhoid bacillus outside the body does not commonly occur, and is a negligible factor in the causation of the disease.

Cholera. — Early investigators, as Nicati and Rietsch, working with sterilized soil and water, found that cholera spirilla would live outside the body sometimes as long as 2 months. But all the more recent workers agree that under natural conditions, in unsterilized materials, the life of the organism is quite short. Loesner[1] recovered the germs from dead bodies, which had been artificially injected, as late as the twenty-eighth day. Houston[2] says that they usually die off in the surface layers of the soil in 12 days, though they may be kept alive longer if the soil is watered with liquid manure. Though Heiser[3] states that the spirillum was found in the quiet water in the bends of the Passig river, no evidence was presented to show that it grew there. Gotschlich[4] states that the spirillum is rarely found in feces for more than three days, and quotes Abel and Draer, Claussen and Dunbar, and refers to Koch, as stating that it dies in dirty canal water in 24 to 30 hours. In unsterilized milk it may live from 1 to 2 days, but dies as soon as the milk becomes sour. All these agree that there is not the slightest evidence that the cholera spirillum can increase in numbers outside of the body. On the other hand, Emmerich and Gemünd[5] claim that it does increase in numbers in the soil, and may be found for two and one-half months. Paladino-Blandini[6] also states

[1] Loesner, Arb. a. d. k. Gsndhtsamte. Berl., 1896, XII, 448.

[2] Houston, Rep. Med. Off. Local Gov. Bd., Lond., 1898–9, XXVIII, 413.

[3] Heiser, Philippine J. Sci. (Med.), 1908, III, 92.

[4] Kolle u. Wassermann, Handbuch [etc.], Jena, 1904, IV, 108.

[5] Emmerich and Gemünd, München med. Wchnschr., 1904, LI, 1089, 1157.

[6] Centralbl. f. Bakteriol. [etc.], I, Abt. Ref., Jena, 1905, XXXVI, 53.

that it may grow in polluted soil. Koch[1] says that it grows only in the human body.

Cholera and Soil. — There is certainly a great deal of clinical evidence that it does not increase in the soil, but on the contrary speedily dies out. The epidemic of cholera in Europe in 1885 was very widespread in Italy and Spain. How extensively it prevailed and what a great number of towns and villages were infected are well shown in the excellent report prepared by Shakespeare.[2] Nevertheless by the succeeding year it had entirely disappeared from Spain, and largely from Italy. Turkey had a similar experience.[3] We know that with the sanitary conditions prevailing in those countries at that time the soil must have been infected with cholera in countless places. But cholera rarely recurred, and when it did, it was in large cities, where, the most probable explanation is, it was maintained during the interval by mild unrecognized cases or latent infections. The extensive epidemic in the United States in 1873 was not followed by a recurrence in the succeeding year. Not only is epidemiological evidence strongly against the saprophytic existence of cholera in temperate climates, but it is equally so for tropical regions. The great outbreak in the Philippine Islands in 1902–3 attacked hundreds of villages, and soil infection was universal, yet the disease speedily died out all over the islands.[4] In 1905 there was a similar experience.

In the Philippine Islands during the latter outbreak it was believed that the cooked food offered for sale in the streets was a frequent vehicle of cholera germs, and a number of samples, particularly of boiled rice, were found to contain the spirilla.[5] The rice was probably contaminated by the

[1] Koch, Die Bekämpfung des Typhus, Berlin, 1903, 14.

[2] Shakespeare, Rep. on Cholera in Europe and India, U. S. Gov. Print. Off., Wash., 1890.

[3] Clemow, Tr. Epidemiol. Soc., Lond., 1904, n. s., XXIII, 223.

[4] Woodruff, J. Am. M. Ass., Chicago, 1905, XLV, 1160.

[5] Maus, Med. News, N. Y., 1902, LXXXI, 318.

hands of sellers or purchasers. Whether the spirilla increased in numbers is not known.

Mediterranean Fever. — Mediterranean or Malta fever has long been recognized as endemic at various points on the shores of the Mediterranean, particularly on the island of Malta. It shows all the characters of "endemic" disease, being confined to certain areas and exhibiting little tendency to pass to other parts of the world, or to extend by contagion. The micrococcus, *M. melitensis*, which is its cause, was discovered by Bruce in 1887 and has been very carefully studied by an English commission acting under the supervision of the Royal Society. This commission, as have independent observers, has given much study to the vitality of the specific organism of the disease outside of the body. The evidence seems to be that it tends, like other disease germs, to perish when removed from the body and deprived of nourishment and moisture and exposed to light and heat, but it may retain its vitality for weeks and even months under certain conditions, behaving in this respect much like the typhoid bacillus.[1] No direct experiments seem to have been made to determine whether it ever maintains a saprophytic existence in the soil, but its habits of life are such that it is a fair inference that it can rarely do so, and that such saprophytic growth, if it ever takes place, is of no greater practical importance than is the saprophytic growth of typhoid germs. The micrococcus was carefully sought for in water and in dust, but was never found.[2] The disease is referred to in this connection because, on account of its localization and slight apparent contagiousness, it was believed by many medical men, as well as the laity, to spring from the soil. Yet the work of the English investigators has conclusively shown that the chief source of the disease is the herds of infected goats. It is by the infected milk of these that the disease is transmitted to human beings. It is barely possible that

[1] Report of Commission of Royal Society, 1901, Pts. I and II.

[2] Bruce, Nature, Lond., 1908, LXXVIII, 40.

the fever may be spread to some extent by contact with infected urine either of goats or of men, just as typhoid fever frequently extends by contact infection, but the fact that thousands of infected men have been invalided home to England without any extension of the disease in that country would indicate that such occurrence is extremely rare.

Bubonic Plague. — The germ of bubonic plague is not so resistant as is that of typhoid fever, nor yet is it of such feeble vitality as that of cholera. It is rather susceptible to disinfectants, to high temperature and to drying, but in a moist condition, particularly at low or moderate temperatures, may remain alive for some months.[1] The endemicity of the disease in many localities has led some to assume that it develops in the soil, but the most careful students see no necessity for assuming soil infection to account for its diffusion, and there is ample positive evidence that plague is derived from other sources. Yet, in view of the fact that soil infection has been so much discussed, it is rather remarkable that so few actual experiments have been made to test the theory. Perhaps it is because such experiments are difficult and those who are most competent to make them have thought their time better occupied with work giving better promise of positive results. Elliot [2] found that soil naturally infected would cause the disease in rats after an interval of a month, and Watkins-Pitchford [3] in some careful experiments found that inoculated soil retained its virulence for four weeks, but not for five weeks. The soil was not sterilized. Gladin [4] found the bacillus alive in unsterile moist earth after 2

[1] Rosenau, U. S. Pub. Health and Mar. Hosp. Serv. Hyg. Lab. Bull. No. 4, 1901. See also Simpson, A Treatise on Plague.

[2] Elliot, Lancet, Lond., 1905, I, 1562.

[3] Watkins-Pitchford, Rep. Gov. Bacteriologist, Pietermaritzburg, 1903 [Report on Plague, 31].

[4] Gladin, Centralbl. f. Bakteriol. [etc.], I, Abt. Orig., Jena, 1898, XXIV, 588.

months, and Rosenau[1] kept it alive a long time in cool moist garden earth, and the Indian Plague Commission, 1901, did the same in moist sterile cow dung. Other experiments by Mackie and Winter in Bombay, cited in the Journal of Hygiene,[2] were with grossly infected cow dung from the floor of a native house. No pest bacilli were recovered by culture on inoculation after 96 hours. Further careful experiments have been made by the Indian Commission of 1905. Their conclusions are as follows:

"Floors of cow dung grossly contaminated with the bacillus of plague remain infective for 48 hours; floors of a sort of native cement for 24 hours, the infectivity being tested in each case by inoculation. The floors were infective to animals allowed to run on them for only half the above time."

Thus there appears to be no bacteriological evidence that the bacillus of plague grows outside of the bodies of living animals, and a great deal of evidence that when separated from the body it tends to die off more or less rapidly and frequently very rapidly. The Indian Plague Commission considers that reports of soil infections are unworthy of credence unless continuous and careful observations on the presence of rats and fleas have been made.

Dysentery Bacillus. — One form of dysentery is caused by a bacillus belonging to the colon group, and it has a number of sub-varieties. It is not quite so resistant as the typhoid bacillus, but it has been known to survive all winter in damp earth.[3] It is said that in Japan local outbreaks often persist longer than do outbreaks of cholera, perhaps due to the higher resistance of the germ.[4] The bacilli appear to be easily de-

[1] Rosenau, U. S. Pub. Health and Mar. Hosp. Serv. Hyg. Lab. Bull. No. 4, 1901, 9.

[2] J. Hyg., Cambridge, 1906, VI, 511.

[3] Schmidt, Centralbl. f. Bakteriol. [etc.], I, Abt. Orig., Jena, 1902, XXXI, 522.

[4] Eldridge, U. S. Pub. Health and Mar. Hosp. Serv. Pub. Health Rep., 1901, 1.

stroyed by other bacteria, for they can rarely be found in feces after two days.[1]

Dysentery Amebæ. — One form of tropical dysentery is caused by an ameba, a protozoan, not a bacterium.

There has been much dispute concerning these amebæ, but it is now, however, believed by the best observers that *Entameba coli*, commonly found in the intestines, and elsewhere, is a harmless parasite, but that *E. histolytica* and *E. tetragena*, and perhaps *E. minuta* and *E. nipponica*, are true parasites and pathogenic. Craig[2] in recent work shows that in all probability the amebæ which cause disease in man do not grow readily, if at all, outside of the body. As most convincing evidence he alleges the inability to grow in cultures the pathogenic forms in regions where there are no saprophytic forms to contaminate the cultures and deceive the observer.

Bacteria of Suppuration. — The formation of pus in wounds, abscesses, or elsewhere, is practically always the result of infection by bacteria. Many varieties of bacteria may cause suppuration, but a few species such as the *Micrococcus aureus*, *M. albus* and *M. citreus*, and *Streptococcus pyogenes*, are by far the most common cause of this process. According to a résumé given by Gotschlich[3] they are constantly found growing in the skin and on the mucous surfaces. References are of course given in his article to numerous original investigations, but among more recent observations may be mentioned those of Ruediger,[4] Gordon[5] and Hess.[6] These bacteria are also found in the tonsils and

[1] Kruse, Deutsche med. Wchnschr., 1901, XXVII, 370, 386.

[2] The Parasitic Amœbæ of Man, Phila., 1911, 58.

[3] Gotschlich, Kolle and Wassermann, Handbuch [etc.], Jena, 1902, I, 147.

[4] Ruediger, J. Am. M. Ass., Chicago, 1906, XLVII, 1172.

[5] Gordon, Rep. Med. Off. Local Gov. Bd., Lond., 1904–5, XXXIV, 387.

[6] Hess, Centralbl. f. Bakteriol. [etc.], I Abt. Orig., Jena, 1907, XLIV, 1.

lymph glands, apparently remaining latent for long periods of time, i.e., not causing suppuration. Bacteria such as the above, which are the constant parasites, or perhaps rather commensals of man, are naturally to be looked for in the vicinity of man and on the surfaces of the body, on clothing, utensils, furniture; and the dust and dirt of all places frequented by human beings are found to contain more or less of them. They may also be found in polluted waters. But whether under natural conditions they are commonly able to maintain a saprophytic existence is another matter. Judging from what I have read in the text-books I should suppose that the pus organisms are not so limited as to the conditions of their growth as are most disease-producing bacteria. They are not so dependent on a high and even temperature or on the composition of the medium on which they grow. I should suppose that they would be more likely to maintain a saprophytic existence than most other pathogenic organisms, yet I do not know that such existence for them has ever been demonstrated. In fact Gotschlich[1] says that they are not saprophytes. *Bacillus pyocyaneus* has, however, been found, by Gorham, growing in a heap of moist rags at a paper mill.

Diphtheria.— Diphtheria was not so very long ago believed to be a "filth disease," that is, its germs were supposed to have a habitat outside of the body in various forms of "dirt." This theory was common during my medical-school days, and when I began health-department work in 1884, I tried to fit the facts as I saw them to this theory. But they did not fit, and the impression continued to grow that diphtheria was a purely contagious disease. The life habits of the diphtheria bacillus indicate that while it is more resistant than some other disease-producing organisms next to be mentioned, and somewhat easier to cultivate, it is very unlikely that it is able to propagate itself outside of the body, except at times in milk. Houston,[2] while he does not consider his

[1] Gotschlich, Kolle and Wassermann, Handbuch [etc.], Jena, IV, 173.

[2] Houston, Loc. Gov. Bd. Rep. of Med. Off., 1898–9, XXVIII, 413.

experiments conclusive, believes that the bacillus of diphtheria dies off very quickly in unsterilized soils of various kinds. Graham-Smith[1] cites a number of writers concerning the vitality of the organism in water and milk. According to Seiler and Stoutz, it multiplies in sterilized water for a while, but Montefusco and D'Espine and Marignac found no evidence of multiplication even in distilled water, and in polluted water it dies in 6 days. Schottelius reported, contrary to general experience, that the bacillus multiplies more rapidly in raw than in sterile milk, while Montefusco found no multiplication in raw milk after 3 days, and Rubinstein found that the bacilli died in 24 hours. Eyre showed that in milk drawn in as sterile a condition as possible the diphtheria like the typhoid bacillus undergoes rapid multiplication. Kersten,[2] on the other hand, reports that diphtheria bacilli will persist in raw milk for 72 days, and though they undergo no increase at first, do so later. Montefusco found that they died in fresh bread in 24 hours. Except in fairly fresh milk at room temperature, it is unlikely that the bacilli of diphtheria multiply outside of the body.

Other Diseases. — Tuberculosis, pneumonia, influenza, cerebro-spinal meningitis, gonorrhea and syphilis are caused by organisms which are difficult to cultivate, and I think all bacteriologists agree that it is futile to seek for their habitat outside of the bodies of men or other animals. As for the protozoan diseases, such as malaria and sleeping sickness, such a habitat is still more improbable. It is only recently, and after laborious experiment, that any of this class of organisms have been cultivated in the laboratory. That they grow outside of the body under ordinary conditions is in the highest degree improbable. There is one protozoan, however, the dysentery ameba, which, if recent observations are correct, does live outside of the body. But this organism belongs

[1] Nuttall and Graham-Smith, The Bacteriology of Diphtheria, Cambridge, 1898, 171.

[2] Kersten, Arb. a. d. k. Gsndhtsamte., Berl., 1909, XXX, 341.

to an entirely different class from the blood parasites, and while the facts so far known render it not improbable that the ameba does grow outside of the body, the facts in regard to blood parasites are against any such hypothesis.

Summary of Laboratory Evidence.—It appears, then, that so far as experimental evidence is concerned there is no warrant for assuming a source for the common infectious diseases outside of animal bodies. It is only with extreme difficulty that a few of the blood parasites belonging to the protozoa can be cultivated, and the cultivation of many bacterial forms is strictly limited, so that it is hardly possible to imagine their maintaining a saprophytic existence. It is true that the bacteria of typhoid fever and perhaps cholera, dysentery, and diphtheria may be conceived of as growing outside of the body under natural conditions, but such growth, if it ever occurs, must be rare.

Lack of Epidemiological Evidence. — Nevertheless during the larger part of the nineteenth century it was common to seek such an outside source for most of the infectious diseases. The filth theory of disease, the vogue of which was largely due to Chadwick, Murchison and Pettenkoffer, assumed that the specific poison of many of our common infectious diseases, and particularly of typhoid fever and cholera, developed in a contaminated soil, or in other forms of filth. There was at that time no knowledge of the micro-organisms which cause disease, and the theories of the origin of disease, so far as they had any basis at all, depended on clinical or epidemiological evidence. There was, it is true, some epidemiological evidence for believing that typhoid fever and cholera could develop in filth, for both of these are excrement-borne diseases, and it was difficult to decide without any knowledge of the bacteria which cause them whether they developed in filth or were merely transmitted in filth. But as regards typhus fever, smallpox, scarlet fever, measles, diphtheria and similar diseases, there is really no epidemiological evidence to suggest that they develop outside of the body. If a disease does have its source in the outer world, we should expect to find it localized, attached to a definite locality, endemic, as it was formerly called. The somewhat well-defined infected area we should expect to maintain its infection for some time, and we should expect persons coming into the area to become infected. But if we watch the outbreaks, especially the smaller outbreaks, of such diseases as measles, smallpox, scarlet fever, diphtheria, etc., which occur in different sections of cities, or in villages, we find nothing to indicate place infection. A "pin map" of these diseases in a city shows first one or two pins, indicating infected houses, then more appearing day by day in the surrounding section, until there are ten or twenty or a hundred cases within the radius of a block or a few blocks or half a mile. The scattered groups of houses are of a somewhat circular form, a little denser nearer the center. The outbreak lasts a few weeks, or two or three months, and then disappears, only to reappear in another part of the city. In village outbreaks contagion is usually more clearly traced. The importation of the disease and the sequence of the earlier cases are often made out. The outbreak lasts only for a moderate time, and then the disease disappears, usually not to return for a considerable time, often for years. There is nothing to indicate soil infection. If these diseases really come from privy vaults, sink drains and garbage heaps, we should expect a very different distribution in the house from what is actually found. The ground floor is not oftener infected than the upper floor, nor (for some might say that rising currents carry disease germs to the top of the house) the upper than the lower. But what is most important, when one family in a house is attacked with such a disease as diphtheria, we should expect the other families to be usually attacked also, if the disease is a disease of locality. But in Providence statistics for the last twenty years show that in scarlet fever and diphtheria in only about seven per cent of the houses does the disease extend from one family to another. In most of these cases of extension, direct contact between members of the families is shown to have taken place.

In such important diseases as smallpox, measles and scarlet fever, the germs of which have not been isolated, as well as in typhus fever, diphtheria and whooping cough, epidemiological evidence of an extra-corporal origin is entirely lacking. Epidemiological and laboratory evidence are against the growth of disease germs outside of the body under ordinary circumstances. The notion still common, even among physicians and health officers, that these infectious diseases are filth diseases, as that term is ordinarily understood, is absolutely without foundation.

Typhoid Fever and Cholera. — Typhoid fever and cholera not infrequently appear in small contact outbreaks very similar to those of scarlet fever and diphtheria, but being excrement-borne, contact infection is not so common as in the latter, while infection by water and food is more common. Some outbreaks of typhoid fever may undoubtedly be interpreted as due to soil infection, but they can also be explained otherwise, and the bacteriological evidence is so strongly against the soil hypothesis that we are not justified at present in assuming it. There is no evidence that cholera finds a habitat in the soil of temperate climates, and the most careful observers in the tropics are, I think, agreed that it is not different there. The same is true of bubonic plague.

Yellow Fever and Malaria. — There is a class of diseases for which there seemed, at one time, to be very strong evidence that the cause which produced them had its origin outside of the body. I refer to yellow fever, malaria, sleeping sickness and the blood-parasite diseases of cattle. Malaria is one of the best defined, oldest, and best understood of diseases. I suspect that for twenty-five hundred years what has been known of malaria has decidedly colored prevailing views as to the nature and source of many other infectious diseases. Malaria is a typical endemic disease. Its localization can scarcely be better illustrated than in my own neighborhood. During the latter half of the nineteenth century the southern part of New England suffered from extensive outbreaks of malarial disease. The whole country was by no means affected, but well-defined limited areas of infection were to be noted all over the region, and in different portions of some of the cities. Infection in many of these persisted from year to year. People moving into them became sick, and malaria was escaped by moving away. Most of these areas were in close proximity to swampy land and marshes, others were some little distance removed, but usually in the direction of the prevailing winds. Thus there was presented a perfect picture of place infection. We were justified, in the then existing state of knowledge, in assuming that the malarial poison developed in the wet and marshy places which were closely connected with these infected spots. We now know that this assumption was incorrect, though it was very near the truth, and that the germs of malaria do not develop in the marshes, but that the mosquitoes which carry the germs from one person to another do breed there. As far as sanitation was concerned the error was not serious. The new facts have simply enabled us to work more economically, by determining accurately just what wet places are dangerous. But the apparent certainty that the malarial virus developed outside of the body had enormous influence in encouraging the belief that other disease poisons also had an extraneous origin. The history of yellow fever is somewhat similar to that of malaria. It is eminently a place disease. So are sleeping sickness and Texas cattle fever and a number of other diseases. All of this group we now know are transmitted by insects, and it is the insects which have an extraneous existence and not the parasite of the disease. The mico-organisms which cause these diseases do not grow outside of the bodies of human beings or other animals which serve as hosts, or of the insects which serve as carriers.

Review of Evidence. — In reviewing this subject we are forced to the conclusion that while it is possible that the anthrax and tetanus bacilli and the pus-forming bacteria may develop in the soil, there is no evidence that they commonly do so. It is also possible that the typhoid bacilli, and to a still less extent the bacteria of cholera, dysentery and plague, maintain a limited saprophytic existence, but this is probably very unusual. There is ample epidemiological evidence that in temperate climates such a source for these diseases must be an almost infinitesimal factor in their development. Probably the diphtheria bacillus never has a saprophytic growth of any significance, unless possibly very rarely in milk. As for tuberculosis, pneumonia, influenza, cerebro-spinal meningitis, scarlet fever, typhus fever, smallpox, whooping cough, gonorrhea and syphilis, malaria, yellow fever and sleeping sickness, there is not the slightest reason for supposing that they ever develop outside of the bodies of animals.

Changes in Present Theories and Practice. — If these facts are correct—and I can scarcely believe that any will seriously contend that we have any evidence that an appreciable amount of our common infectious diseases arises in the external world—prevailing notions as to the sanitary functions of the state should be decidedly modified. The laity and the lay press still believe that most of the infectious diseases have their origin outside of the body, in filth, or if admitting contagion, attach equal importance to external sources of infection. And even very many health officials and some teachers and writers on sanitation hold the same view. Municipal sanitation and municipal cleansing are still synonymous terms to many health officers. It is true enough that two or three diseases, as typhoid fever and cholera, the germs of which are found in human excrement, have markedly diminished as a result of improved methods of excrement disposal, or because of the introduction of water supplies uncontaminated with human excrement. It is also doubtless true that whatever promotes municipal cleanliness tends to promote personal cleanliness, and real personal cleanliness, as we shall see, is doubtless an important factor in the prevention of contagion. Intelligent and effective control of excreta disposal, of the mosquito nuisance in certain regions, of the rat nuisance in the presence of plague, and perhaps of the fly nuisance, are of great importance in the prevention of certain diseases. In the northern parts of the United States typhoid fever and dysentery and perhaps diarrhea are the only diseases likely to be effected by nuisance inspection and only when it is directed along certain lines. Except for a few diseases or except for very indirect effects, the cleansing of streets, alleys, and back yards, of dwellings and stables, the regulation of offensive trades, and the prevention of nuisances generally, have, so far as we can see, no effect on the general health, nor any value in the prevention of specific diseases. While municipal improvements such as the above are desirable, there is little more real reason why health officials should work for them than there is that they should work for free transfers, cheaper commutation tickets, lower prices for coal, less shoddy in clothing or more rubber in rubbers—all good things in their way and tending towards comfort and health.

CHAPTER II.

CARRIERS AND MISSED CASES.

A Recent Discovery. — That there are occasionally seen mild cases of the infectious diseases difficult or impossible to recognize, has long been known. That such cases are rare has always been generally believed. That the germs of disease can maintain themselves and increase in number in a person without causing any symptoms at all, was until recently scarcely thought possible, and the idea that such latent infections are extremely common would have been scouted as preposterous. Even to-day the facts are denied by many sanitary officials, and there are comparatively few who recognize the frequency with which mild atypical forms of disease and healthy " carriers " of germs are found, or realize the tremendous importance which such cases have in the spread of the contagious diseases. Undoubtedly the most fruitful medical discovery of the last century, and perhaps of all time, was the discovery of the parasitic nature of the infectious diseases. Probably the most important discovery bearing on preventive medicine since the demonstration of the bacterial origin of disease, is that disease germs frequently invade the body without causing disease. The succeeding pages will be devoted to a consideration of some of the data available concerning the existence of mild cases and carriers. The term " carrier " is applied to those persons in whom pathogenic micro-organisms exist, but who, nevertheless, show no symptoms. Such carriers are rarely found by the health officer, and the very mild cases also naturally escape notice and are hence called by the English " missed cases," i.e., cases which fail of recognition.

Typhoid Fever not an Intestinal Disease. — Bateriologists and pathologists now consider typhoid fever essentially an infection of the blood, rather than a disease of the intestines. Houston [1] urged this view in his report of a urinary carrier in 1899, and it was also set forth by Horton-Smith in 1900.[2] The latter considers that the bacilli probably pass through the intestinal wall without causing changes there and proliferate in the mesenteric glands, whence they pass into the circulation. Pyer's patches are secondarily infected from the blood stream. A number of instances are recorded in which the bacilli pass through the blood into the fetus, causing a systemic infection but without intestinal lesions. It is a fact that in adults the intestinal lesions are frequently slight, and often the bacilli are few in number in the feces, and sometimes they cannot be found at all. Semple and Greig [3] report a case of typhoid fever in which the bacilli were found in the blood from July 20th to September 20th, but were never once found in the feces or urine.[4] So far as we know, the typhoid bacillus may enter the lymph and blood from any portion of the alimentary canal, and Semple and Greig, Lentz, Forster, Kayser and others believe that it frequently enters through the tonsils; and Pratt, Peabody and Long [5] say that there is no more evidence of entrance through the intestines than through the tonsils. Indeed, Lentz [6] says that he has shown, by the finding of bacilli in the tonsils, that the latter may be the portal of infection. He states that tonsillitis is of common and early occurrence in typhoid fever and quotes Drigalski as finding it in 40 per cent of all cases.

[1] Houston, Brit. M. J., Lond., 1899, I, 78.

[2] Horton-Smith, Brit. M. J., Lond., 1900, I, 827.

[3] Semple and Greig, Sc. Memoirs, Med. and San. Dept., Gov. of India, 1908, XXXII, 9.

[4] See also Opie and Bassett, cited by Pratt, Peabody and Long.

[5] Pratt, Peabody and Long, J. Am. M. Ass., Chicago, 1907, XLIX, 846.

[6] Lentz, Brit. M. J., Lond., 1910, II, 1501.

In any event, the bacillus is soon found in the blood, and continues in this fluid through the acute stages of the disease. Typhoid fever is, then, essentially a bacteremia. Audibert [1] has recently shown that this at times presents a subacute type. The bacillus may migrate from the blood to any organ. As has been shown by Pratt, Peabody and Long, a favorite habitat is the gall bladder. Pratt found it in the gall bladder in 21 out of 30 cases. Kelly [2] says that typhoid bacilli were found in 7 of 74 gall-bladder operations, and he states that in many cases there is no evidence of intestinal infection. Primary cholecystitis has also been reported by many others. Recently Elmer [3] reports a case, occurring in a small milk outbreak, in which the only symptoms were cholecystitis. The distended gall bladder was drained with immediate relief of the symptoms. The bacillus may also infect the bones,[4] kidneys,[5] ovaries and cerebro-spinal fluid.[6]

It would appear from the pathology that typhoid infection deviating from the intestinal type is by no means uncommon.

Typhoid Bacilli in the Feces. — Typhoid bacilli were first sought for and found in the feces, and it was then thought that they freely developed in the intestinal contents. It is now believed that, while some of the bacilli in the feces may have their origin in the intestine itself or its contents, the greater number come into the gut with the bile. It was long known that they could be found in the bile, but the importance of this fact and the relation of these bacteria to the gall bladder was not recognized until the carrier question came to the front. From the evidence furnished by a considerable number of animal experiments, as

[1] Audibert, Le Processus Éberthien, Masson et cie, Paris, 1911.
[2] Kelly, Am. J. M. Sc., Phila., 1906, n. s., CXXXII, 447, 744.
[3] Elmer, Arch. Pediat., N. Y., 1911, XXVIII, 217.
[4] Sultan, Deutsche med. Wchnschr., 1894, XX, 675.
[5] Greaves, Brit. M. J., Lond., 1907, II, 75.
[6] Lavenson, Univ. Penn. Med. Bull., 1908–9, XXI, 55. Silberberg, Berl. klin. Wchnschr., 1908, XLV, 1354.

well as by pathological studies on human beings, it seems probable that the bacilli reach the gall bladder by way of the blood stream. Once there, they may merely lead a saprophytic existence, increasing to enormous numbers in the bile and passing with it into the intestine, whence they are discharged in the feces. At other times the mucosa of the gall bladder is attacked and becomes inflamed, and nests of bacilli are found in the tissue. Such nests are not confined to the gall bladder but are found in the hepatic ducts, which fact must be taken into account when it is proposed to cure intestinal carriers by the washing out or removal of the gall bladder. Indeed, Ledingham refers to cases in which this operation did not prevent the subsequent discharge of bacilli in the feces.

Loele [1] opened the gall bladder in a convalescent typhoid case which was excreting bacilli, but no trace of them could be found in the gall bladder.

Typhoid bacilli are not rarely found in gallstones and it is thought by some that they make their way into the stones after they are formed, but the general opinion is that they are the nuclei around which the stones develop.

The bacilli are by no means constant in the intestines, even during the course of the disease, and indeed they are sometimes entirely absent, as in Semple and Greig's case previously mentioned. With improvements in technique they are more frequently found than formerly. The following figures from Gaehtgens and Brückner in 1910 [2] give the highest percentages.

	Cases.	Bacilli found.	Percentage.
1st week	21	12	57
2nd week	32	17	53
3rd week	13	10	77
4th week	4	2	50
5th week	2	2	100

[1] Loele, Deutsche med. Wchnschr., 1909, XXXV, 1429.

[2] Centralbl. f. Bakteriol. [etc.], I Abt. Orig., Jena, 1910, LIII, 559.

Typhoid Bacilli in Urine. — Typhoid bacilli were noted in the urine as early as 1886 by Hueppe,[1] and similar findings were reported in succeeding years by many other observers. The first extensive study of this condition was made by Richardson in 1898.[2] The bacilli are usually not found in the urine until the later stages of the disease, but are occasionally observed earlier, as by Connell,[3] on the seventh day. They are usually in large numbers and often in pure culture. Richardson found them present in about 23 per cent of all cases examined, and earlier and later observers give about the same figures. Thus Connell tabulated 621 reported examinations, of which 24 per cent were positive. The bacilli generally continue in the urine for a while after recovery, but usually disappear within three months. Oftentimes the presence of the bacillus is not accompanied by symptoms referable to the urinary tract. Often, however, cystitis develops, which may persist an indefinite time, accompanied by the presence of the bacilli in the urine. The pelvis of the kidney may also be attacked by the bacilli, and foci of infection may be found in the kidneys themselves. As early as 1889 Konzajeff [4] reported finding in the kidneys infarctions containing typhoid bacilli.

Marchildon [5] has recently reported two cases in which the presence of typhoid bacilli in the urine was due to their growth in the seminal vesicles and the prostate, and Gould and Qualls[6] found the bacilli in the prostatic fluid of 1 of 19 convalescents.

Typhoid Bacilli in the Sputum. — Pratt, Peabody and Long, previously quoted, cite several observers as finding

[1] Hueppe, Fortschr. d. Med., 1886, IV, 448.

[2] Richardson, J. Exper. M., N. Y., 1898, III, 349; 1899, IV, 19.

[3] Connell, Am. J. M. Sc., Phila. and N. Y., 1909, n. s., CXXXVII, 637.

[4] Konzajeff, Centralbl. f. Bakteriol. [etc.], Jena, 1889, VI, 672.

[5] Marchildon, Am. J. M. Sc., 1910, CXL, 74.

[6] Gould and Qualls, J. Am. M. Ass., Chicago, 1912, LVIII, 542.

the bacillus in the bronchial secretions of typhoid fever patients, and state that Dieudonné found it for seven weeks after recovery. Richardson [1] also reports finding it in the sputum on three successive days. That this is not a common condition is probable from the investigations of Tenney,[2] who examined 53 typhoid fever patients without finding the bacilli in the sputum. A few of the cases had bronchial symptoms. He found that the bacilli would grow and survive in sputum for 125 days.

Typhoid Carriers. — Though typhoid carriers seem to have been first observed in England, their epidemiological importance was not realized until, under the direction of Koch, the active campaign against the disease in southwest Germany was begun in 1903. During the next few years extensive observations of carriers were made in this and other portions of Germany.

Since the first edition of this book appeared, J. C. G. Ledingham [3] has published a most valuable study of typhoid carriers, and in addition to the data presented in my first edition, I have made free use of his material in the following pages.

A typhoid " carrier " is a person without signs of illness in whom typhoid bacilli are living and increasing in numbers. Some of these carriers have had typhoid fever, others so far as can be learned have not. In a large proportion of cases the carrier condition follows convalescence and lasts only for a few weeks or months. Some cases, on the other hand, become chronic carriers. Again, persons may be carriers for a period, perhaps usually short, before the disease develops. Various names have been applied to the different kinds of carriers, both by the Germans and by the French, and a formal classification has been suggested. In

[1] Richardson, J. Bost. Soc. M. Sc., 1897, II, 21.

[2] Tenney, Bost. M. & S. J., 1910, CLXIII, 124.

[3] Ledingham, Rep. Med. Off. Local Gov. Bd., Lond., 1909–10, XXXIX, 249–384.

Germany carriers who excrete bacilli for less than 3 months are generally called *Bazillenträger*, and those who remain carriers over that time are *Dauerträger*. The English equivalents are "temporary" or "transitory" carriers, and "chronic" carriers. Sacquépeé [1] names the excretors of bacilli in the incubation stage as "precocious" carriers, those who have had the disease and who continue to excrete bacilli for less than 3 months as "convalescent" carriers, those who excrete them over three months as "chronic" carriers, and those who have never been sick as "healthy carriers," or "well carriers."

For the present purpose interest attaches chiefly to the frequency of the carrier state, the length of time it continues and the liability of carriers to cause disease in others. Some carriers excrete bacilli in the feces, some in the urine, and some in both. Only one sputum carrier has been reported.

Carriers during Incubation. — Cler and Ferazzi,[2] during a food outbreak, found 6 of 39 persons who had eaten the food and who, though exhibiting no symptoms, were carrying the bacilli in their intestines. These "precocious" carriers may become sick later, and sometimes the period of incubation, so called, may be three or four weeks, or even longer.[3] Indeed, it is not rare to find typhoid bacilli in the feces during the period of incubation. Conradi noticed this, and considers it an important factor in the spread of the disease.[4] Ravenel and Smith [5] have reported an outbreak of forty cases due to contact with a case before the symptoms had developed. Prigge [6] discovered 3 carriers who developed the disease, 18, 19 and 20 days afterwards.

[1] Sacquépeé, Bull. de l'Inst. Pasteur, Paris, 1910, VIII, 1, 49.

[2] Cler and Ferazzi, Centralbl. f. Bakteriol. [etc.], Jena, I Abt., Ref. 1905, XXXVI, 479.

[3] Griffith, Med. Press and Circ., 1905, LXXIX, 208.

[4] Conradi, Deutsche med. Wchnschr., 1907, XXXIII, 1684.

[5] Ravenel and Smith, J. Am. M. Ass., Chicago, 1909, LII, 1635.

[6] Prigge, Klin. Jahrb., Jena, 1909, XXII, 245.

G. Mayer [1] reports 3 cases. One of these was a boy whose stools contained the bacilli 8 days before the symptoms arose. According to Ledingham, Klinger concluded that of 812 cases of contact infection studied by him, 33 acquired the disease from a case in the first week of incubation and 150 during the second week. He assumes two weeks as the average period of incubation, though he found it in 60 cases, in which its duration was pretty well determined, to vary from 5 to 45 days, the average being 16 days. During the Spanish war many cases of typhoid fever were attributed to exposure to cases in the incubation stage.[2]

Convalescent Carriers. — Drigalski [3] was the first to study the persistence of typhoid bacilli in the feces of convalescents. Of 64 patients, he found that 7, or 11 per cent, continued to excrete them from 8 to 10 weeks, and 3 for over 3 months. One of these was later, at 9 months, found to be still a carrier. Klinger [4] at Strassburg examined 482 cases of typhoid fever during convalescence and 63, or 13.1 per cent, were carriers, of whom 8, or 1.7 per cent, continued so for a period of over 6 weeks. Later [5] he reported that of 604 convalescents, 80, or 13.2 per cent were temporary carriers, 70 intestinal and 10 urinary. G. Mayer [6] found that 232, or 24.9 per cent, of 930 typhoid fever cases became carriers during convalescence. Graham, Overlander and Dailey [7] found the bacilli in the feces of 11, or 16.9 per cent, of 65 patients after defervescence and previous to their discharge from the hospital. Including the

[1] Mayer, Centralbl. f. Bakteriol. [etc.], Jena, I Orig., 1910, LIII, 234.

[2] Abst. of Rep. on Origin and Spread of Typhoid Fever in U. S. Military Camps during Spanish War of 1898, Wash., 1900, 178.

[3] Drigalski, Centralbl. f. Bakteriol. [etc.], I Abt., Jena, 1904, XXXV, 776.

[4] Klinger, Arb. a. d. k. Gesundhtsamte., Berl., 1906, XXIV, 91.

[5] Klinger, Arb. a. d. k. Gesundhtsamte., Berl., 1907, XXV, 214.

[6] Mayer, Centralbl. f. Bakteriol. [etc.], Jena, I Abt. Orig., 1910, LIII, 234.

[7] Graham, Overlander and Dailey, Bost. M. & S. J., 1909, CLX, 38.

urinary carriers there were 15, or 23 per cent. Semple and Greig[1] report that 16, or 18.8 per cent, of 86 typhoid convalescents continued to excrete bacilli after their temperature became normal.

Ledingham[2] gives a table and chart taken from Klinger's account (1909) of the anti-typhoid work in Germany, which shows the age and sex distribution of transitory and chronic carriers. Of 211 of the temporary carriers, 35 were between 5 and 10 years of age, the period showing the maximum number of cases. The age period of greatest incidence for the 220 chronic carriers was between 40 and 45, at which period there were 30 cases. Among the transitory carriers the proportion of females to males was 1.4 to 1, while among the chronic carriers it was nearly 5 to 1. Prigge[3] shows two diagrams, on one of which the maximum age of female cases is given as 15 to 20 years and the average age of female carriers as 40 to 45 years.

Chronic Carriers. — The larger number of convalescent carriers cease excreting bacilli at varying intervals after their recovery. A certain number remain carriers for an indefinite period, sometimes for many months, sometimes for years, and perhaps occasionally for a long lifetime. The earliest and most extensive series of observations as to the number of typhoid fever patients who become chronic carriers was made by the men carrying on the campaign against this disease in Germany. According to Ledingham, of 6708 typhoid fever cases observed during the years 1904 to 1906, 166, or 2.47 per cent, became chronic carriers. Of 3867 cases in 1906 and 1907, 38, or 1 per cent, proved to be chronic carriers. In the Bavarian Pfalz from 1904 to 1907, there were observed 930 cases, of which 78, or 8.1 per

[1] Semple and Greig, Scient. Mem., Med. and Surg. Dept., Gov. of India, 1908, XXXII, 9.

[2] Ledingham, Rep. Med. Off. Loc. Gov. Bd., Lond., 1909–10, XXXIX, 267.

[3] Prigge, Klin. Jahrb., Jena, 1909–10, XXII, 245.

cent, continued to excrete bacilli for over three months. Park [1] examined the feces of 52 cases eight months after recovery and found bacilli present in 2; in one of them, however, it was present in only one of three tests. Of 16 other persons who had the disease six months previously, 2 were carriers. He thinks that 2 per cent of all typhoid fever cases became permanent carriers, and these may be found in the population at the rate of about one to five hundred. Brückner [2] states that of 316 persons who had the disease, 12, or 3.8 per cent, became carriers, or omitting the 104 children, only 1 of whom was a carrier and who rarely become such, 5.2 per cent continued to excrete bacilli. Semple and Greig, before referred to, found nearly 4 per cent of typhoid patients remained carriers for over three months. Aldridge,[3] also working in India, reports that 6 of 190 convalescents, or 3.1 per cent, remained carriers for longer than six months. Tsuzuki [4] found 3 of 51 convalescents, or 5.8 per cent, to be chronic carriers. Recently Hamilton,[5] following out the suggestion of Gaehgtens, tested the opsonic index of 25 persons who had gall-bladder trouble and found 7 with an abnormally high index. All 7 proved to be carriers. She hopes that this will prove a simple means of discovering carriers.

In Washington [6] 380 persons who had had typhoid fever during the years 1904 to 1909 were in 1909 examined and 8, or 2.8 per cent, found to be carriers.

Klinger found that of 220 chronic carriers 30, or 13.6 per cent, had gallstones. There is no doubt that the presence of typhoid bacilli in the bladder and gallstones are definitely associated.

[1] Park, J. Am. Ass., Chicago, 1908, LI, 981.
[2] Brückner, Arb. a. d. k. Gesundhtsamte., Berl., 1910, XXXIII, 435.
[3] Aldridge, J. Roy. Army Med. Corps, Lond., 1909, XIII, 221.
[4] Tsuzuki, Arch. f. Schiffs-u. Tropen-Hyg., Cassel, 1910, XIV, 147.
[5] Hamilton, J. Am. M. Ass., 1910, LIV, 704.
[6] U. S. Pub. Health and Mar. Hosp. Serv., Hyg. Lab. Bull. No. 77, 171.

There is little doubt that the percentage of carriers both convalescent and chronic is considerably larger than is indicated by the above figures. Owing to the very marked intermittency with which bacilli are excreted in the feces of many carriers, an intermittency which is also shown by the urinary carriers, though to a lesser extent, it is certain that more extended examination of the excreta would discover many more carriers. It must be remembered that most studies of this subject have been based on not more than two or three examinations.

Carriers among Contacts. — Persons brought into intimate relation with the sick may become infected without exhibiting any symptoms whatever. Drigalski and Conradi [1] found the infection in 4 well persons in contact with typhoid cases, Liefmann and Nieter [2] found 7 carriers out of 252 persons examined in an insane asylum, some of whom it was believed were carriers and the causes of the outbreak in the institution, but some of them, however, were true contacts. Scheller [3] examined 40 persons who drank milk which had been handled by a typhoid carrier. Of these 5 were sick, and 13 others, who had no symptoms, were yet found to be excreting typhoid bacilli in either feces or urine or both. All of them became free from germs within a few weeks.

Ledingham states that at the St. Brieuc garrison in 1909, Billet and others found 1 carrier among 53 men who lived in rooms where the cases had been most numerous.

Typhoid Bacilli in Persons Never Sick. — Not only are persons who have had typhoid fever found to be "carriers" of the germs, but persons who have never had the disease, and who give no history of contact, may be infected.

[1] Drigalski and Conradi, Ztschr. f. Hyg. u. Infectionskrankh., Leipz., 1902, XXXIX, 283.

[2] Liefmann and Nieter, München med. Wchnschr., 1906, LIII, 2097.

[3] Scheller, Centralbl. f. Bakteriol. [etc.], I Abt. Orig., Jena, 1908, LXVI, 385.

Allowance must, however, be made for failure to recognize and remember mild atypical attacks, and some of the chronic carriers who are said never to have been sick may have forgotten an attack of "grip" or "malaria" years before. Soper's case so far as known had never had the disease. Houston's case, which had the bacilli in the urine for three years, had not been sick. One of the carriers, the source of several cases, discovered by Semple and Greig, had never had typhoid fever so far as known. Roscoe [1] reports an outbreak of twelve cases in an insane asylum due to contact with a carrier who had never had the disease. Jundell [2] notes a series of twenty-two cases on an estate in Sweden occurring at intervals since 1854. The grandmother of the family, who had never had typhoid fever, was shown to be excreting the bacilli from 1904 until the time of the report, 1908. According to Ledingham, Prigge found that 8 of 84 carriers studied by him had never had the disease. Of 431 carriers reported by Klinger, 163 gave no history of having had typhoid fever.

Carriers among the Public. — There have been a few studies to determine the number of carriers in the general population. Minelli [3] found 1 carrier in 250 prisoners in Strassburg. The most extensive investigation has recently been carried on in Washington,[4] where the feces from 986 well persons were examined bacteriologically. Only one test was made for each person, and 3 carriers were found. These were subsequently re-examined and two proved to be negative.

Much more evidence is needed as to the number of carriers to be found, both among the general public and among

[1] Roscoe, Lancet, Lond., 1909, II, 1137.

[2] Jundell, Abst. J. Am. M. Ass., Chicago, 1909, LII, 388.

[3] Minelli, Centralbl. f. Bakteriol. [etc.], Jena, I Abt. Orig., 1906, XLI, 406.

[4] U. S. Pub. Health and Mar. Hosp. Serv., Hyg. Lab. Bull. No. 52, 145.

contacts. Extensive investigation ought to be made in different parts of the world and among different classes of people.

Duration of Infection. — The bacilli may be found in the urine and feces of carriers, often in enormous numbers, for years. Not so very many cases have been followed bacteriologically for a great length of time, though in one instance the positive examinations lasted four and one-half years. Tsuzuki followed several cases over a year. Mayer, before referred to, reports the following duration of infectivity: for 6 months, 56; 6 months to 1 year, 38; 1 year to 2 years, 16; 2 years to 4 years, 17.

There is, however, epidemiological evidence for assuming a much longer continuance of the infection. Dean[1] reports the case of a medical man who had had typhoid fever twenty-nine years before, and had since then frequent attacks of biliary colic. Typhoid bacilli were recovered from his feces. It was believed that no one had contracted the disease from him, but he had always been very careful in his personal habits. Huggenberg[2] noted thirteen cases in a household extending over a period of thirty-two years. One woman who had the disease in 1877 was shown to be a carrier in 1908. Scheller[3] reported thirty-two cases extending over a period of fourteen years, all probably due to a carrier who had been sick seventeen years before. Gregg[4] found a woman whose blood gave a positive Widal reaction, and in whose feces bacilli were found, and who had had typhoid fever fifty-two years before. She had presumably infected seven persons. Jundell's case reported above was infectious perhaps for fifty-four years. Chalmers' case[5] had had the disease sixteen years before.

[1] Dean, Brit. M. J., Lond., 1908, I, 562.

[2] Huggenberg, Cor.-Bl. f. Schweiz. Aerzte., 1908, XXXVIII, 622.

[3] Scheller, Centralbl. f. Bakteriol. [etc.], I Abt. Orig., Jena, 1908, LXVI, 385.

[4] Gregg, Boston M. & S. J., 1908, CLIX, 80.

[5] Chalmers, Rep. of Med. Off. Health, Glasgow, 1907, 61.

Frosch [1] reports that evidence was presented to the commission appointed by the Prussian Government to study this subject as follows: That fourteen carriers had been infective four to nine years, six for ten to twenty years, and five for from twenty-one to thirty years. Soper's case has now been infectious for ten years, and a number of other writers report instances of carriers who were presumably excreting bacilli more or less constantly for periods of from four to eight years.

Intermittent Excretion. — From what has been said about the carrier state and the existence of nests of typhoid bacilli in the tissue of the gall bladder, the hepatic ducts and in the tissues of the urinary tract, it might be surmised that excretion of bacilli is not in all cases continuous. That there have been reported considerable periods in which the feces and urine of carriers remain free from bacilli is not surprising. G. Mayer [2] claims to have been the first to note this intermittent excretion in 1905, but the matter did not receive much consideration until Davies and Hall [3] called attention to the marked intermittency of bacillus excretion in their case, reported previously by Davies, and which will be again referred to. This patient had been infectious at times for four years, particularly in the spring, and on one occasion she was herself sick.

Davies and Hall laid considerable stress on this presumed seasonal intermittency, but Ledingham, who with Thompson afterwards followed up their case and also six others, considers that the evidence is not convincing, though certainly their carriers gave many more positives during the first than during the last half of the year. Semple and Greig report 18 instructive cases which they followed daily for a considerable period. One of their cases gave only negative

[1] Frosch, Klin. Jahrb, Jena, 1908, XIX, 537.

[2] Mayer, Centralbl. f. Bakteriol. [etc.], I Abt. Orig., Jena, 1909–10, LIII, 234.

[3] Davies and Hall, Lancet, Lond., 1908, II, 1585.

tests for thirty-one days, followed by a positive, another carrier remained free from bacilli, as shown by daily examination, for a period of seventy-five days, and other cases for lesser periods. Scheller noted considerable intermittency in the excretion of bacilli. Of 108 examinations of urine and feces from 18 carriers, 48 only were positive.

Instances of marked intermittency have been noted by others, as Brückner, Kayser, Nieter & Liefmann, Eccard and Prigge. The latter, according to Ledingham, noted intermittent periods lasting from one to two and one-half years. Eccard, in an effort to check typhoid fever prevailing in an asylum, discovered three carriers who were effectually isolated. The disease, however, continued, and on three subsequent examinations, made several months apart, fresh carriers were found who before had given only negative results, in one instance five times. The disease ceased on the isolation of this carrier. This experience of Eccard illustrates how greatly intermittency interferes with all preventive work based on the discovery and control of carriers. An instructive table showing the marked intermittency of carriers in an insane asylum is given by Neisser.[1]

Carriers Cause Disease by Contact. — Perhaps one of the most convincing instances of contact infection from a carrier is the celebrated case of "Typhoid Mary," so well investigated by Soper.[2] Between August 27 and September 3, 1907, 6 cases of typhoid fever developed in a banker's family of 11 persons at Oyster Bay. All the usual routes of infection were most carefully investigated by Soper and discarded because of the lack of evidence. Convinced that some peculiar event must have occurred in the family about August 1, he sought for it, and the only change that he could discover was a change in cooks. But the cook had left and no trace of her could at the time be found. Soper concluded that she was, in view of the evidence, the most

[1] Neisser, Berl. klin. Wchnschr., 1910, XLVII, 2142.
[2] Soper, J. Am. M. Ass., Chicago, 1907, XLVIII, 2019.

likely source of the trouble, and he made every effort to locate her, but was unsuccessful until she had figured in two more outbreaks. No information was ever obtained from her as to her wanderings, but in various ways Soper learned that a case developed in a family in Mamaroneck where she lived in 1900, another case in a family in New York in 1901, 7 in a family of 9 persons at Dark Harbor, Me., in 1902, 4 in a family at Sands Point in 1904, and 7 cases at Oyster Bay in 1906. After leaving Oyster Bay she went direct to Tuxedo, N. J., a locality free from typhoid fever for several years, but where the laundress developed the disease fourteen days after the cook's arrival. "Mary" went to a family in New York in December and within a few weeks 2 cases developed in this family. No wonder that with this evidence extraordinary means were taken to obtain specimens of her excreta, and it can be no surprise to any epidemiologist that she proved to be a carrier. She was confined in a hospital in New York for a long time and her release was refused by the courts, but she was after a while discharged, though still a carrier, and has recently brought suit against the city for $50,000. I am inclined to the opinion that few even of the scoffers at the "carrier theory" would care to employ Mary Wallon as cook.

Hilgermann [1] narrates an instance in which new servants coming to a certain house soon developed typhoid fever. Cases were reported in 1895, 1900, 1902, 1903, 1905 and 1907, in all 15 cases. Suspicion fell upon a woman of 71 years who had had typhoid fever in 1894. She was found to be a carrier. This is the complement of Soper's case, where a moving carrier infected persons in successive houses. Here a stationary carrier infected a series of arrivals at her home. G. Mayer, before quoted, shows a genealogical tree of 195 cases occurring in a certain district in Bavaria during the course of about five years. In this tree are 13 carriers,

[1] Hilgermann, Klin. Jahrb., Jena, 1908, XIX, 463.

and from 8 of them the disease extended, that is, without them the "tree" would have had many less branches. Of these 13 carriers 2 had a recurrence of the disease. During the years in which his observations were made, of 495 endemic cases of typhoid fever 160 were traced to 91 carriers. O. Mayer [1] has traced several "contact chains" from carriers. Sumacher,[2] after a careful investigation in the village of Crov, reported that he could trace 26.6 per cent of the cases to direct contact with carriers and 44.4 per cent to indirect contact.

The following case came under my own observation in 1911: A girl 15 years old, whom we will call A, was reported as going to bed with typhoid, March 3. On April 12 the family went to their farm for a few days, and again they were at the farm on April 29 and 30. At this time two friends of A, Miss B and Miss C, were also of the party. There were no servants at the farm and the family prepared the food. On May 7 two other members of the family were taken sick with typhoid fever, and on May 6 Miss C went to bed with the same disease and on May 9 Miss B. On May 17 the father came down with typhoid fever, and a few days later the mother. The evidence pointed to infection at the farm, and of course the family suspected milk and water. The former was from the cow of a neighbor, where there had been no sickness, and the latter was found to be excellent. Further evidence acquitting the farm and farmer's family was furnished by the fact that another member of the family, a student at Bryn Mawr, had 6 of her college friends at the farm from March 22 to April 2 and none of them developed typhoid fever. On the other hand, every one of the party who went to the farm with the convalescent, April 29–30, later had the disease. The city milk supply was beyond suspicion. I naturally suspected that the girl A, the one first sick, was a

[1] Mayer, München. med. Wchnschr., 1908, LV, 1782.

[2] Sumacher, Klin. Jahrb., Jena, 1909–10, XXII, 263.

carrier, and had infected the food at the farm on April 29 or 30, thus causing the sickness of her brother and sister and two friends. The sickness of father and mother might also have been derived from A, but more likely from the later cases which they helped to care for. No examinations were made of excreta until June 28, when A was found to be a carrier, as I at first suspected. Typhoid bacilli were again found in the excreta on July 29.

Davies and Hall [1] report the case of a cook who, after discharge from a hospital, where she had had typhoid fever, went to her home, where 4 cases developed in the family. Besides these, 4 other cases occurred in three other locations; in all 8 cases in about three years.

Carriers Cause Disease in Institutions. — Typhoid fever not infrequently appears in institutions; and in insane asylums especially, owing to the difficulty in controlling the habits of patients, such outbreaks are apt to occur. Sometimes the source is to be found in a sick person and sometimes in a carrier. A. & J. C. G. Ledingham [2] report an instructive and long-standing institutional infection of this kind. The asylum in 1908 held 92 male and 53 female patients. Cases of typhoid fever had developed in every year between 1893 and 1907, except four. In all there were 31 cases, of which 24 were women. Drainage and water supply could be eliminated as causes. All of the female patients were examined and 3 carriers were found. These were isolated in November, 1907, and since then no cases of the disease have developed in the institution.

Ledingham quotes Eccard in regard to typhoid fever in a large asylum at Frankenthal. Most of the cases, however, occurred in a female block containing 110 " unclean, stupid and noisy women." From 1901 to 1906 there had been 21 cases. Repeated search for carriers was made in

[1] Rep. Med. Off. Health, Bristol, 1909, 61.

[2] A. & J. C. G. Ledingham, Rep. Med. Off. Local Gov. Bd., Lond., 1909–10, XXXIX, 304.

1903 and in 1906 and 1907. In the latter years some were discovered whose examination in earlier years had been negative, owing probably to intermittent excretion. Since 1906 no cases of typhoid fever have developed. Other instances of asylum typhoid due to carriers have been reported by Liefmann and Nieter, Levy and Kayser, Friedel, Dehler,[1] C. Neisser,[2] Roscoe [3] and Ledingham.[4] Dehler [1] removed the gall bladder from two carriers who were found to be the cause of the outbreak, and their feces were afterwards free from bacilli.

A very convincing instance of carrier infection was reported by Davies [5] of Bristol, England. A woman, Mrs. H, 50 years old, had had typhoid fever in 1901. In May, 1904, she went to a home for girls at Brislington to work in the kitchen. From that time until September, 26 persons in the institution developed typhoid fever. From September, 1904, to March, 1905, Mrs. H was in private service. She was then cook in a children's home for some months. The one case which developed here may have had no significance. In April, 1906, she was employed in the kitchen of the Inebriate Reformatory in Bristol. In the autumn of that year 4 cases developed among users of institution milk. There was no typhoid fever in the neighborhood, nor had there been any in the institution since it was opened. There was another outbreak in May, 1907, and up to November 4 of that year there had been 23 cases. Apparently the milk was at fault, and if so was infected after sterilization. Evidence pointed to Mrs. H, who handled the milk after it had been sterilized, and it was discovered by Davies that she was a carrier. She was then removed from contact with the food and there were

[1] Dehler, München. med. Wchnschr., 1907, LIV, 779, 2134.
[2] C. Neisser, Psychiat.-neurol. Wchnschr., Halle, 1908–9, X, 37.
[3] Roscoe, Lancet, Lond., 1909, II, 1137.
[4] Ledingham, Brit. M. J., Lond., 1908, I, 15.
[5] Davies, Proc. Roy. Soc. Med., 1908, I, Epidemiol. Sec., 175.

no more cases. Davies and Hall [1] by following up this case showed that the excretion of bacilli was markedly intermittent. They report also that the woman had what might be called a slight relapse in May, 1908, probably a cholecystitis, and in July a woman with whom she shared her lunch developed typhoid fever.

Carriers Cause Disease through Milk. — In typhoid outbreaks due to milk, water or food, the large number of cases, massed closely together in point of time, often furnish far more certain evidence as to causation than do smaller and less marked outbreaks due to contact infection. There have now been quite a number of milk outbreaks reported as due to carriers, and some of these are very striking. The following outbreak was reported by Lumsden and Woodward.[2] Fifty-four cases of typhoid fever were reported on the routes of two milk dealers in Washington during the autumn of 1909. The outbreak was localized in that part of Washington still known as Georgetown. This section of the city was served by about thirty milk dealers. Of the 54 patients, 33 took milk from dealer A and 21 from dealer B. Dealer A, it was found, received 40 gallons of milk daily from the farm of Mrs. X, and dealer B received 20 gallons daily from the same source. The rest of Mrs. X's milk was peddled direct to eleven families nearby. Among these were 3 cases, not seen by a physician, which quite likely also were typhoid fever. The age distribution of the cases and all the other features of the outbreak pointed to milk infection, with its source on the farm of Mrs. X. No recognized cases of typhoid fever, or illness likely to be mistaken for it, had occurred on the farm, and naturally a search was made for carriers. Mrs. X herself was found to be excreting typhoid bacilli in her feces, and conditions were such that infection of the milk from her was very possible. If a well-defined case of

[1] Davies and Hall, Lancet, Lond., 1908, II, 1585.

[2] Lumsden and Woodward, J. Am. M. Ass., Chicago, 1909, LII, 749.

typhoid fever had been found on this farm, it is improbable that any epidemiologist would for a moment hesitate to attribute the outbreak to that case, even if no examination were made to show the presence of the bacilli in the excreta. When now a person is found actually discharging bacilli in large numbers, I can see absolutely no reason for not considering her in all probability the source of the trouble. The fact that the woman had typhoid fever as long as 18 years before, and had not, so far as known, previously been a cause of disease, is urged by some as a reason for not admitting her to be the source of infection at this time. We know in the first place that many carriers are markedly intermittent in the excretion of bacilli, and, what is more to the point, it is by no means as easy to cause infection of persons or things as has generally been believed. Plenty of cases of typhoid fever have occurred on milk farms without doing harm, and numberless cases of scarlet fever, diphtheria and smallpox, as well as of typhoid fever, are most carelessly cared for, yet fail entirely to spread disease.

Bigelow [1] reports that in Worcester in 1910 there were only 295 reported cases of typhoid fever. Of these, 204 were the customers of a single dealer. The facts pointed to four farms as possible sources. No cases of the disease were found on the farms, and blood tests gave a positive Widal test from only one person, who daily assisted in the milking. He had had typhoid fever 26 years before, and about two weeks before the outbreak he had a slight attack of diarrhea with a little blood in the stools, and accompanied by some headache. He was on two occasions shown to be a urinary carrier.

During February, 1910, there was an outbreak of typhoid fever in New York City in a section corresponding to the route of a large milk dealer. Of the 48 cases, 41 used this milk. The infected milk was traced to a distant farm in

[1] Bigelow, J. Am. M. Ass., Chicago, 1911, LVII, 1418.

Vermont, where a carrier who was doubtless the source of the trouble was found. It is worthy of note that a laboratory assistant while pipetting a culture of the bacillus from this carrier drew some of it into her mouth and two weeks later developed a typical attack of typhoid fever.[1]

Bolduan and Noble [2] report an outbreak of several hundred cases in New York City in 1909 which was traced to that portion of the milk of a large dealer which came from Camden, N. Y. There had been a case of typhoid connected with a creamery there, and also a case on farm X, the milk from which was supposed not to go to the creamery, both cases becoming sick at about the time of the city cases. But it was found that farmer X did send a part of his milk to the creamery and thence to New York. It was also learned that there had been much typhoid in Camden for several years, and that of 27 cases in 1908–09, 20 were on the milk route of X. It was also found that on the farm of X during the years 1878 to 1909 there had been 7 cases of what was probably typhoid fever. Mr. X himself had had typhoid fever in 1863–64. He was, on two occasions, a month apart, found to have typhoid bacilli in his feces.

The Abundance of Evidence. — Only a very few though striking instances of the rise of sickness from carriers have been selected for the purpose of illustration. Within the past three or four years a great mass of similar material has appeared in the medical press,—material already too abundant for satisfactory compilation. Articles are constantly appearing in the medical journals of all lands reporting instances of apparent infection by carriers. It is true that in many instances the evidence is by no means conclusive, often, indeed, only warranting a surmise. In many cases, on the other hand, — and the number is rapidly increasing, — the evidence which leads to the discovery of the carrier is

[1] Bolduan and Noble, N. York M. J., 1911, XCIV, 1313.

[2] Bolduan and Noble, J. Am. Med. Ass., Chicago, 1912, LVIII, 7.

as good, and often better, than that on which, with unquestioning confidence, outbreaks are traced to recognized cases. The evidence which implicates the carrier is the same, and is as convincing as that which determines the contagiousness of the disease.

Evidence against Carriers. — While the evidence is thus seen to be very strong that typhoid carriers are an important factor in the spread of this disease, some facts are presented which apparently point the other way. Thus Linossier[1] says that at least 10,000 persons with biliary lithiasis must visit Vichy each year. From what is known of this condition, it seems probable that a large proportion of these must be typhoid carriers, though no systematic examinations have been made to determine this. If this is so, typhoid fever ought to prevail in Vichy, but as a matter of fact there is very little. Linossier explains this as perhaps due to the fact that most visitors to Vichy are beyond the age of marked susceptibility to the disease, and in part also because they are mostly well-to-do and of cleanly habits.

T. Thomson[2] also finds the conditions after extensive water outbreaks somewhat puzzling. He says that in Worthing after the outbreak of 1893, in which 8 per cent of the population of 17,000 were attacked, there was, for some years, less typhoid fever than before. After the outbreak in Maidstone in 1897, involving 6 per cent of 33,000 persons, there was somewhat more typhoid fever for about four years; and in Lincoln, after the outbreak in which 2 per cent of 52,000 persons were sick, the amount of typhoid fever remained about the same. As we could expect the outbreaks to have left 39, 57 and 30 chronic carriers in the three towns respectively, Thomson says that one would naturally look for an increase in the disease over the pre-epidemic years. Such, however, does not seem to have

[1] Linossier, Bull. Acad. de méd., Par., 1909, 3 S. LXII, 627.
[2] Proc. Roy. Med. Soc., Lond., 1910–11, IV, Epidemiol. Sect., 1.

taken place. While this is somewhat paradoxical, the problem is so complicated by the development of acquired immunity, and the generally falling incidence of typhoid fever, that the apparent innocuousness of hypothetical carriers under such conditions should not be allowed to weigh too heavily against the very clear and abundant evidence on the other side.

Neisser [1] calls attention to the danger of attributing too much importance to the reports from certain insane asylums that endemic typhoid fever has ceased after the isolation of carriers. He shows that in other institutions typhoid-free years have occurred without any control of carriers. He also states that in four institutions where there were outbreaks involving 79 cases, 21 attendants were attacked, while of the attendants on carriers he can find only 3 attacked. He considers the danger from carriers less than is generally believed, yet he thinks it sufficient to warrant the examinations of all newcomers at Benzlau and their isolation under the care of immune attendants.

Atypical Typhoid Fever. — There can be no question that mild unrecognized cases of typhoid fever are extremely common. Greater care in diagnosis has made an apparent increase in the number of reported cases of this disease, and a decrease in fatality. Thus in my own city the reported fatality from typhoid fever has during the last twenty years been reduced from 50 to 12 per cent; and it is probably really considerably less than that. I have noticed that in milk and water outbreaks, when public attention is directed strongly towards the disease, the case fatality is often very low, which merely means that most of the cases have been recognized. In the Spanish War the committee of investigation believed that the number of cases actually existing amounted to 20,738, while the number reported by the army surgeons was only 10,428.

[1] Neisser, Berl. klin. Wchnschr., 1910, XLVII, 2142

Recently Bates[1] has reported a series of mild atypical typhoid fever cases in Panama Canal Zone, and states that such cases are quite common there, and are the chief factor in the extension of the disease. At the time Koch made his investigation of the four Trier villages there were 8 recognized cases, but a thorough bacteriological investigation of suspects discovered 64 more. Of these 49 were children.[2] These mild unsuspected walking typhoid cases not rarely result in death. Velich[3] notes 36 such cases, and a number of others are reported by Curschmann, and they also have been seen by the writer. I have recently investigated two milk outbreaks, in one of which the cause was apparently a mild unrecognized case, and in the other either a convalescent or a carrier associated with him. Neufeld[4] devotes considerable space to this class of cases.

Lemoine[5] for three years examined the blood of every case of gastro-intestinal disturbance and jaundice in his service at the military hospital at Val-de-Grâce and found typhoid bacilli in 40 per cent, although there was little to lead him to suspect typhoid fever. Ledingham quotes Billet, etc., who report an outbreak of typhoid fever of 142 cases in a regiment at St. Brieuc. Besides these, there were 57 other atypical cases which doubtless would not have been recognized except for the epidemic. Brückner[6] reports three outbreaks, all originating in mild missed cases. He finds that children are very susceptible, the most susceptible age being 11 to 15 years, and that in them the disease is apt to run an atypical course. More recently[7] he has reported an outbreak in an institution for boys in which

[1] Bates, J. Am. M. Ass., Chicago, 1908, L, 585.
[2] Koch, Die Bekümpfung des Typhus, Berl., 1893, 14–15.
[3] Velich, Arch. f. Hyg., München u. Leipz., 1904, XLIX, 113.
[4] Kolle u. Wassermann, Handbuch [etc.], Jena, 1903, II, 271.
[5] Lemoine, Presse méd., Par., 1910, XVIII, 113.
[6] Brückner, München med. Wchnschr., 1910, LVII, 1213.
[7] Brückner, München., med. Wchnschr., 1911, LVIII, 1008.

three-fourths were attacked, many cases running an atypical course and only discovered by the use of the thermometer. Chamberlain [1] says that a third of all cases among both American and Philippine soldiers can only be detected by laboratory methods.

The Spanish War investigation showed that most of the volunteer regiments were infected when they came to camp, that is, they must have contained carriers or mild cases, and it was by extension from these that most of the true typhoid fever later developed.[2] The distinction between a case of true typhoid fever of mild type and a carrier often cannot in practice be made. There is no sharp line of demarcation, but infection by typhoid bacilli may result in a series of cases presenting gradation from the most severe symptoms to none at all. It is most unwarranted to assume, as some appear to do, that a mild unrecognized walking typhoid case may start up an outbreak, but that a true carrier cannot do so.

Paratyphoid Fever. — It is generally admitted that agglutination does not afford a reliable means for differentiating the various members of the typhoid group of bacilli. Recent English writers, however, as Dean, Bainbridge and Firth, believe that this can be satisfactorily accomplished by means of complement fixation. According to Bainbridge,[3] *B. suipestifer*, *B. enteritidis* (Gärtner), *B. partyphosus A* and *B. paratyphosus B* can be differentiated in this way. The first two of the above-mentioned bacilli are connected with disease in the lower animals or are at least found in such animals and have been definitely connected with outbreaks of sickness in man due to the use of infected food. *B. paratyphosus A*, on the other hand, is said by Bainbridge

[1] Chamberlain, Philippine J. Sc., 1911, VI, Med., 299.

[2] Abst. of Rep. on the Origin and Spread of Typhoid Fever during the Spanish War of 1898, Wash., 1900, 168–175.

[3] Bainbridge, Proc. Roy. Soc. Med., Lond., 1911, IV, Epidemiol. Sect., 51; Lancet, Lond., 1912, I, 705.

to be a human parasite, just as is *B. typhosus* (the ordinary typhoid bacillus). The disease caused by *B. paratyphosus A* is said by Firth [1] to be very common in India. It is milder in type, with a more irregular fever and a more sudden onset, and is accompanied by more headache. It may very frequently be recognized clinically. Grattan and Wood [2] say that one-third of all cases of uncertain fever are due to this bacillus. This type of enteric is not, according to these authors, and to Bainbridge, common either in England or the United States, though perhaps its apparent rarity is due partly to lack of careful investigation. Grattan,[3] however, could not find this bacillus in 48 cases of enteric fever studied by him in London. But in India Grattan and Wood studied 157 cases of this disease. Of these 10 became carriers, but in only one case did the bacilli persist for as long as 5 months. They believe that these acute carriers are a greater factor in the spread of disease than are typhoid carriers in ordinary typhoid fever. These authors [4] report an outbreak of 9 cases of this type of paratyphoid fever in barracks at Benares, probably due to a man who was discovered to be a carrier. A similar outbreak of 8 cases due to a carrier was reported by Grattan.[5]

B. Paratyphosus B. — Bainbridge and O'Brien [6] consider that *B. paratyphosus B* as well as *A* has its habitat in man. Carriers are frequently found, and such may infect food and thus cause food outbreaks of the disease. They did not find this bacillus in 300 typhoid convalescents, but

[1] Firth, Roy. Army Med. Corps., Lond., 1911, XVII, 136.

[2] Grattan and Wood, J. Roy. Army Med. Corps., Lond., 1911, XVII, 143.

[3] Grattan, J. Roy. Army Med. Corps., Lond., 1910, XIV, 385.

[4] J. Roy. Army Med. Corps., Lond., 1911, XXII, 131.

[5] Grattan, J. Roy. Army Med. Corps, Lond., 1911, XVI, 9.

[6] Bainbridge and O'Brien, J. Hyg., Cambridge, 1911, XI, 68; also Brit. M. J., Lond., 1910, II, 1503.

they did find it in 6 cases of fever in which it was apparently the causative agent, also in 4 convalescent carriers and in 3 healthy persons. According to Bainbridge, carriers of *B. paratyphosus B* were first noted by Lentz and later by Hamilton, Gaehtgens, Brückner, Mayer and Prigge and Sachs-Müke. But if Bainbridge's contention is correct, and if these Germans, as he states, have not made use of complement fixation to differentiate the bacilli, their data cannot be relied upon. It is not unlikely, however, that some of these were really carriers of *B. paratyphosus B*. Of those noted by Prigge and Sachs-Müke,[1] 4 were in connection with a food-poisoning outbreak. One of the carriers was under observation in a hospital for 2 years. Another, a well person, was found to be a carrier during a food-poisoning outbreak, and 6 months later, after an intermission of excretion for 3 months, finally became sick and the bacilli were found in the feces.

Bainbridge and Dudfield [2] report a contact outbreak of 13 cases in a boarding house at Paddington. It was thought probable that it was due to a carrier, but none was found. At Wrexham in 1910 over 100 cases of food poisoning occurred which were traced to pork pies. The meat was not infected when received, as other portions sent to other places did no harm. Apparently infection took place during the making of the pies. It was found that the head cook, who did not eat the pies and who was not sick, had the bacilli in the feces and was therefore presumably the carrier who infected the pies, though she claimed not to have had anything directly to do with the making of the pies. She had another typhoid-like bacillus in her urine, and these too were found in the pies. Sacquépeé and Bellot [3] also report the case of a cook who had an abortive attack and while continuing at work infected 19 persons in

[1] Sachs-Müke, Klin. Jahrb., Jena, 1909–10, XXII, 237.

[2] Bainbridge and Dudfield, J. Hyg., Cambridge, 1911, XI, 24.

[3] Sacquépeé and Bellot, Prog. méd., Par., 1910, 3. s. XXVI, 25.

a garrison of 250. G. Mayer [1] writes of a man who became a carrier from eating meat and later caused the infection of another. An outbreak of 38 cases was due to eating vegetables fertilized with the contents of a privy vault used by a man with "liver trouble," who had paratyphoid *B* bacilli in his feces.

Cholera Spirilla in Convalescents. — Usually the germs of cholera disappear from the feces early in convalescence, and until recently chronic carriers were unknown. Pfeiffer [2] reviews the literature, and cites Simond's observation that the average duration of infection is only about 6 days, and that the longest seen by him was 18 days. Of 117 cases reported to Rumpel, not one carried the germs over 24 days. Abel and Claussen found the average of 17 cases to be 5 or 6 days, and Pfeiffer the average of 39 cases 10 days, though in 2 the infection persisted 23 days. Other writers have made similar observations.

Zirolla [3] found 29 convalescents excreting bacilli from 6 to 40 days. Zlatogoroff [4] followed 255 cases until three negative examinations were made. In 134 the spirilla disappeared by the fourteenth day, and in 22 they persisted after 21 days, in one case lasting for 56 days. Burgers [5] found the average duration of infection in a small outbreak was about 3 weeks from the beginning of sickness, but in one case the spirilla persisted for 69 days. According to Kolle,[6] cholera spirilla are sometimes found in the intestines of convalescents as long as 48 days. Rommelaere [7] reported a

[1] G. Mayer, Centralbl. f. Bakteriol. [etc.], Jena, I Abt. Orig., 1910, LIII, 234.

[2] Pfeiffer, Klin. Jahrb., Jena, 1908, XIX, 483.

[3] Abst., Med. Officer, 1911, VI, 84.

[4] Zlatogoroff, Centralbl. f. Bakteriol. [etc.], I Abt. Orig., Jena, 1911, XLVIII, 14.

[5] Burgers, Hyg. Rundschau, Berl., 1910, XX, 169.

[6] Kolle, Ztschr. f. Hyg. u. Infectionskrankh., Leipz., 1895, XVIII.

[7] Rommelaere, J. de méd., Brux., 1892, XCIV, 837.

case retaining the infection 47 days. Forrest [1] found the germs remaining 6 weeks. Kirchner [2] says that the spirilla are sometimes carried for weeks or months.

Zlatogoroff says that Jakowleff found the germs in the feces 56 days after the attack, and Zeidler 93 days. Zlatogoroff himself found them for 56 days.

Chronic and Intermittent Carriers. — Until recently it was thought that cholera carriers were always of the "temporary" type, and that propagation of the spirilla was confined to the intestinal contents. It was believed that they did not invade the gall bladder or other organs as do typhoid bacilli. Observations by Kulescha, however, show that the spirilla can be found in the gall bladder in 10 per cent of the cases, sometimes producing lesions and propagating in the biliary passages. Consequently it is not surprising that Kulescha reports a case which was discharged from the hospital in January, 1909, after having had the spirilla in the feces for 57 days, and which re-entered the hospital in October of the same year with hepatic trouble and soon died. Cholera germs were found in the biliary passages. McLaughlin,[3] who takes these facts from Kulescha, states that Gaffky reports a cholera convalescent who was a carrier for 6 months. Adami, Vallée and Martineau [4] have published notes of a case which arrived in Quebec from Russia 16 November, 1910. The man had perhaps had a slight attack of cholera on the steamship. At any rate cholera germs were found in his feces, and he remained a carrier until the next May. The spirilla were identified by agglutination.

Intermittent Excretion of Spirilla. — Intermittent excretion, which at first was not suspected, is now known to occur. Zirolla states that 2 cases observed by him showed

[1] Forrest, J. Trop. M. [etc.], Lond., 1908, XI, 321.
[2] Kirchner, Klin. Jahrb., Jena, 1908, XIX, 483.
[3] McLaughlin, Boston M. & S. J., 1911, CLXV, 561.
[4] Adami, Vallée and Martineau, Canad. M. Ass. J., 1910, I, 697.

a germ-free period of 1 month and 20 days respectively. During such a period attacks of indigestion or the administration of salts caused the spirilla to reappear in the feces. Creel [1] reports the case of a carrier under observation at quarantine in New York for 54 days. Of 12 examinations of the feces, 6 were positive and 6 negative.

Spirilla in Healthy Persons. — Dunbar [2] was the first to note the occurrence of cholera spirilla in the feces of healthy persons. He discovered 28 healthy carriers in Hamburg in 1892–93. Rommelaere noted such a carrier in 1892, and carriers are by Koch considered an important factor in the spread of the disease. In 1905 cholera seemed to have been brought down the rivers from Russia into Germany by raftsmen, and Kirchner says that of 27 persons on one raft 2 were carriers. Pfeiffer states that in this outbreak there were 174 cases of the disease, and that 38 other carriers were discovered. He cites Frosch as discovering 16 carriers, of whom 12 were children, and Friedheim as finding 51. In one family observed by Pfeiffer 4 died, 1 was very sick, 1 was mildly sick, and 2 were carriers. He says that there are very many mild cases of the disease which can only be recognized bacteriologically. Burgers [3] discovered 6 carriers connected with an outbreak of 30 cases in East Prussia. In Madeira in 1910,[4] of 600 contacts, 37 proved to be carriers. Of these, 12 later developed the disease. The average duration of infection was 6 to 8 days. In a convalescent it continued for 5 weeks. McLaughlin[5] found 17, or 6.44 per cent of 264 prisoners in Manila, to be carriers, and in the city 27, or 7.18 per cent of 376 persons examined.

During the summer of 1911 there was some cholera in

[1] Creel, J. Am. M. Ass., Chicago, 1912, LVIII, 187.
[2] Dunbar, Mod. Med., Osler, Phila. & N. Y., 1907, II, 720.
[3] Burgers, Hyg. Rundschau, Berl., 1910, XX, 169.
[4] Franca, Bull. Soc. path. exot., Par., 1911, IV, 358.
[5] McLaughlin, J. Am. M. Ass., Chicago, 1909, LII, 1155.

the Philippines but only 1 case in Manila. Of 7 persons brought in close contact with this case all were shown to be carriers.[1] While during an outbreak, as stated above, 6 per cent of the population may be found to be carriers, McLaughlin[2] states that between outbreaks thousands of stools may be examined without finding a single carrier. That carriers increase as the number of cases increase is a phenomenon common to other diseases as well as cholera. It will be shown in the following pages to be true for cerebro-spinal meningitis and for diphtheria. Jakowleff, Zabolotny, Zlatogoroff and Kulescha[3] state that in St. Petersburg the feces from 2440 apparently well persons were examined, all of whom had been more or less in contact with cholera cases. Of these 125 showed the cholera spirillum, of whom 40 proved to be mild unrecognized cases, 25 were incubating the disease, and 60 were true carriers.

During nearly four months of the summer of 1911, while cholera was prevailing in certain parts of Italy, bacteriological examination of the feces of immigrants was largely made use of to prevent the introduction of the disease into the United States. A sharp watch was kept by the steamship companies and by the United States officials on the other side to prevent the embarkation of possibly infected persons, and indeed all immigrants from infected districts were kept under observation for five days. Many also were subjected to bacteriological examination. According to a letter from Dr. John F. Anderson, of about 20,000 so examined in Italy, 41 were found to be carriers. Of about 25,000 immigrants examined at American ports, 27 were shown to be carriers. All of these were discovered early

[1] U. S. Pub. Health and Mar. Hosp. Serv., Pub. Health Rep., 1911, 1493.

[2] McLaughlin, N. York M. J., 1911, XCIII, 115.

[3] Jakowleff, Zabolotny, Zlatogoroff and Kulescha, Bull. Soc. path. exot., Par., 1909, II, 276.

in the season while the control of embarkation was not so strict.

Gotschlich[1] examined pilgrims returning from Mecca, and though cholera had not so far as known prevailed among them, he found several Russian and Turkish pilgrims who proved to be carriers of the spirilla. According to Pfeiffer, these spirilla of Gotschlich have been carefully studied by a number of observers and show slight variations from the type, and have probably lost their virulence.

Atypical Cases of Cholera. — While perhaps most cases of cholera are readily recognized, atypical and mild cases occur, and they are particularly frequent among children. McLaughlin [2] says that cholera in children simulates acute and chronic enteritis and meningitis, and is often thus wrongly diagnosed by practicing physicians. By means of examination of the feces he raised the proportion of cholera cases reported among children from 22 to 35 per cent of the total cases.

Cholera Derived from Carriers. — Cholera spirilla from carriers have according to Zlatogoroff and others been shown to be as virulent for animals as those from cases, but this perhaps ought not to be taken as an indication of their virulence for man. While Pfeiffer gives several instances in which cholera was spread by carriers, the number of definite cases recorded in medical literature is not large. A very striking one, however, is reported by Macrae.[3] In a hospital in Calcutta, 10 nurses, 3 patients and a sweeper developed cholera within 4 days. An examination of 127 articles of food and drink demonstrated spirilla in 14 samples of water and milk, all of which had been handled by the servants. An examination of 12 servants

[1] Gotschlich, Ztschr. f. Hyg. u. Infectionskrankh., Leipz., 1906, LIII, 281.

[2] McLaughlin, Philippine J. Sc., Manila, 1909, IV, Sec. B, 363.

[3] Macrae, Indian M. Gaz., Calcutta, 1909, XLIV, 361.

showed that 2 were carriers, and spirilla were recovered from their hands.

Since the possibility of the spread of cholera by carriers has been recognized, outbreaks of the disease have occurred in Russia and Germany, and both Russian and German observers consider that carriers afford the best explanation of many of the phenomena of cholera outbreaks. The repeated occurrence of the disease in the Philippines, since the occupancy of the islands by the United States, has given a splendid opportunity for the study of cholera epidemiology, which has been well taken advantage of by our officials. Heiser and McLaughlin are firmly convinced that carriers are a most important factor in the spread of the disease. Indeed, McLaughlin says that their importance can hardly be overestimated. He has no doubt that cholera is often spread from village to village by carriers, and that intervals between local outbreaks are bridged over by the same means. There is no evidence that the spirilla maintain a saprophytic existence in the soil or water of the islands.

Chantemesse [1] says cholera was introduced into Italy in 1910 by a party of gypsies who arrived at Brindisi, July 27, from Batum. They then went to Trani, where the disease developed August 7. None of the party were sick. Cases developed in October in Marseilles after the arrival of immigrants from the East, though there was no recognized sickness among them. On October 7 cholera developed on a ship which carried Russian emigrants from Southampton 30 days after the latter had left Russia. The baggage in all these cases had been disinfected and the emigrants themselves had been examined several times by physicians, who failed to find recognizable cholera.

In 1911 there were five cases of cholera in the United States, of which only one had any connection with a previous case. Shall we assume that dried and dying germs

[1] Chantemesse, Bull. Acad. de méd., Par., 1911, LXXV, 113.

on clothing caused them, or living germs from a carrier? In 1893, at a time when a cholera ship lay in the harbor several miles from New York, a number of unconnected cases occurred in that city. Were they caused by flies, by floating mattresses or clothing, as was then supposed, or were they derived from a carrier from some other ship? Similarly, "sporadic" cases occurred in England at the same period. In 1873, at least three local outbreaks in the United States were traced to immigrants recently arrived from Europe at points in the interior. Then it was thought that the germs were brought in the baggage. To-day do not carriers seem a more likely explanation? In 1866, New York was the starting place of an extensive epidemic. From May to July there were only a few cases in the city not directly connected with any imported cases, nor often with each other. The epidemiologists of the day attributed these cases to fomites, or the feces of recovered cases. Our present-day knowledge shows us how much more likely the latter is as a cause than the former, and vindicates the judgment of the men of that day who without the help of bacteriology surmised the existence of the "carrier." McLaughlin[1] says that in the Bilibid prison at Manila the food and water were so well controlled that the only entrance for cholera was by means of carriers. As soon as carriers were sought for and isolated the disease was stamped out.

Bacillary Dysentery. — There are two forms of dysentery, one caused by bacilli, the other by amebæ. The dysentery bacilli form a group of closely allied types, as the Shiga, the Flexner and the Harris types. Certain of the group are called pseudo-dysenteric but yet are pathogenic. What is commonly called dysentery may be caused by a number of different pathogens, and the dysentery bacilli may cause diarrheal symptoms quite different from typical dysentery. For the present purpose the whole dysentery

[1] McLaughlin, N. York M. J., 1911, XCIII, 115.

group of bacilli may be referred to without distinction. Collins [1] and Goodwin [2] have studied the occurrence of the bacillus in well persons. According to Collins, Flexner, Wollstein and others failed to find it in healthy persons. Duval [3] found it in 2 instances, and Charlton and Jehle [4] in 2 of 10 cases examined. Collins found it in 2 of 30 normal persons, and in 1 three weeks after an attack of dysentery, and in another child who had had a few mucous stools. Goodwin found the Flexner-Manila type of the bacillus in 1 of 59 well persons examined. Kruse [5] says that all types of the bacilli have been found in well persons, and that these carriers are an important cause of the disease. Though carriers have fewer bacilli in their feces, which are also less in volume, they come in contact with a larger number of persons than do the sick. There are also many mild atypical cases. Kruse has found the bacilli in relapses after two years,[6] and says that Drigalski and Lentz have made similar observations. He also cites Ford as finding 10 carriers among 50 persons examined. In an asylum outbreak Heuser [7] found 3 carriers. Conradi,[8] while studying a contact outbreak near Metz, found several carriers. Küster [9] isolated bacilli from a carrier who had probably been excreting since an attack years before. Kruse cites Kriege as saying that about 4 of 36 cases of dysentery become chronic, but usually the infection lasts only 2 to 6 weeks. Conradi found that in 4 of 27 cases the bacilli persisted up to the end of the fourth week, while in 11 cases they disappeared by the middle of the second week.

[1] Collins, Rep. Dept. Health, City of New York, 1904, I, 428.
[2] Goodwin, Rep. Dept. Health, City of New York, 1904, I, 423.
[3] Duval, Studies from Rockefeller Inst., 1904, II, 42.
[4] Charlton and Jehle, Tr. Ass. Am. Physicians, 1904, XIX, 405.
[5] Kruse, Med. Press & Circ., 1908, LXXXV, 175.
[6] Kruse, Klin. Jahrb., Jena, 1908, XIX, 529.
[7] Heuser, Deutsche med. Wchnschr., 1909, XXXV, 1694.
[8] Conradi, Festschrift v. Robert Koch, 1903, 555.
[9] Küster, München med. Wchnschr., 1908, LV, 1833.

Shiga[1] says that the bacilli generally remain 1 or 2 weeks, and that perfectly normal persons sometimes harbor the germs. Aveline, Boycott and McDonald[2] failed to find the bacillus in 27 contacts in an asylum.

Cameron[3] also, and Macalister,[4] rarely found bacilli in perfectly healthy contacts. The latter writer found that 26 per cent of the cases studied by him in a certain asylum developed a mild chronic state or had relapses, and that these conditions only could be regarded as dangerous. These he considers as practically carriers, and says their importance cannot be overestimated.

O. Mayer[5] has reported finding entirely healthy carriers, and one of these later became sick. The bacillus found was of the "pseudo-" type *Y*. In convalescents he found them persisting up to 202 days. The average persistence is 3 to 7 months. In healthy persons they were not found over 30 days. Intermittency of excretion was noted in both convalescent and healthy carriers.

Chronic Plague in Rats. — Bubonic plague is a disease which attacks not man alone but many other species of animals, particularly the rat. In fact it may be considered primarily a rat disease, and without doubt the rat is the most important agent in its diffusion. That mild cases and chronic cases exist among rats which superficially appear not to be sick, seems to be proved. Simpson[6] says chronic plague was observed in some of the animals experimented on in Hong Kong, and by Albrecht and Ghon in guinea pigs, and in rats for months by Kolle and Martini. The Indian Plague Commission (1905)[7] found eleven of the

[1] Shiga, Philippine J. Sc., Manila, 1906, I, 485.

[2] Aveline, Boycott and McDonald, J. Hyg., Cambridge, 1908, VIII, 309.

[3] Cameron, Brit. M. J., Lond., 1911, I, 973.

[4] Macalister, Brit. M. J., Lond., 1910, II, 1506.

[5] Mayer, Münch. med. Wchnschr., 1910, LVII, 2566.

[6] Simpson, A Treatise on Plague, Cambridge, 1905, 129.

[7] J. Hyg., Cambridge, 1907, VII, 379.

rats which they had fed with plague bacilli to be infected, although they appeared to be perfectly well. While chronic plague has been seen in laboratory animals, several observers in Bombay and Sydney have failed to find it under natural conditions, as also did Blue in San Francisco.[1] But Hunter found rats with chronic plague in Hong Kong, and the Indian Plague Commission (1905) found a number of rats infected with plague at a time when no rats with acute plague could be discovered, and when there was no outbreak among human beings. The infected rats showed no sign of sickness.[2] Later observations discovered similar instances of chronic rat infection in animals caught in a number of different places. The pathological conditions indicated a slowly resolving rather than a true chronic process. Watkins-Pitchford[3] found the bacillus in convalescent rats and guinea pigs. It is evident that such chronic "carriers" may be an important factor in the maintenance and extension of the disease.

Atypical Human Plague. — Among human beings mild cases of the glandular type are by no means uncommon. But fortunately these are rarely dangerous, for without suppuration there is no escape of bacilli. But in certain instances, later suppuration may take place, or lung symptoms develop, so that the individual may become a focus of infection.[4] Rat "carriers," on the other hand, are always dangerous, for they may at any time suffer accidental death, and their carcasses may then readily infect other animals and even man.

Plague Bacilli in Convalescents. — In the pneumonic type in human beings the bacilli are thrown off in large numbers

[1] Blue, J. Hyg., Cambridge, 1909, IX, 1.

[2] J. Hyg., Cambridge, 1906, VI, 530–535; 1907, VII, 373.

[3] Watkins-Pitchford, Rep. of Bacteriologist, Pietermaritzburg, Natal, 1903 [Rep. on Flague, 31].

[4] Gotschlich, Kolle u. Wassermann, Handbuch, Jena [etc.], 1904, IV[1], 69.

from the lungs. Martin,[1] Gotschlich [2] and others have found them in the sputum up to 76 days after the attack, or 42 days after recovery. Gaffky[3] cites Vagedes as reporting pulmonary infection lasting 2 months in a case in Oporto, and bacilli in an abscess persisting more than 2 months, and Vages one lasting 4 weeks in Paraguay. The latter also isolated the bacilli from a man who later became sick with the disease. Shottelius found the germs in the bronchial secretion of mild ambulant cases. It is thus very probable that mild cases and true carriers among both rats and human beings may play a considerable part in the dissemination of this disease.

White Diarrhea of Chicks. — One form of diarrhea common among young chickens appears to be due to a bacillus, *B. pullorum*. The nature and mode of spread of this disease were well worked out by Rettger and Stoneburn.[4] It affects young chickens three or four days old and spreads among them by contact or infection of their food with excreta. Many of the survivors become carriers of the bacillus until after they have become mature hens. Such hens show few or no symptoms. The eggs which these carriers lay become infected in the oviduct, and chicks hatched from them develop the disease, though they never come in contact with frank cases. Similar observations have been made by Gage.[5] Note is made of this disease here not because it is transmissible to human beings, for so far as is known it is not, but because it is an excellent illustration of latency, and shows how efforts to suppress a disease are doomed to failure unless account is taken of the part played by carriers. No amount of isolation of chicks sick with this form of diarrhea can ever be successful in stamping out the disease.

[1] Martin, Ann. de l'Inst. Pasteur, Par., 1900.

[2] Gotschlich, Ztschr. f. Hyg. Infectionskrankh., Leipz., 1899, XXXII, 402.

[3] Gaffky, Klin. Jahrb., Jena, 1908, XIX, 491.

[4] Rettger and Stoneburn, Storrs, Agric. Ex. Sta., Bull. 60 and 68.

[5] Gage, J. Med. Research, Bost., 1911, n. s., XIX, 491.

It is also interesting to note the analogy to ophthalmia neonotorum, which in many cases is due to mild, long-standing and unrecognized infection of the genital tract of the mother with the gonococcus.

Mediterranean Fever.—Mediterranean fever, like plague, appears to be a disease of the lower animals, only secondarily affecting man. The germ which is its cause may, like so many other pathogenic organisms, develop in the body without giving rise to symptoms. Goats appear to be the chief source of human infection. In 1905 there were 363 cases among the garrison at Malta, but in 1906, presumably owing to the cutting off of the supply of goat milk, there were only 35 cases;[1] and in 1907 it was practically exterminated.[2] An interesting account is given of an outbreak of the disease on a steamship, among persons who drank the milk of a herd of goats that were being brought to America.[3] The goats were not sick. Horrocks[4] shows that probably one or more animals in every herd are excreting the germs in the milk and urine, and that 50 per cent give evidence by serum reaction that they are, or have been, infected. Other investigations show that as high as 10 per cent of milch goats have the germs in their milk, although they present no symptoms of the disease. Carriers are also common among human beings. Shaw[5] found that 10 of 525 well persons were excreting the germs in the urine. Ross,[6] of Port Said, found the bacillus not constant in either milk or blood.

Meningococcus in Nose. — While the germ of epidemic cerebro-spinal meningitis (*Micrococcus meningitidis*) has been

[1] Hewlett, Practitioner (Lond.), 1908, LXXX, 222.

[2] Bruce, Nature, Lond., 1908, LXXVIII, 39.

[3] U. S. Pub. Health and Mar. Hosp. Serv. Hyg. Lab. Bull. No. 41, 203.

[4] Horrocks, Rep. of Commission of Roy. Soc., 1905–6, Pts. III, IV.

[5] Shaw, J. Roy. Army Med. Corps, Lond., 1906, VI, 638.

[6] Ross, J. Roy. Army Med. Corps, Lond., 1911, XI.

known for many years, it is only very recently that any explanation has been forthcoming as to the mode of infection. The finding of the organism in the nose of patients suggests the possibility that infection may pass to the brain from this point. It is theoretically possible for infection to take place through the cribriform plate of the ethmoid bone, or, as suggested by Westenhoeffer,[1] by the lymphatics from the pharyngeal tonsils, or as some think, by absorption from the alimentary canal and passage through the lymph channels or the general circulation. The organism is certainly found in the blood in a considerable number of cases.[2] What the exact route to the brain is, however, has not yet been determined.

That the germ of this disease is found in the nose of the sick is now generally recognized, though considerable doubt has been thrown on the accuracy of some of the earlier observations, as this organism is not readily distinguished from the cocci frequently found in the normal nose. Culture and agglutination tests are now recognized as the only valid methods of differentiation. Among those who have certainly isolated it in a considerable number of instances from the nasal mucous membrane of cerebro-spinal meningitis cases may be mentioned Dunham,[3] Weichselbaum and Gohn,[4] Lingelsheim,[5] Goodwin and von Sholly [6] and others.

Causes Rhinitis.—That this micrococcus is frequently found in the nose of contacts, and other persons showing no symptoms of the disease, is now well established. An interesting case is that of Kiefer,[7] who while working with a culture in the laboratory developed a severe rhinitis and succeeded in

[1] Westenhoeffer, Berl. klin. Wchnschr., 1905, XLII, 737.

[2] Birnie and Smith, Am. J. M. Sc., Phila., 1907, CXXXIV, 582, and Simon, J. Am. M. Ass., Chicago, 1907, XLVIII, 1938.

[3] Dunham, J. Infect. Dis., Chicago, 1906 [Suppl. No. 2], 10.

[4] Weichselbaum and Gohn, Wien. klin. Wchnschr., 1905, XVIII, 625.

[5] Lingelsheim, Klin. Jahrb., Jena, 1906, XV, 373.

[6] Goodwin and von Sholly, J. Infect. Dis., Chicago, 1906 [Suppl. No. 2], 21.

[7] Kiefer, Berl. klin. Wchnschr., 1906, XXXIII, 628.

recovering the micrococcus from his nose. A similar case was reported to me by P. E. Rauschenbach, at the time working in a hospital at Newark. Ford[1] also had a case of this kind.

Meningococcus in Contacts. — Among those who have found the organism in well persons may be mentioned Weichselbaum and Gohn,[2] who obtained it in 3 of 24 persons examined. Ostermann[3] found it in 17 of 24 contacts in Breslau, but his methods of employing the agglutination test have been called in question. One well child in whose nose the germs were found was taken sick three days later and died the next day. Many of the carriers had pharyngitis and rhinitis. Of 49 children in schools where these carriers attended, 2 showed the meningococcus, and one of these had been playing with a carrier. Ostermann failed to find it in 50 persons who had not come in contact with cerebro-spinal cases. Goodwin and von Sholly, in New York, obtained it in 5 of 45 contacts, and a similar coccus which did not agglutinate, in 2 of 55 medical students not contacts. Bolduan[4] found the organism in 10 per cent of 150 contacts. Lingelsheim,[5] during an extensive outbreak in Beulen, Prussia, found the organism in the nose of 26, or 9 per cent of 289 contacts. Later he found it in 4 of 56 school children, but all 4 came from families where there had been cases of the disease. In 2 of the 4 cases no agglutination test was applied. In the cases of the disease examined by Lingelsheim the micrococcus disappeared by the fifth day in 66 per cent, and by the sixth to tenth day in 24 per cent. In 4.39 per cent of the cases it persisted over three weeks, and in 1 case it was found three months from the beginning of the attack.

[1] Quoted by Councilman, J. Am. M. Ass., 1905, XLIV, 999.

[2] Weichselbaum and Gohn, Wien. klin. Wchnschr., 1905, XVIII, 625.

[3] Ostermann, Deutsche med. Wchnschr., 1906, XXXII, 414.

[4] Bolduan, Med. Times, N. Y., 1908, XXXVI, 193.

[5] Lingelsheim, Deutsche med. Wchnschr., 1905, XXXI, 1017, 1217; Klin. Jahrb., Jena, 1908, XIX, 519.

Infection in the Family. — Bruns and Hohn[1] found that the proportion of carriers decreased as the outbreak decreased. This is shown in the following table:

	Reported Cases.	No. of Families	No. of Well Persons Examined.	No. of Carriers.	Per cent of Carriers.
March	148	7	23	14	61
April	278	39	135	67	50
May	327	42	172	81	47
June	188	23	93	34	36
July	146	21	67	18	27
August	68	22	119	10	8.5

They found that of the fathers in these families 60 of 113 carried the germs; of the mothers, 39 of 114; of children in the families, 118 of 360; and of other members of the families 7 of 22 were carriers.

Persistence of Infection. — Bruns and Hohn give for the duration of the infection the following:

For 8 days	28 cases	For 5 weeks	4 cases
2 weeks	18 cases	6 weeks	3 cases
3 weeks	13 cases	7 weeks	3 cases
4 weeks	10 cases	8 weeks	1 case

Selter, in Bonn,[2] has observed a very much longer persistence of the infection. In the case of a mother and daughter who recovered from the disease, the cocci persisted from February 3 to June 4. The father in this family, who had not been sick, yielded positive findings in May, June, July and August, and had in all probability been infective for seven months. In another family where the disease appeared, the 6 well persons were carriers at one time or another from February 18 to June 5, during which period

[1] Bruns and Hohn, Klin. Jahrb., Jena, 1907–08, XVIII, 285.
[2] Selter, Klin. Jahrb., Jena, 1908–09, XX, 457.

they were examined twelve times. Sometimes the examinations were positive and sometimes negative, which is just what occurs in the examination of typhoid and diphtheria carriers. This apparent intermittency may be due in part to faulty technique, and in part to the temporary absence of the bacteria. In the 69 examinations of the family above referred to, 49 were positive and 20 negative. Selter could find no difference between the cocci found in the sick and in the carriers, but he was not able to trace a case of sickness to any of his known carriers. Kirchner,[1] in Hamburg, found 22, or 9.7 per cent, carriers, out of 237 well members of infected families, but in 3 families all the members were carriers, and in 10 other families 75 per cent were. Most of these were adults. In two instances the infection persisted 44 and 66 days respectively. Vagedes[2] reports 3 cases in barracks at Charlottenburg. Of 58 hospital attendants, etc., there, 4 were carriers, and of 593 of the soldiers 10 only were carriers. On a second examination five days later 1 only was found, and nineteen days later none. By the isolation of carriers the disease was "stamped out," but it will be noticed that the infection was not widely diffused before it was recognized. Bochalli,[3] in certain barracks where the disease prevailed, found 10 of 16 roommates of the sick, or 62 per cent, to be carriers. Of 485 in other companies, 42, or 8.6 per cent, were infected. Usually the germs quickly disappeared, but in one case they persisted for four and a half months. In another instance a nurse, going to a district where there was no meningitis, was attacked about one month later. Similar observations have been made in several places during the recent outbreak in Scotland. Buchanan,[4] in Glasgow, found the micrococcus in 81, or 26.3 per cent of 308 con-

[1] Kirchner, Klin. Jahrb., Jena, 1908, XIX, 473.

[2] Vagedes, Deutsche mil.-ärztl. Ztschr., Berl., 1907, XXIII, 647.

[3] Bochalli, Ztschr. f. Hyg. u. Infectionskrankh., Leipz., 1908, LXI, 454.

[4] Buchanan, San. Rec., Lond., 1907 n. s., XI, 245.

tacts in 74 families. Most of them were over fifteen years of age. In 14 families he obtained it from more than one person, in 2 instances from five. In 4 instances it was found in the nose two years, one year, one year, and three months, respectively, after an attack. He quotes Arbuckle, medical officer of health of Partick, as finding 23.1 per cent of 230 contacts infected. In Leith, Fraser and Comrie [1] found it in 10, or 14 per cent, of 69 contacts. Of these 5 were adults whose children were sick, and all of whom had worked on a ship in the air of whose engine room meningococci were found. Bethge,[2] immediately after the appearance of the first case in a certain institution, found that of 187 persons 66 were carriers.

Found only in Those near Sick. — The micrococcus which is the cause of this disease, while frequently noted in contacts, is rarely found in those not exposed to the disease. Ostermann, when there were no cases about, failed to find the germ in 50 children and in many adults. Bolduan did not find it in 150. Kolle and Wassermann[3] recovered the germs from 2 of 114 persons, but one had been in contact with the disease, and the other shortly became sick. Bochalli found none in 40 men in a non-infected regiment, Lingelsheim[4] none in 129 persons otherwise sick, and none in 184 non-exposed children, and he cites Droba and Kucera as finding none among 210 children living where there was no meningitis. In 23 persons not exposed to the disease and examined by Fraser and Comrie none of these organisms were found. Arkwright[5] failed to find them in 54 well persons, and Flexner[6] could find none in 50 persons in Philadelphia at a time when the disease was not present in the city.

[1] Fraser and Comrie, Scot. M. & S. J., Edinb., 1907, XXI, 18.
[2] Bethge, Deutsche med. Wchnschr., 1910, XXXV, 66.
[3] Kolle and Wassermann, Klin. Jahrb., Jena., 1906, XV, 507.
[4] Lingelsheim, Klin. Jahrb., Jena, 1906, XV, 373.
[5] Arkwright, J. Hyg., Cambridge, 1907, VII, 145.
[6] Flexner, J. Exper. M., N. Y., 1907, IX, 105.

As Lingelsheim says, it appears that the nearer we approach cases of the disease the more numerous carriers are, and the more extensive the outbreak the more numerous they are. Adults are more commonly infected than children. Flügge thinks that carriers are ten to twenty times as numerous as cases, and that is doubtless true.

Infection by Carriers. That carriers are the chief source of the disease is the opinion of those Germans who have lately had experience in severe outbreaks, and it is shared by the Scotch health officers. Lingelsheim says that there is no bacteriological or epidemiological evidence to show that the sick are more dangerous than the well, otherwise the cases would occur in groups. On the contrary the carriers mingling freely with the public are the most dangerous. Jehle [1] states that 23 cases occurred in children in the families of miners. None of the miners were sick, but when they were transferred to another mine, children there soon began to develop the disease. Their parents were doubtless carriers. Meyer [2] reports an instance where carriers gave rise to three cases. At Leith, Buchanan[3] says that the first few cases could be traced to carriers, and Thomson[4] makes a similar statement regarding the early cases in Lanarkshire. Flatten[5] gives the details of numerous instances of the transmission of the disease by well persons.

Carriers explain Spread of Disease. — Previous to the discovery of the presence of the specific organism of cerebrospinal meningitis in the nose, and particularly in the nose of contacts, the mode of extension of the disease was a mystery. Though certainly an infectious disease, and appearing in epidemics, often quite severe, it was apparently only slightly if

[1] Jehle, cited by Warrington, J. Roy. San. Inst., Lond., 1907, XV, 656.
[2] Meyer, Centralbl. f. Bakteriol. [etc.], I Abt. Orig., Jena, 1909, XLIX, 305.
[3] Buchanan, Brit. M. J., Lond., 1907, II, 852.
[4] Thomson, Med. Press & Circ., Lond., 1908, n. s., LXXXVI, 344.
[5] Flatten, Klin. Jahrb., Jena, 1906, XV, 265.

at all contagious. Personally, out of over a hundred cases, I have only twice seen two cases in the same family, and have, except in those instances, never been able to trace connection between any two cases. Cases are frequently treated in considerable numbers in general hospitals all over the world, and infection of others has rarely, if ever, taken place. In New York a greater degree of contagiousness has been noted than in most places.[1] Of 1500 consecutive cases, 112, or 7 per cent, were secondary cases in the family. It is said that when more than one case occurs in a family they all are usually taken sick at about the same time,[2] but this was not so in New York. The following shows the date at which the secondary cases appeared in that city:

Where First Cases were removed to Hospital.		Where First Case remained at Home	
No. of Secondary Cases.	Interval.	No. of Secondary Cases.	Interval.
14	1–7 days	3	1 day
5	1–2 weeks	4	2 days
4	2–3 "	1	3 "
3	3–4 "	1	5 "
2	4–5 "	1	6 "
3	5–6 "	4	7 "
2	7–8 "	1	9 "
1	3 mos.	1	11 "
34		1	21 "
		1	30 "
		18	

The 34 cases which developed after the removal of the primary case to the hospital indicate either that the germ of the disease remained in the house, on fomites, which is highly improbable, as its powers of resistance are extremely

[1] Am. Pub. Health Ass. Rep., 1905, XXXI, 359.
[2] Bolduan and Goodwin, Med. News, N. Y., 1905, LXXXVII, 1222.

slight, or that unrecognized carriers, persons with the coccus growing in the nose, remained behind, a supposition which is entirely in accord with bacteriological findings. In Glasgow,[1] of 194 cases, 7, or 4.1 per cent, were secondary cases in the family. Some of these occurred after disinfection. It is not unlikely that the more extensive the outbreak the more numerous will be the "secondary" cases in the family. In Oppeln, where there was a very severe outbreak, Flatten[2] found the number of secondary cases as follows in successive months of the outbreak:

	No. of Families.	No. of Cases.
January	71	79
February	143	163
March	257	296
April	310	368
May	349	414
June	374	439

If, as appears, the meningococcus is frequently found in the nose of sick persons and of contacts, the mode of extension of the disease becomes apparent. Observations indicate that a very considerable number of persons who come in contact with cases of this disease carry the organism on their mucous membrane. Yet very few of these persons ever become sick. It appears that the development of the cerebrospinal symptoms, that is the disease as we know it, is really a rather unusual accident of a not uncommon harmless infection of the nasal passage. We can therefore understand how the disease, though apparently showing little contagiousness, is nevertheless a strictly contagious disease. It extends almost entirely through the agency of carriers. Sometimes, as was previously stated, these carriers can be discovered, particu-

[1] Rep. Med. Off. Health, Glasgow, 1906, 89.
[2] Flatten, Klin. Jahrb., Jena, 1906, XV, 228.

larly early in an outbreak. The appearance of cases in different localities in a community, and at varying intervals, is readily explained by, and is almost a proof of, the existence of a considerable number of undiscovered carriers.

Meningitis an Accident of Infection.—The growth of the germs in the nose cannot properly be considered the "incubation" of the disease. Inoculation experiments[1] indicate that the nervous symptoms develop in a very few hours after the specific bacteria are injected into the meninges. There is much evidence, as given above, to show that the germs may grow on the surface of the nasal mucous membrane for days, weeks and perhaps months, but when they once gain access to the meninges the symptoms of the disease speedily develop.

Meningitis also occurs as a result of infection by the pneumococcus. The disease thus caused is not essentially different from the epidemic form. The number of well carriers of the pneumococcus is enormously greater, and is much more constant than is the number of carriers of the meningococcus, and the chance of the former invading the meninges and causing sickness is small, very much less than the chance of the latter doing so. In either case it may be considered an unfortunate accident of a usually benign infection.

Inutility of Isolation of Meningitis. — If these views are correct, little can be done by means of isolation to prevent the spread of the disease. When an outbreak occurs, there is certain to be a large number of carriers that cannot be found or isolated. To isolate the sick, and even those in immediate contact with the sick, will probably never make any appreciable difference in the progress of the disease, that is if the findings of to-day are confirmed by more extended observations. By the time several cases have developed in a community, there will probably usually be a considerable number of carriers who cannot be found. Stringent isola-

[1] Lingelsheim, Deutsche med. Wchnschr., 1905, XXXI, 1017, 1217; Flexner, J. Exper. M., N. Y., 1907, IX, 142.

tion of the families of known cases will accomplish little, and will work much hardship and injustice.

Diphtheria Bacilli in Well Persons. — Loeffler [1] himself in 1884 found diphtheria bacilli in a person who was not sick, and in 1889 Roux and Yersin [2] called attention to the persistence of diphtheria bacilli on the mucous membranes of convalescents, and their observations were at intervals substantiated by others. In 1894 Park and Beebe [3] examined the throats of 330 healthy persons who had not, so far as known, been in contact with diphtheria cases, and found diphtheria bacilli in 24, or 7.3 per cent, but of these only 8, or 2.4 per cent, of the 330 were virulent. These authors minimized the danger to be apprehended from these carriers, and although for some time similar observations were reported, they were generally, and are even now by many, considered of little importance. It seems to me otherwise, and therefore a considerable number of these observations are here summarized. Müller [4] examined in routine 92 children sick with diseases other than diphtheria, in Heubner's clinic, and reported that 12, or 13 per cent, were infected with diphtheria, but only 6 of the 12 were tested on guinea pigs. Later 18 children in the same institution, who had negative cultures on admission, were found to harbor the bacilli. Kober [5] in Breslau found that of 600 school children 2.5 per cent were carriers of diphtheria bacilli, but in only 0.83 per cent of the 600 were they virulent. At Baltimore,[6] in 1899, during an exceptional prevalence of diphtheria in a number of schools, cultures were taken from 4068 pupils apparently well, and of these 157, or 3.8 per cent,

[1] Loeffler, The Bacteriology of Diphtheria, Nuttall and Graham-Smith, Cambridge, 1908, 31.

[2] Roux and Yersin, Ann. de l'Inst. Pasteur, 1890, IV, 385.

[3] Park and Beebe, Med. Rec., N. Y., 1894, XLVI, 385; Sci. Bull. 1, Dept. Health N. Y. City, 1895.

[4] Müller, Jahrb. f. Kinderh., 1896, XLIII, 54.

[5] Kober, Ztschr. f. Hyg. u. Infectionskrankh., Leipz., 1899, XXXI, 433.

[6] Baltimore, Rep. Com. of Health, 1899, 96; 1900, 85.

showed diphtheria bacilli. The next year, of 351 examined, 23, or 6.6 per cent, were positive.

Varieties of Bacilli found. — Reports of the finding of diphtheria bacilli in well persons would have more value if it were made clear what was meant by the term diphtheria bacilli. The bacillus varies greatly in form, and those who have studied it most carefully are by no means agreed as to what should or should not be properly so called. Fortunately Wesbrook's classification of all these varieties, both admitted and questioned, renders it possible to interpret properly the reports of all who will take the trouble to use his nomenclature, and it is to be regretted that more do not use it. Again, diphtheria bacilli are quite as frequently found in the nose as in the throat, but few observers state whether the cultures were taken from throat or nose or both. For the purpose of securing definite data from a large number of cases, a collective investigation was undertaken by the Massachusetts Association of Boards of Health.[1] The number of persons examined was 4250 in different parts of the United States. Most of them had probably not been directly exposed to diphtheria except in Minnesota, where most of the cultures were taken from schools and institutions where there had recently been cases of the disease. The majority of the persons examined were adults, and cultures were taken from both throat and nose. Of all persons examined, 2.89 per cent had "granular" forms of diphtheria bacilli, i.e., those showing polar staining with methylene blue. If "barred" and other aberrant types are to be considered as diphtheria bacilli, as they are by some, the number of cultures to be reported positive would have been more than doubled. Referring only to the typical granular types, 1.46 per cent of all persons showed throat infection (either with or without concurrent nose infection) and 2.07 per cent showed nose infection (either with or without concurrent throat infection). In the different cities the percentage of infected persons varied from 0.43 in Provi-

[1] J. Mass. Ass. Bds. Health, Bost., 1902, XII, 74.

dence, where particular care was taken to avoid contacts, most of the cultures being taken from schools where there had been no diphtheria for at least two years, to 3.66 in the Willard State Hospital, and 6.03 in Minnesota, in both of which localities there had recently been diphtheria in the institutions examined. There were 47 tests for virulence, of which 8, or 17 per cent, were positive. Recently cultures were taken from school children in Brighton (Boston) by Slack.[1] Of over 4000 children examined by throat and nose culture on two occasions, 1.93 per cent showed diphtheria bacilli. Of these 8 were tested for virulence, of which all proved to be non-virulent. Most of these children were excluded from school until free from bacilli, but all of them had, of course, been carrying bacilli in school for a longer or shorter period. No case of clinical diphtheria was traced to any of these carriers, either in school or out of school. These facts have been advanced as evidence that the danger from such carriers is a negligible factor in contrast with the danger from convalescents whose bacilli are usually virulent. But in Providence in 1908, 73 convalescents carrying diphtheria bacilli were admitted to school, and it is not known that they were in any instance the source of new cases in the school, and in all but two or three instances it is certain that they were not. Forbes [2] cites Meikle as reporting 27 carriers discharged from the hospital without any return case. These facts merely indicate that the amount of danger from a single focus of infection is much less than is generally believed.

Value of Bacteriological Findings. — Neumann[3] could not find any diphtheria bacilli in 111 perfectly normal throats and noses, but did find them in 8 of 95 cases suffering from catarrhal inflammation of the mucous surfaces. He does not think that they are found in normal throats, but certainly all who have had any experience in taking cultures have seen

[1] Slack, Arms, Wade and Blanchard, J. Am. M. Ass., 1910, LIV, 951.
[2] Forbes, Brit. M. J., 1909, II, 522.
[3] Neumann, Ztschr. f. Hyg. u. Infectionskrankh., Leipz., 1902, XL, 33.

numberless cases where diphtheria bacilli were found in throats which, so far as appearances go, were perfectly normal. When diphtheria bacilli are found on a reddened or slightly inflamed mucous surface, the abnormal condition may not in every individual case be due to their presence, for certainly " catarrhal " inflammations of nose and throat, due to other causes than the presence of diphtheria bacilli, are extremely common. The evidence is that at present, in cities, from 1 to 2 per cent of the population are infected with diphtheria bacilli. The presence of diphtheria bacilli in an inflamed throat may be, then, in 1 or 2 per cent of the findings merely a coincidence. It is safe to assume that in all but 1 or 2 per cent the presence of diphtheria bacilli stands in causative relation to the inflammation of the surface on which they are found.

Diphtheria Bacilli in Children. — In Bristol, Heaven[1] examined 704 children (throat and nose) connected with schools where there had been considerable diphtheria, and found diphtheria bacilli in 24, or 3.4 per cent. Of 758 cultures taken from schools in London where there had been occasional cases of diphtheria, 58, or 7.6 per cent, showed the bacilli.[2] Pennington[3] examined 375 well children in Philadelphia schools, in some of which there had been more or less diphtheria, and of 37 positive cultures from these, 24 were more or less virulent. Of 125 pupils from four other schools 10.4 per cent gave positive cultures, about half of which were virulent. But Pennington found that of 25 cultures from convalescents 22 were virulent. In the city of Mexico, of 300 school children 10, or 3.3 per cent, showed diphtheria bacilli.[4] Von Sholly[5] examined 1000 tenement-house children in New York, taking cultures only from those whose throats appeared normal. The

[1] Heaven, Pub. Health, Lond., 1902–03, XV, 516.
[2] Rep. Med. Off. Health, Lond., 1904, Appendix III, 25.
[3] Pennington, J. Infect. Dis., Chicago, 1907, IV, 36
[4] Fabela, Rep. Am. Pub. Health Ass., 1906, XXXII, Pt. 2, 199.
[5] Von Sholly, J. Infect. Dis., Chicago, 1907, IV, 337.

children for the most part were those brought to hospitals and dispensaries for treatment, but all cases were excluded which had any suggestion of sore throat, nasal discharge, etc. Of these 1000 cases 5.6 per cent showed diphtheria-like organisms, of which, however, only 1.8 per cent (of the 1000 cases) proved to be virulent. In 50 of the cases nose cultures also were taken, and one of these proved to have virulent bacilli. During a very severe outbreak of diphtheria in Christiania, Ustvedt[1] examined 4277 school children, and found diphtheria bacilli in 191, or 4.5 per cent. Of these, 10 afterwards developed diphtheria. Of 7 cultures tested for virulence 4 were positive. In one school in which the percentage of positive cultures was 9.2 during the outbreak, it was 3.2 some months later. In a school in the country where there had been no diphtheria for years, no bacilli were isolated from 86 pupils. Ruediger[2] found diphtheria bacilli in 3 of 51 normal throats. Gross[3] took two throat and nose cultures from 314 children (without diphtheria) on admission to the Children's Hospital in Boston, and isolated diphtheria bacilli from 26, or 7.9 per cent. Five were tested for virulence, 4 of which were positive. Hewlett and Murray[4] found that 58, or 15 per cent, of 385 children on admission to the Victoria Hospital for Children in London, were diphtheria carriers, and that in children under two years of age the percentage was 21. Cobbett[5] at Cambridge reported diphtheria bacilli in 2.9 per cent of 650 well persons, many of whom were contacts. Some had mild sore throat.

Diphtheria Bacilli in Scarlet Fever. — While the presence of diphtheria bacilli in scarlet fever cases sheds little light on their prevalence in normal throats, it is of much interest

[1] Ustvedt, Ztschr. f. Hyg. u. Infectionskrankh., Leipz., 1906, LIV, 147.

[2] Ruediger, J. Am. M. Ass., Chicago, 1906, XLVII, 1173.

[3] Gross, Univ. M. Mag., Phila., 1896–7, IX, 45.

[4] Hewlett and Murray, Brit. M. J., Lond., 1901, I, 1474.

[5] Cobbett, J. Hyg., Cambridge, 1901, I, 242.

from an epidemiological standpoint. The exudation which frequently covers the tonsils in scarlet fever is often mistaken clinically for a sign of diphtheria, and such cases are, before the appearance of the eruption, often reported as diphtheria, so that there is a popular impression among physicians that the two diseases are frequently combined, and that the presence of scarlet fever predisposes to diphtheria. While bacteriological examinations tend to show that diphtheria infection on scarlet fever is not so common as is often assumed, and that many cases reported as a combination of the two diseases are not really such, yet diphtheria bacilli are frequently found in cases of scarlet fever, more frequently than they are found in the general public from whom the scarlet fever cases come.

In Providence during the past four years cultures have been taken from 92 scarlet fever cases in their homes, of which 6, or 6.5 per cent, were positive. Of 245 cultures in the hospital, 26, or 10.6 per cent, were positive. During the preceding three years 116 cultures were taken, but it was not recorded whether they were from hospital or home cases, and of these, 5, or 4.3 per cent, were positive. The excessive percentage of positive findings in the hospital was due to infection after admission. Both throat and nose cultures were taken in nearly every case. In the Western Fever Hospital of London,[1] of 1019 throat swabs taken from the same number of scarlet fever patients on admission, 7.86 per cent were positive; at another hospital 5.41 per cent of 203 cases, and at another 6.8 per cent of 87 cases. Of the 939 cases at the Western Hospital which did not have diphtheria bacilli on admission, 6 later developed diphtheria, ranging from the ninth to the fiftieth day after admission, and 28 more acquired diphtheria bacilli without being sick. Of the 80 cases that entered infected, 4 developed clinical diphtheria on the fourth, fifth, seventh and thirty-first days. Soerensen[2] found that of 1547 scarlet fever cases examined on admission, 38, or

[1] Cumpston, J. Hyg., Cambridge, 1907, VII, 598.

[2] Soerensen, Ztschr. f. Hyg. u. Infectionskrankh., 1898, XXIX, 250.

2.5 per cent, carried diphtheria bacilli. During a service of two years 32 cases of diphtheria occurred in the scarlet fever wards among about 1500 patients, and 208 others were found to be infected but not sick. Ruediger[1] found diphtheria in 4 of 75 scarlet fever throats, or 5.3 per cent. Garratt and Washbourn[2] found diphtheria germs in 8, or 1.2 per cent, of 666 scarlet fever cases. In Croydon,[3] 37, or 17.3 per cent, of 213 cases of scarlet fever were shown to be infected with diphtheria bacilli on admission to the hospital. In Brighton,[4] in 1905, 33, or 25.9 per cent, of 166 cases of scarlet fever had diphtheria bacilli present, and all but one were infected on admission; in 1907, 21 of 340 were infected. In Bristol,[5] of 202 scarlet fever patients in the hospital in 1904, 75 per cent had positive cultures on admission. In 1905, of 476 cases, 21, or 4.4 per cent, were positive, besides 3 others which showed symptoms of the disease. In Philadelphia, of 700 scarlet fever admissions, 11 per cent showed diphtheria bacilli.

Percentage of Diphtheria Carriers. — The evidence thus far adduced tends to show that diphtheria bacilli are quite widely distributed in the urban population of Europe and America. Perhaps on the average 1 or 2 per cent harbor the germs of this disease in mouth or nose; but observations also indicate that the less diphtheria there is in a community, and the farther removed the persons examined are from cases of the disease, the less likely they are to be infected. Thus in Christiania during an outbreak, 9.2 per cent of the pupils in a certain school were infected, while some months later the ratio was only 3.2. The Massachusetts Association of Boards of Health report an infection of 6.03 per cent of the school children recently exposed to diphtheria in Minneapolis, while in schools in Providence where there had been no diph-

[1] Ruediger, J. Am. M. Ass., Chicago, 1906, XLVII, 1173.
[2] Garratt and Washbourn, Brit. M. J., Lond., 1899, I, 893.
[3] Rep. Med. Off. Health, Croydon, 1904, 68.
[4] Rep. Med. Off. Health, Brighton, 1905, 42; 1907, 22.
[5] Rep. Med. Off. Health, Bristol, 1904, 100; 1905, 71.

theria for a long time the ratio was only about one-half of 1 per cent.

Percentage among Contacts. — There are numerous observations made on persons brought more or less closely in contact with the sick, which show that under such conditions

Percentage of Carriers in Diphtheria Families, Providence, 1897–1901.

Ages.	Persons examined.	Number of Carriers.	Percentage of Carriers.
Under 1 year	119	17	14.2
1 "	112	15	13.3
2 years.....	97	23	23.7
3 "	112	25	22.3
4 "	116	31	26.7
5 "	120	17	14.1
6 "	137	42	30.6
7 "	130	30	23.1
8 "	119	25	21.0
9 "	113	23	20.3
10 "	139	26	18.7
11 "	79	11	13.9
12 "	127	28	22.0
13 "	86	15	17.4
14 "	88	13	14.7
15 "	70	5	7.1
16 "	64	9	14.0
17 "	57	9	15.7
18 "	57	6	10.5
19 "	45	4	8.8
20 "	34	4	11.7
Adults...........	2505	277	11.0
Totals.........	4526	655	14.4

the number of carriers may be very high. For several years in Providence[1] cultures were taken from all the wage earners in the family at the time the case was reported, and from all the members of the family for release, that is, to determine

[1] Rep. Supt. Health, Providence, 1901, 44.

the end of isolation. Only throat cultures were taken. Of 4526 such contacts examined 14.4 per cent were found to be infected. If nose as well as throat cultures had been taken, and if cultures had been taken from the whole family about midway in the course of the disease, I imagine the percentage would have been several times greater. The preceding table shows the percentage infected at different ages. The women in the family were infected very much oftener than the men. It was noticed that in about 10 per cent of the cases some well member of the family remained infected after the patient was entirely free from germs. In Glasgow,[1] of 2305 contacts in infected families 9.2 per cent were carriers.

Percentage of Carriers in Infected Schools. — In a certain school in Minnesota,[2] of 263 well children, 129, or 49 per cent, were infected with the granular and barred types of the bacillus. In Bristol[3] during a school outbreak in 1907, of 190 well children, 12.5 per cent were carriers. At the Willard Hospital for the Insane during an outbreak, of 1423 well persons, 189, or 13 per cent, were carriers. At the State Hospital in California, 11.6 of 1115 persons were infected.[4] In Providence during an outbreak of diphtheria in an infant asylum, of 175 children and adults, 116 or 66.2 per cent, proved to be infected at one time or another, but this was only after many repeated cultures extending over a period of some months. Many of them were persistent carriers, one of them remaining infected for twenty-two months. Crowley[5] in a school outbreak found 42 of 93 children infected, or 45 per cent. In Bermondsey, London,[6] the children in diphtheria families have a single throat culture taken, and of 597 children so

[1] Rep. Med. Off. Health, Glasgow, 1908, 71.

[2] Wesbrook, St. Paul M. J., St. Paul, Minn., 1900, II, 219 [p. 6 of reprint].

[3] Rep. Med. Off. Health, Bristol, 1907, 51.

[4] Rep. Calif. St. Bd. Health, 1906–08, 201.

[5] Crowley, J. Roy. San. Inst., 1904–05, XXV, 807.

[6] Rep. Med. Off. Health, London, 1904, 31.

examined 64, or 10.8 per cent, were found to be infected. Of 115 well children in an institution in Minneapolis, Corbet [1] found 29, or 25.2 per cent, infected. In several instances the bacilli presented atypical forms, but many of these were virulent. In a school in the same city, where there had been some diphtheria, he found that 20, or 14.3 per cent, of 140 cultures showed the presence of typical bacilli.[2] Ustvedt,[3] in Christiania, found 17 per cent of contacts infected. In a school at Oakland, California,[4] 25 per cent of the pupils were carriers. In Glasgow,[5] of 322 well members of diphtheria families 10.5 per cent were infected. In the Duke of York's school, London, of 536 well pupils 117, or 20 per cent, showed diphtheria bacilli, and of these 10 later had diphtheria, while only one of the "free" boys developed it. Of 13 cultures from the well boys, 7 were virulent, though mildly so, but the bacilli from the sick also showed a low virulence. It is worthy of note that the disease recurred in this school for two or three years.[6] von Sholly [7] found bacilli in 20 of 202 contacts, or about 10 per cent, and of these 14 were virulent. Buchanan [8] in Glasgow found that the bacilli were virulent in 66 per cent of 21 healthy carriers, and that bacilli recovered from 56 cases of the disease proved virulent only in 74 per cent. Aaser [9] found 19 per cent of contacts in cavalry barracks infected, and 20 per cent of children in a scarlet fever ward. Hellström [10] in Stockholm, of 786 soldiers who had been more

[1] Corbet, Rep. Com. Health, Minneapolis, 1905, 7.

[2] Rep. Com. Health, Minneapolis, 1903, 16.

[3] Ustvedt, Ztschr. f. Hyg. u. Infectionskrankh., Leipz., 1906, LIV, 147.

[4] Bull. Calif. St. Bd. Health, November, 1906.

[5] Rep. Med. Off. Health, Glasgow, 1906, 135.

[6] Arkwright, J. Hyg., Cambridge, 1908, VIII, 48; Rep. Med. Off. Health, Lond., 1906, 36.

[7] von Sholly, J. Infect. Dis., Chicago, 1907, IV, 337.

[8] Buchanan, Brit. M. J., Lond., 1909, II, 519.

[9] Aaser, Deutsche med. Wchnschr., 1895, XXI, 357.

[10] Hellström, cited by Kober, Ztschr. f. Hyg. u. Infectionskrankh., Leipz., 1899, XXXI, 433, and by Fibiger, Berl. klin. Wchnschr., 1897, XXXIV, 753.

or less in contact with diphtheria, found 151, or 19.2 per cent, infected. Goadby,[1] in 586 pupils in a school where there had recently been 21 diphtheria cases, found that 190, or 34.1 per cent, were carriers, and he quotes Meade Bolton as finding 45.5 per cent of 214 contacts infected. Of the children examined by Goadby 262 had enlarged tonsils and 196 abnormal throats. In another school where there had been no reported cases, 18 of 100 were infected.

Berry and Washbourn[2] report 17, or 11.9 per cent, of infected contacts in a school of 142 girls. Lister[3] found 48 per cent of 125 contacts in Shadwell Hospital infected. Twenty-four of them had nasal discharge. Park and Beebe[4] in a foundling asylum obtained virulent bacilli and one non-virulent form from 5 of 55 contacts. Fibiger,[5] during a school outbreak of diphtheria, recovered the bacilli in 22, or 16.4 per cent, of 134 children. Denny[6] found 11 per cent of 200 children infected, in a school where there had recently been 4 cases of diphtheria, and Graham-Smith,[7] 10.4 per cent of 519 school children. Gabritschewsky[8] in the Russian military service found, during the prevalence of diphtheria, that 20 per cent of the well persons examined were carriers, and in a school in Moscow, at a time when there was much diphtheria, 21 of 66 well children showed diphtheria bacilli.

Atypical Diphtheria. — The old notion was, and I fear that very many physicians and not a few health officers so believe to-day, that diphtheria is a well defined disease with characteristic symptoms. They cannot imagine diphtheria without

[1] Goadby, Lancet, Lond., 1900, I, 236.

[2] Berry and Washbourn, Brit. M. J., Lond., 1900, I, 198.

[3] Lister, Brit. M. J., Lond., 1898, II, 1338.

[4] Park and Beebe, Med. Rec., N. Y., 1894, XLVI, 385.

[5] Fibiger, Berl. klin. Wchnschr., 1897, XXXIV, 753.

[6] Denny, Bost. M. & S. J., 1900, 515.

[7] Graham-Smith, J. Hyg., Cambridge, 1903, III, 216.

[8] Gabritschewsky, Ztschr. f. Hyg. u. Infectionskrankh., Leipz., 1901, XXXVI, 45.

serious illness. There always have been, however, some acute clinicians who thought otherwise. Jacobi in New York was among the foremost. He recognized that the disease often presented a mild type and that diagnosis was impossible. He said in 1884:[1]

"The symptoms are often but few. A little muscular pain and difficult deglutition are, perhaps, all that is complained of. Women will quietly bear it; men will go about their business. . . . There is as much diphtheria out of bed as in bed; nearly as much out of doors as indoors. Many a mild case is walking the streets for weeks without caring or thinking that some of his victims have been wept over before he was quite well himself. . . . Diphtheria is contagious. Severe forms may beget severe or mild forms. Mild cases may beget mild or severe cases."

Under Jacobi's teaching I early learned to look for such mild cases, and I remember seeing an outbreak in a children's home during the early eighties, in which there were many very mild sore throats and walking cases. Mild diphtheria of this type does not usually come to the notice of a physician, and when it does is frequently not recognized. How frequent such cases are it is difficult to determine, but they must be very numerous. In a general hospital at Chelsea[2] (London), where there had been considerable trouble from outbreaks of diphtheria, it was determined to take cultures from all patients admitted who showed any symptoms of sore throat. Of 815 persons so examined 65, or 7.3 per cent, gave positive cultures. In New York City[3] the school inspectors were directed to take cultures from all children showing slight redness of the throat or hypertrophied tonsils. Of 11,451 cultures 757, or 6.7 per cent, were positive. These children were not in any sense considered as ill, yet the percentage

[1] Quoted by Solis-Cohen, J. Am. M. Ass., Chicago, 1907, XLIX, 32.

[2] Parkes, Pub. Health, Lond., 1902–03, XV, 538.

[3] Letter from Dr. Cronin, N. Y. Bd. Health, Sept. 23, 1904.

infected is certainly much higher than would be looked for among the general school population. In Hartford[1] during the years 1900–1903 cultures were taken from 2038 mild sore throats seen in the schools. Of these, 591, or 29 per cent, were positive. These children might be said to have a decided sore throat, though they were all well enough to be in school. They were all excluded from school. During the same period there were reported in Hartford 1537 cases of diphtheria, so that the cases found in the manner described equaled one-third of the total cases. In Indianapolis,[2] at a time when there were 60 reported cases of diphtheria in the city, a diligent search for, and taking of cultures from, sore throats among the school children revealed the presence of 46 other cases. Every one knows how extremely common sore throat and tonsillitis are, and even if only a very small proportion, much less than 29 per cent, of these, are true diphtheria, the number in the aggregate must be very large. I think I am well within bounds when I assume that for every recognized case of diphtheria there is at least one sore throat which is also diphtheria though unrecognized. Judging from the proportion of mild cases in institution outbreaks, the proportion of unrecognized, mild, but yet clinical cases, must be much greater than that. Careful medical inspection often discovers that these missed cases have been the source of reported cases. For example, the Report on the Health of the City of Manchester (England), 1906, gives a list of 29 cases caused in this way during that year.

Rhinitis and Otitis. — Diphtheria sometimes assumes a chronic form with few symptoms. Indeed some, as Neumann, believe that long persistence of diphtheria bacilli in throat and nose is always accompanied by local disturbance. That such is often the case in the nose, and that subacute chronic rhinitis may be a form of diphtheria, and may give rise to typical pharyngeal cases, is generally recognized.

[1] Reps. Bd. Health, Hartford, 1900 to 1903.
[2] Rep. Dept. Pub. Health & Charities, Indianapolis, 1908, 8.

Park,[1] Abbott,[2] Ravenel,[3] Schaps,[4] Treitel and Koppel,[5] DeStella,[6] Ballin[7] and many others report cases of chronic rhinitis due to the presence of the diphtheria bacillus. The middle ear sometimes suppurates in diphtheria, as it does in scarlet fever, though less frequently, and this discharge may remain virulent for long periods.[8] I happen to have such a case under observation at the present time.

A Real Danger. — There can be no doubt, then, that mild and unrecognized cases of diphtheria are very common, that convalescents long harbor the bacilli, and that contacts and other carriers are very numerous; in fine, that these sources of infection far outnumber the cases of recognized sickness. But are these really sources of infection, or are they, as so many believe, an imaginary danger evolved in the brain of the laboratory worker? It is well again to emphasize the fact that long before Klebs and Loeffler identified the bacillus of this disease a few able clinical observers like Jacobi believed that evidence pointed clearly to the great danger of these unrecognized sources of infection. The bacteriologists have not raised the bugaboo of carrier infection, they have simply explained the facts which observing men have long recognized.

Carriers cause Disease. — A little perusal of medical literature will show that many cases are reported of what is apparently the distribution of diphtheria by carriers.

Peck[9] reports an instance where a young man who was

[1] Park, Med. Rec., N. Y., 1892, XLII, 121.

[2] Abbott, Med. News, Phila., 1893, LXII, 505.

[3] Ravenel, Med. News, Phila., 1895, LXVI, 537.

[4] Schaps, Arch. f. Kinderh., Stuttg., 1905, XL, 80.

[5] Treitel and Koppel, Arch. f. Kinderh., Stuttg., 1895–96, XIX, 107.

[6] DeStella, Arch. internat. de laryngol. [etc.], Par., 1903, XVI, 970.

[7] Ballin, Jahrb. f. Kinderh., 1903, LVIII, 412.

[8] Newsholme, Rep. Med. Off. Health, Brighton, 1906, 13; Address at Victoria Univ., Manchester, March 9, 1904, 21.

[9] Peck, Brit. M. J., Lond., 1895, I, 971.

perfectly well but was a carrier, probably gave diphtheria to another young man with whom he slept.

In 1897 a mother whom I saw, stayed for a few days in a house on a neighboring street taking care of a diphtheria case. Soon after her return home her son was taken sick with diphtheria, and when cultures were taken from her throat she also was found to be infected.[1] In 1905 a child who was sent to the hospital for some surgical lesion developed scarlet fever and was removed to the scarlet-fever ward. Three days after his return home another child in the family was taken sick with diphtheria, and a few days later a culture taken from the first child was positive.[2] Wesbrook[3] reports: " Two always well children carrying bacilli sent home. Diphtheria broke out shortly after their arrival. No other source of infection discovered. One always well girl carrying diphtheria bacilli went to her home. Stepmother and children developed diphtheria within a few days. This family was practically isolated in the country."

Hellström,[4] during a diphtheria outbreak in a cavalry regiment, noted two instances in which perfectly well soldiers who had diphtheria bacilli on their mucous membrane carried the disease to others. Aaser [5] reports a child with diphtheria germs taking the disease home from a scarlet-fever ward where there was a diphtheria outbreak.

In 1906 at Birmingham [6] there was a milk outbreak of diphtheria of 13 cases due to infection of the milk by the milk handlers, who had diphtheria bacilli in their throats, but were not sick. As soon as they were isolated the outbreak ceased. Similar milk outbreaks caused by infected well per-

[1] Rep. Supt. Health, Prov., 1897, 21.

[2] Rep. Supt. Health, Prov., 1905, 32.

[3] Prelim. Rep. on Diphtheria in Well Persons, J. Mass. Ass. Bds. Health, Bost., 1901, XI, 10.

[4] Hellström, cited by Fibiger, Berl. klin. Wchnschr., 1897, XXXIV, 753.

[5] Aaser, Deutsche med. Wchnschr., 1895, XXI, 357.

[6] Rep. Med. Off. Health, Birmingham, 1906, 40.

sons have been reported from Fitchburg,[1] Lowell,[2] Brookline,[3] Montclair, N. J.,[4] Oroville, Cal.,[5] Australia[6] and other places.

At the Willard State Hospital[7] a watchman, who lived with his son-in-law in the village, who had diphtheria, was never sick but was a carrier. He played cards with two clerks, and they all drank from the same pitcher. The clerks, who had not been exposed to diphtheria, were a week later taken sick with the disease. Four other instances of infection by carriers occurred during the same outbreak, and a similar instance some years before.

In Lagrange Co., Ind.,[8] in 1902, there were three outbreaks in a school, apparently caused by the teacher, in whose nose diphtheria bacilli were found, and who had shown no symptoms but a slight cold. In Boston[9] a boy who had recovered from diphtheria, escaped from isolation and went to Brockton, and within four days three clinical cases developed in the house where he visited. Fischer[10] reports an outbreak traced to a restaurant in which were several carriers and mild sore throats. Solberg[11] had a boy who caused several cases of the disease. He had been kept in the hospital for several months, but was finally discharged with the bacilli present. Cobbett's[12] outbreak in Cambridge was due to a boy apparently

[1] Prelim. Rep. on Diphtheria in Well Persons, J. Mass. Ass. Bds. Health, Bost., 1901, XI, 9.

[2] Rep. Bd. Health, Lowell, 1904, 24.

[3] Prelim. Rep. on Diphtheria in Well Persons, J. Mass. Ass. Bds. Health, Bost., 1901, XI, 9.

[4] Pediatrics, N. Y., 1901, XII, 366.

[5] Rep. St. Bd. Health, Cal., 1906–08, 198.

[6] Armstrong, Austral. M. Gaz., Melbourne, 1908, XXVII, 350.

[7] Report of Epidemic of Diphtheria at Willard State Hospital by Russell and Salmon [Rep. State Com. on Lunacy, XVI], 35 of Reprint.

[8] Letter from Dr. H. N. Hurty, Sec. Ind. St. Bd. Health, 1907.

[9] Prelim. Rep. on Diphtheria in Well Persons, J., Mass. Ass. Bds. Health, Bost., 1901, XI, 9.

[10] Fischer, München med. Wchnschr., 1906, LIII, 250, 314.

[11] Solberg, quoted in Pub. Health, Lond., 1902–03, XV, 515.

[12] Cobbett, J. Hyg., Cambridge, 1901, I, 229.

well, but who for some weeks had had a slight nasal discharge in which diphtheria germs were present. Williams[1] notes a case in which a teacher was infected with clinical diphtheria by the nasal discharge of a pupil containing atypical bacilli.[2] Newsholme[3] saw a case of diphtheria in February, 1901, which had ear discharge for a short time only. Suppuration recurred April, 1904, and diphtheria germs were present. Three cases of the disease occurred in the family soon after. The ear again discharged in March, 1906, with bacilli present, and a sister apparently contracted the disease from this source. Newsholme had a similar case in 1907. Vance[4] states that a nurse had diphtheria in June, and after one negative culture from the throat, went home and infected 3 persons. In August she returned to the hospital and infected 4 other persons, at which time a culture from throat and nose was negative. Subsequent cultures proved positive, and continued so until late in November. Strain[5] also reports a nurse in whose nose diphtheria bacilli were found intermittently for nine months, but they were never present in the throat. Edsall[6] notes five outbreaks due to carriers, and Solis-Cohen[7] seven such outbreaks. Cameron[8] reports that in 70 instances cases of scarlet fever discharged from the London hospitals carried diphtheria to their homes, and that in many of these carriers diphtheria bacilli were shown to be present.

Similar cases in which clinical diphtheria is apparently contracted from perfectly well convalescents or carriers, or from slight unnoticed sore throat, or from rhinitis, are found scat-

[1] Williams, J. Laryngol., Lond., 1905, XX, 591.
[2] Wesbrook's D^1D^2.
[3] Newsholme, Rep. Med. Off. Health, Brighton, 1906, 13.
[4] Vance, Intercolon. M. J. Australas., Melbourne, 1908, XIII, 152.
[5] Strain, Lancet, Lond., 1908, II, 1143.
[6] Edsall, J. Am. M. Ass., Chicago, 1909, LII, 125.
[7] Solis-Cohen, J. Am. M. Ass., Chicago, 1909, LII, 111.
[8] Cameron, Rep. to Asylums Bd. on Return Cases of Scarlet Fever in London, 1901–02, 41.

tered through medical literature, and a number of such have been collected by the Massachusetts Association of Boards of Health,[1] Nuttall and Graham-Smith,[2] Newsholme,[3] Sittler,[4] Niven,[5] Schneider,[6] myself [7] and others.

Chronic Diphtheria. — Diphtheria sometimes assumes a chronic form, with few constitutional symptoms, and little that is noticeable, and nothing that is characteristic in the fauces. This condition may continue for months, and is sometimes accompanied by considerable antitoxin in the blood. Such cases may cause typical diphtheria.[8]

Glanders. — According to veterinary writers [9] the infection of glanders often remains latent, and also many mild chronic cases occur which are the source of considerable outbreaks. The Bureau of Animal Industry [10] reports an instance where a horse was apparently infectious for eight years without manifesting any symptoms which would lead even an expert to suspect the infection. Another instance was given of a year-long infection of an apparently well animal.

Influenza. — The rapidity with which epidemic influenza spreads, its sudden contemporaneous appearance at many distant points, and the difficulty of tracing the route of infection, render it almost certain that there must in this disease be many mild atypical cases, and many persons infected, but showing no symptoms. That the disease is not carried by

1 Prelim. Rep. on Diphtheria Bacilli in Well Persons, J. Mass. Ass. Bds. Health, Bost., 1901, XI, 9.

2 Nuttall and Graham-Smith, The Bacteriology of Diphtheria, Cambridge, 1908, 311.

3 Newsholme, Address at Victoria Univ., Manchester, Mar. 9, 1904, and Med.-Chir. Tr., Lond., 1904, LXXXVII, 549.

4 Sittler, München med. Wchnschr, 1906, LIII, 863.

5 Niven, Rep. on the Health of Manchester, 1908, 204.

6 Schneider, Ztschr. f. Med.-Beamte, Berl., XX, 698.

7 Rep. Supt. Health, Prov., 1897, 19; 1898, 23; 1905, 32.

8 Neisser and Kahnert, Deutsche med. Wchnschr., 1900, XXVI, 525, and Neisser, Deutsche med. Wchnschr., 1902, XXVIII, 719.

9 Law, Text-Book of Veterinary Medicine, Ithaca, 1902, IV, 235.

10 U. S. Dept. Agric., Bu. An. Ind., Circ. No. 78. 4.

the air over long distances, as has been urged by many, but is invariably transmitted by persons, has been shown by Parsons, Schmid and others. That these persons often show no symptoms, and are not suspected of being carriers, also seems certain.

There is some bacteriological evidence of this, but the bacteriologists have not given to the study of this disease the attention which it deserves. Finkler found the bacillus in the sputum a year after the beginning of an attack. Lord,[1] during non-epidemic periods, in examining cases of what appeared ordinary cough, found influenza bacilli present in 60 per cent of the cases. Later,[2] in 186 non-tuberculous cases, mostly bronchitis, he found the bacillus frequently present, often in almost pure culture. Boggs[3] has also found chronic cases somewhat simulating tuberculosis, in one instance lasting for a year. Holt,[4] in the Babies' Hospital in New York, obtained 112 positive cultures out of 312 taken from 198 persons. Of 48 healthy persons 16 yielded positive cultures. I have found scarcely any other reports of the examination of well persons for this organism, but the frequency with which it is found in those sick with other diseases is evidence of the widespread distribution of the bacillus. Wollstein,[5] by swabbing the throat, found the bacillus in 16 of 37 cases of pneumonia, in 11 of 34 of bronchitis, in 8 of 18 cases of measles, in 8 of 16 of tuberculosis, but only 5 times in 65 cases of other diseases. Davis[6] found influenza-like bacilli in normal throats, and in 61 of 68 cases of whooping cough and in 13 of 23 cases of measles. Inoculated on the mucous surface of a healthy young man, fever and catarrhal symptoms developed. Both Davis and Wollstein consider that the so-called

[1] Lord, Boston M. & S. J., 1902, CXLVII, 662.
[2] Lord, Boston M. & S. J., 1905, CLII, 574.
[3] Boggs, Am. J. M. Sc., Phila., 1905, n. s., CXXX, 902.
[4] Holt, Am. J. Obst., N. Y., 1909, LX, 343.
[5] Wollstein, J. Exper. M., N. Y., 1906, VIII, 681.
[6] Davis, J. Am. M. Ass., Chicago, 1907, LXVIII, 1563.

pseudo-influenza bacilli in their different forms are of the same "species" as the typical forms. Others have found the bacillus in other infectious diseases, as Leibscher [1] and Auerbach,[2] the latter of whom obtained it in 5.4 per cent of 700 cases of diphtheria, scarlet fever, etc.

The Coccus of Pneumonia. — That the pneumococcus is present in the saliva of normal mouths was early recognized by Pasteur, Sternberg, Welch and others, and is, of course, a now well-established fact. Recently a number of careful observations have been made to determine the frequency of its occurrence, its virulence, and variations in form and habits of growth. Buerger[3] found it present in 50 per cent of 78 normal mouths, and in 34.8 per cent of 204 normal throats not so carefully examined. He also found that it could be recovered for weeks from convalescents. Of the cultures from normal mouths 79 per cent proved virulent. Hiss[4] found it in 14 of 22 persons, and Duval and Lewis[5] in all of 24 persons about the laboratory. Longcope and Fox[6] obtained it in 40 per cent to 50 per cent of mouths examined. It was more often found and more virulent in winter. Frost, Divine and Reineking[7] found it in 36 per cent of healthy mouths, 23 per cent in autumn, 43 per cent in winter and 50 per cent in the spring. The organism may persist in the same individual for months. Park and Williams [8] report the pneumococcus as prevalent both in city and country, as do others, but note that germs from normal mouths are less virulent for rabbits

[1] Leibscher, Prag. med. Wchnschr., 1903, XXVIII, 85.

[2] Auerbach, Ztschr. f. Hyg. u. Infectionskrankh., Leipz., 1904, XLVII, 259.

[3] Buerger, J. Exper. M., N. Y., 1905, VII, 497.

[4] Hiss, J. Exper. M., N. Y., 1905, VII, 547.

[5] Duval and Lewis, J. Exper. M., N. Y., 1905, VII, 473.

[6] Longcope and Fox, J. Exper. M., N. Y., 1905, VII, 430.

[7] Frost, Divine and Reineking, J. Infect. Dis., Chicago, 1905 [Suppl. No. 1], 298.

[8] Park and Williams, J. Exper. M., N. Y., 1905, VII, 403.

than those from cases of pneumonia. Wells [1] found pneumococci in the throat or upper respiratory passages in 45 per cent of 135 persons, and Besser [2] found them in 14 per cent of the noses of 57 well persons, and Hasslauer [3] in 24 of 111 normal noses. Ruediger [4] got positive results in 90 per cent of 51 normal throats, in 91.4 per cent of 71 scarlet fever throats, in 12 of 14 cases of measles, and in 8 of 9 cases of tonsillitis, or pharyngitis.

Gonorrhea. — That gonorrhea assumes a latent form in both men and women, showing no signs whatever for considerable periods, and relapsing into a subacute or even acute condition after it was supposed to be cured, has long been known. But it is only since the discovery of the gonococcus that the latency of this infection, as well as its persistence, has been fully appreciated, just as it has only been the recognition of this coccus which has shown the serious pathological changes in important organs which often follow gonorrhea. There has also been demonstrated recently the frequent innocent transmission of the disease among young children. All the text-books and monographs dealing with gonorrhea dwell on these facts, and refer to the finding of the germ in cases long supposed to be well, and to its persistence for long periods of time.[5] A physician told me of a case lasting from the third year of life to the twenty-eighth. Some striking instances of the latency of gonorrhea are given by Chapman,[6] and he has shown me records of many more in which unsuspected infection had lasted for many years. The same author states that the gonococcus may be encysted

[1] Wells, J. Am. M. Ass., Chicago, 1905, XLIV, 361.

[2] Besser, Beitr. z. path. Anat. u. z. allg. Path., Jena, 1889, VI, 331.

[3] Hasslauer, Centralbl. f. Bakteriol. [etc.], 1st Abt. Ref., Jena, 1905, XXXVII, 1.

[4] Ruediger, J. Am. M. Ass., Chicago, 1906, XLVII, 1171

[5] Wertheim, Arch. f. d. Geburtsh., Jena, 1902, XLII, 192.

[6] Chapman, Fiske Fund Prize Essay, Providence, 1905, The Sequelæ of Gonorrhea, etc., 31.

or dormant in tubal or ovarian tissue indefinitely. Rathbun and Dexter[1] from a clinical and careful bacteriological study of cases show that infection often persists long after the patient is apparently cured, and that such uncured cases are far more common than is generally believed. Hamilton[2] refers to the difficulty of demonstrating the coccus in mild and chronic cases, and states that such cases are very common. Nottshaft[3] followed 120 cases of gonorrhea and obtained the gonococcus from 73 per cent during the second six months. During the fourth six months the percentage fell to 18, and in the third year the gonococci still persisted in 6 per cent of the cases. This latency is the chief cause of innocent marital infections. It is also one reason why the medical supervision of prostitution can never have much effect in restricting the disease. No practicable amount of inspection would ever guarantee freedom from infection.

Tubercle Bacilli in Mouth and Nose. — There are two conditions under which tubercle bacilli may exist in human beings without appreciable symptoms.

First, they may be found on the mucous surfaces of mouth, throat, or nose. Straus[4] examined the nose of 29 well persons, orderlies, nurses and physicians about tuberculosis wards, and recovered tubercle bacilli from 9. Cornet found them in his own nose.[5] Jones,[6] by inoculating animals with mucus from the nose of 31 persons not brought into particularly close contact with consumptives, demonstrated the presence of tubercle bacilli in 11. Similar results have been

[1] Rathbun and Dexter, N. York M. J. [etc.], 1909, XC, 241.

[2] Hamilton, J. Infect. Dis., Chicago, 1908, V, 134.

[3] Nottshaft, Die Chronische Gonorrhea der Mänsliche Harnröhre, Leipzig, 1905.

[4] Straus, Arch. de méd. expér. et d'anat. path., Par., 1894, VI, 633.

[5] Cornet, Nothnagels Encyclopedia, Phila. and Lond., 1907, Tuberculosis, 152.

[6] Jones, Med. Rec., N. Y., 1900, LVIII, 285.

reported by Möller [1] and Bernheim.[2] Persons in the vicinity of consumptives must, unless great care be taken, receive a certain number of tubercle bacilli upon their mucous surfaces. Whether they increase in numbers in such a location is not shown by the observers quoted, but unless they do it seems rather surprising that they can be demonstrated in such a proportion of cases. On the other hand, it does not seem likely that conditions in the mouth and nose are favorable for the growth of this bacillus, and the weight of evidence seems to be that the tubercle bacillus does not, to any extent at least, develop on the normal mucous membrane of the throat or nose of well persons.

Blair [3] reports finding tubercle bacilli in the nose of various wild animals in captivity.

Latent Tuberculosis. — That the tubercle bacilli invade the tissues and, creating little disturbance, remain latent for a considerable period of time, has been amply demonstrated. While there are not many who believe that this latency is so universal or so persistent as does von Behring, yet it is certainly not a rare phenomenon. L. Rabinowitsch[4] in a recent article gives a short résumé of the work of various observers, and Harbitz [5] has also discussed it in an article on tuberculosis of children. Harbitz, in 142 autopsies of children who were clinically free from tuberculosis, and in whose glands no macroscopic or microscopic signs of the disease could be seen, nevertheless was able by inoculation to demonstrate the presence of virulent tubercle bacilli. Rabinowitsch reports four cases of virulent bacilli in lymph glands that had undergone calcareous degeneration, thus indicating a long-standing latency. Many similar observations by other

[1] Möller, Ztschr. f. Hyg. u. Infectionskrankh., Leipz., 1899, XXXII, 205.

[2] Bernheim, Clinique, Brux., 1905, XIX, 346.

[3] Blair, J. Comp. M. & Vet. Arch., 1903, XXIV, 278.

[4] Rabinowitsch, Berl. klin. Wchnschr., 1907, XLIV, 35.

[5] Harbitz, J. Infect. Dis., Chicago, 1905, II, 143.

writers are given by those just quoted, and Gaffky[1] has recently reported finding the glands of 11 per cent of 246 well persons as containing living bacilli, demonstrated by inoculation tests. Tubercle bacilli are found in the tonsils as well as in the lymph glands. Lartigau and Nicoll[2] found infected adenoids in 12 of 75 healthy children, and Weichselbaum and Bartel,[3] Goodale[4] and Cornet[5] report similar findings.

Leprosy. — Sticker[6] says that lepra bacilli often remain latent in the nose for long periods.

Bacteria of Suppuration, Latency. — As has been stated on page 20, pus bacteria are normal inhabitants of the skin and mucous surfaces, and may even invade the glands and other deeper tissues and remain latent for long periods of time. They may later, as the result of traumatism, be carried by the circulation to distant organs, there causing suppuration.[7] Among those who have demonstrated the latency of infection with pus-forming bacteria may be mentioned Manfredi and Viola,[8] Kälble,[9] Perez[10] and Hess.[11] Conradi[12] seems to have employed an improved technique in his work, and has demonstrated bacteria in 72 of 162 apparently healthy organs taken

[1] Gaffky, Konferenz Internat. f. Tuberk., Wien, 1907.

[2] Lartigau and Nicoll, Am. J. M. Sc., Phila., 1902, n. s., CXXIII, 1031.

[3] Weichselbaum and Bartel, Wien klin. Wchnschr., 1905, XVIII, 241.

[4] Goodale, Boston M. & S. J., 1906, CLV, 278.

[5] Cornet, Nothnagels Encyclopedia, Phila. and Lond., 1907, Tuberculosis, 158.

[6] Sticker, Arb. a. d. k. Gesndhtsamte., Berl., 1899, XVI, Anlage I.

[7] Soprano, Centralbl. f. Bakteriol. [etc.], 1st Abt. Orig., Jena, 1906, XLI, 601.

[8] Manfredi and Viola, Ztschr. f. Hyg. u. Infectionskrankh., Leipz., 1899, XXX, 64.

[9] Kälble, München med. Wchnschr., 1899, XLVI, 622.

[10] Pérez, Jahresb. u. d. Fortschr. . . . d. path. Mik. Baumgarten, 1897, XIII, 894.

[11] Hess, Centralbl. f. Bakteriol. [etc.], 1st Abt. Orig., Jena, 1907, XLIV, 1.

[12] Conradi, München med. Wchnschr., 1908, LV, 1523.

from 150 healthy animals. Ford[1] and Dudgeon[2] also report finding bacteria, especially pus-forming types, lying latent in healthy organs. Bardley[3] found bacteria pathogenic for rabbits in 196 of 200 atrophied tonsils, and in 101 he demonstrated *Streptococcus pyogenes*.

Latent Tetanus. — Canfora[4] and Vincent[5] have both shown that tetanus spores may be injected into the body and remain latent for some time. Tetanus occasionally develops in an inexplicable manner after surgical operations and under certain other conditions, as following the administration of hypodermic injections of the salts of quinia. Semple[6] has recently studied this subject in a most careful manner. He finds that washed spores of tetanus when injected into test animals do not cause the disease, and may remain latent and virulent for as long as 7 months. Injections of the salts of quinia will in such animals give rise to tetanus by the injurious effects of the solution upon the tissues. It may be that surgical operations may sometimes operate in the same way to favor the development of latent spores. It has been suggested that the relapses which are sometimes noted in tetanus are due to the persistence of foci of latent infection. Semple found tetanus bacilli in the intestines of 4 of 10 healthy human beings, and in 3 they proved virulent for guinea pigs.

Likeness of Scarlet Fever and Diphtheria.—Unfortunately we do not know the nature of scarlet fever virus, hence many important matters relating to the causation of this disease

[1] Ford, J. Hyg., Cambridge, 1901, I, 277.

[2] Dudgeon, Lancet, Lond., 1908, II, 1651.

[3] Bardley, Johns Hopkins Hosp. Bull., Balt., 1909, XX, 88.

[4] Canfora, Centralbl. f. Bakteriol. [etc.], I Abt. Orig., Jena, 1907, XLX, 495.

[5] Vincent, J. de physiol. et de path. gén., Par., 1908, X, 664.

[6] Semple, Sc. Memoirs, Med. and San. Dept., Gov. India, 1911, XLIII.

are in doubt. There are many points of resemblance between this disease and diphtheria, such as the degree of infectiveness, the apparent variation in the period of incubation and duration of infection, the very brief incubation in some cases, the persistence of infection in some instances long after recovery and the contrary fact of the early loss of infectivity in many instances, the prominence of the initial throat symptoms, and the occurrence of albuminuria and middle ear inflammations. We are justified, I think, in looking for a bacterial infection, and the probability is that scarlet fever is in the main, like diphtheria, a local disease of the mucous surfaces, chiefly of the throat and nose. We certainly see many mild atypical cases of scarlet fever just as we do of diphtheria, probably fully as many, and we naturally expect to find also true carriers who exhibit no symptoms at all.

Atypical Scarlet Fever. — As the bacteriologist cannot help us, we have to rely on clinical evidence, which is much more uncertain and difficult to secure. The layman and the inexperienced physician are apt to scoff at the suggestion of scarlet fever unless the patient has a high fever and is as red as a lobster. But all who have seen much of this disease know that it is exceedingly common to see cases with a scarcely discernible indefinite rash lasting for only a few hours, a rise in temperature of only a degree or two lasting also only a few hours, and the merest trace of sore throat. Sometimes the rash may be entirely absent and even the fever may escape the most careful observation.[1] In institutions and families, such cases, considered doubtful at first, or perhaps entirely neglected, prove to be the origin of typical symptoms in others. Every health officer will recall many such cases. They are the missed cases which are such a factor in the maintenance of this disease. There are many references to them in the reports of health officers and in medical literature. Among others who report such atypical cases are News-

[1] Caziot, Bull. et mém., Soc. méd. d. hôp. de Par., 1903, n.s., XX, 799; Semaine méd., Par., 1903, XXIII, 205.

holme,[1] Caziot,[2] Welch and Schamberg,[3] Cameron,[4] Butler,[5] Lesarge,[6] Thresh,[7] Corlett,[8] Lüdke,[9] Kerley,[10] and Thornton and Mäder referred to below. In most of these missed cases there were some slight symptoms, though overlooked or misunderstood at the time. In Manchester, in 1906, there were discovered 229 missed cases, mostly of a mild character. From these 139 other cases had developed.[11]

Number of Atypical Cases. — It is difficult to estimate the number of atypical cases of scarlet fever. Probably it varies according to the extent and severity of the outbreak, and for other reasons. Newsholme[12] has reported a milk outbreak in which the number of sore throats without the presence of eruption was 215, while the number of typical cases of scarlet fever was only 38. Butler,[13] at Wellesden, studied the incidence of sore throat in families where there was reported scarlet fever, and found that 31.2 per cent of 1266 persons in such families had sore throats, while only 2.8 per cent of 1644 persons living in families where there was no scarlet fever had sore throat. In a school with 300 children Thornton[14] found 31 typical cases, 19 cases with no rash and slight sore throat, and 46 cases in which only desquamation

[1] Newsholme, Tr. Med.-Chir. Soc., Glasg., LXXXVII, 549.

[2] Caziot, Bull. et mém., Soc. méd. d. hôp. de Par., 1903, n. s., XX, 799; Semaine med., Par., 1903, III, 205.

[3] Welch and Schamberg, Acute Infectious Diseases, Phila., 1905, 390.

[4] Cameron, Rep. on Return Cases of Scarlet Fever and Diphtheria to Asylums Bd., Lond., 1901–02, 38, 78.

[5] Butler, Proc. Roy. Soc. Med., Lond., 1908, I, Epidemiol. Sec., 225.

[6] Gaz. d. hôp., Par., 1909, LXXXII, 1471.

[7] Med. Officer, 1910, IV, 5.

[8] J. Am. M. Ass., Chicago, 1910, LV, 195.

[9] Med. Klin., Berl., 1911, VII, 127.

[10] Am. J. Dis. Child., 1911, I, 71.

[11] Rep. on Health of Manchester, 1906, 43.

[12] Newsholme, Rep. Med. Off. Health, Brighton, 1906, 48.

[13] Butler, Rep. Med. Off. Health, Wellesden, 1907, 76.

[14] Thornton, Brit. M. J., Lond., 1908, I, 495.

was noticed. Mäder[1] observed 9 typical and 12 very atypical cases in an outbreak in a home for epileptics. Ewart,[2] from an examination of 8000 school children at Middleborough, estimates that there must be at least 3 missed cases annually for each 1000 children. True " carriers," that is, perfectly well persons, are sometimes reported. Thus I have noted an instance where a woman apparently in this way carried scarlet fever to her child. She had been taking care of another child, and after an entire change of clothing, bath and shampoo, visited the first-named child, who was taken sick two days later. Newsholme reports what he thinks are possibly, or even probably, similar cases. Newman,[3] of Finsbury (London), noted 5 carriers among school children, three of whom, though they had never had the disease, transmitted it to others. Kerr[4] also reports 5 such cases. When a diphtheria patient discharged from a hospital carries scarlet fever home to his family, he must in most instances be considered a true carrier, for it is unlikely that symptoms of scarlet fever would often escape notice in the hospital. Ten of this sort of return carriers are reported by Simpson,[5] 30 by Cameron[6] and 44 by Turner.[7]

Smallpox. — There is still doubt as to the specific cause of smallpox. The claims that have been advanced in favor of this or that micro-organism have not as yet been substantiated. Hence there is no " laboratory " evidence that carriers of this disease exist, nor is there much clinical evidence

[1] Mäder, Cor.-Bl. f. schweiz. Aerzte, 1908, XXXVIII, 169.

[2] Ewart, Pub. Health, Lond., 1910–11, XXIV, 275.

[3] Newman, Rep. Med. Off. Health, Lond., 1904, 27.

[4] Kerr, Rep. Med. Off. Education, Lond., 1907, 43.

[5] Simpson, Rep. on Return Cases of Scarlet Fever and Diphtheria to Asylums Bd., Lond., 1898–99, 8.

[6] Cameron, Report on Return Cases of Scarlet Fever and Diphtheria to Asylums Bd., Lond., 1901–02, 43.

[7] Turner, Rep. on Return Cases of Scarlet Fever and Diphtheria to Asylums Bd., Lond., 1902–04, 3.

that perfectly well persons transmit the disease. There are, it is true, scattered through medical literature numerous reports of instances of such transmission. These reports, as often in other diseases, are, as regards the evidence, rather unsatisfactory. There is usually a possibility of such transmission, no actual demonstration. Nevertheless it is quite possible that there may be true carriers of smallpox, and there may be a considerable number of them. Mild cases are often very numerous. This was well illustrated in the recent epidemic in the United States and England. In the United States in the year ending June 30, 1901, the fatality in 38,506 cases was only 1.79 per cent. At such a time great numbers of cases escape recognition. The patients often have no idea that they are sick with a dangerous disease. They may be at their work even during the prodromal stage. There may be only half a dozen, or even fewer, atypical pustules. I have in rather a limited experience seen several such cases. They are also reported by Welch and Schamberg.[1] These authors also state that cases occur where there is no eruption at all. Davies[2] reports a nurse who was exposed to smallpox early in February and who had some fever and headache without any eruption or other symptoms. Twelve days after she returned to her ward work, which was on February 28th, one of her patients in the ward developed frank smallpox. Davies from epidemiological evidence thinks that chronic carriers do not occur in this disease. The step from half a dozen points of eruption to none at all is so slight, and the extremely mild cases at times are so numerous, that a considerable number *sine eruptione* may reasonably be expected. Armstrong[3] recently reports three such cases with some fever and subjective symptoms but no eruption. They occurred in infected families and subsequently proved refractory to vaccination.

[1] Welch and Schamberg, Acute Infectious Diseases, Phila., 1905, 207.
[2] Davies, Rep. Med. Off. Health, Bristol, 1909, 24.
[3] Armstrong, Arch. f. Diagnosis, 1909, II, 126.

Measles.—There is little clinical evidence that "carriers" of measles are common. Most health officers consider that measles is rarely carried by a "third person." It usually has a quite definite clinical picture. In Aberdeen, so Dr. Matthew Hay writes to me, judging from a census taken in certain schools, it was estimated that from 90 to 93 per cent of the children over ten years of age had had a recognized attack of measles. That such a high percentage of children had recognized attacks indicates that atypical cases cannot be very common. Mild, atypical and unrecognized cases of this disease must be far less numerous than are such cases in scarlet fever, diphtheria and typhoid fever. Levy at Richmond[1] investigated 2331 cases during an outbreak. They were all, without exception, traced to previous frank cases of the disease. Levy could find no evidence of infection from either carriers or fomites. His careful work in the study of this outbreak renders his conclusions of the highest value.

Protozoan Diseases. — Although the marks of distinction between animal and vegetable life as seen among the lower forms are ill defined and uncertain, yet it is generally agreed that though the group of organisms known as bacteria have characters belonging to both the vegetable and the animal kingdom, they are more nearly allied to the former, while another group, known as protozoa, are allied to the lower forms of animal life. Although one of the latter class was discovered to be the cause of malaria in 1880, at a time when most of the disease-producing bacteria were unknown, the bacteria have received far more study, and indeed it is only recently that the protozoa as the cause of disease have received much attention. It is known that a number of diseases both of men and of animals are caused by protozoa of various types. As has recently been emphasized by Daniels,[2] latency is a

[1] Richmond Rep. Health Dept., 1910, 38.

[2] Daniels, Brit. M. J., Lond., 1909, II, 767.

common phenomenon of protozoan infection, and is of the utmost importance from an epidemiological standpoint. Not only do the blood parasites maintain long continued infection with few symptoms, but such forms as *Ameba, Balantidium* and *Lamblia* live in the intestines indefinitely, reproducing themselves asexually. A number of the diseases to be referred to do not affect man, but they serve to illustrate the prevalence of latency in protozoan infections.

Texas Cattle Fever. — It has long been recognized that the Texas fever of cattle could be transmitted by apparently healthy animals. The explanation of this fact was not, however, forthcoming until Smith and Kilborne's [1] classical researches in 1893 demonstrated that the disease was due to a blood parasite, a protozoan (*Piroplasma bigeminum*), not a bacterium, and also demonstrated that it is only transmitted from animal to animal by means of a species of tick (*Boöphilus annulatus*), in which the parasite passes through a cycle of changes necessary for the maintenance of the species. This work of Smith and Kilborne's was one of the most important steps in the development of our knowledge of the insect carriage of disease, a knowledge which has been of such inestimable value in connection with malaria, sleeping sickness, yellow fever and other blood diseases. It was soon determined that animals which had recovered from Texas fever and were immune to it, carried the piroplasma in the blood for an indefinite time. In one instance it was known to have remained for thirteen years.[2] Reports from the Philippines [3] show that many of the cattle in those islands are infected with the parasites of Texas fever though showing no symptoms. Slightly different types of this disease occur among cattle in Europe and in Africa caused by different species of piroplasma and spread by carriers.

[1] Smith and Kilborne, U. S. Dept. Agric., Bu. An. Ind., Bull. No. 1, 1893, 57.

[2] U. S. Dept. Agric., Rep. Bu. An. Ind., 1904, XXI, 26.

[3] Bull. 14, Bu. Gov. Lab., Manila, P. I., 1904, 11.

Nagana. — Nagana[1] is an African cattle disease which, like the sleeping sickness, is caused by a trypanosome, *T. brucei*, and is also transmitted by a tsetse fly, *G. morsitans*. Wild herbivora are very generally infected, but because of immunity, probably acquired, they show few or no symptoms. These carriers are the real source of the disease.

Dourine. — This is a contagious disease of horses spread almost exclusively by the sexual act. It is caused by a trypanosome, *T. equiperdum*, found in the secretions,[2] blood and tissues. Although recovery may occur, the trypanosomes remain for months in the sexual organs of apparently cured animals and thus spread the disease.

Malaria. — The most important of the protozoan diseases is malaria. It had always been believed that this disease might remain latent for months and years, but what latency really meant could not be determined until after the discovery of the specific cause of the disease. Many of the protozoa pass through various metamorphoses, or fixed cycles of development, and it was found that in malaria the *Plasmodium*, which is its cause, may in certain stages persist in the blood or organs of the body without causing any characteristic symptoms, or indeed any symptoms at all. Then at any time, from one cause or another, its reproduction may again become active and more or less marked symptoms appear. Thus relapses may occur after a period of several years, when the bodily resistance is from any cause impaired. Thus fever after surgical operation is not rarely due to a latent malaria becoming active, the parasite being found in the blood and the symptoms yielding to quinia. As malaria is a strictly transmissible disease, the plasmodium which causes it being borne from one person to another by mosquitoes, a latent case of the kind described may be, and doubtless often is, the means of introducing the disease into hitherto

[1] Minchin, Gray and Tullock, Proc. Roy. Soc., Lond., 1906; Nature, Lond., 1906, LXXVII, 57.
[2] U. S. Dept. Ag., Bu. An. Ind., Bull. No. 142, 1911.

uninfected localities. Unless such cases drift into hospitals, they are almost certain to be unrecognized. Craig[1] made a careful study of 424 such latent cases found among 1653 soldiers examined in the Philippines. Since I first wrote this chapter Craig's book has appeared in which he discusses in much detail latency and recurrences.[2] He has noted an asexual conjugation of the parasites in the blood cells, which is followed by a resting stage, and which he believes has some relation to the latency of the infection. Where malaria prevails extensively, as in the tropics, it has long been noticed that a large part of the adult population is immune. It is now known that this immunity is to a large extent acquired, and is due to the invasion of the body in infancy by the parasites. This invasion, while sometimes causing symptoms and death, frequently gives rise to few or no symptoms, or if some reaction appears at first, it soon disappears, and the children may seem perfectly well though the parasites are constantly found in the blood. They disappear year by year and infection is rarely found after adolescence. Koch[3] in Africa found large numbers of children infected, even as high as 100 per cent. Plehn[4] found many adults infected though not sick. Christophers and Stephens[5] found the parasites in the blood of 90 per cent of infants examined in one locality on the Gold Coast in Africa, and the Thompson Yates expedition to Nigeria[6] reports finding them in 63 per cent of children under 3 years of age. Ziemann[7] found that in the Cameroon country 37 per cent of children under 5 years of

[1] Craig, J. Infect. Dis., Chicago, 1907, IV, 108.

[2] The Malarial Fevers, N. Y., 1909, 228.

[3] Koch, cited in Thompson Yates' Lab. Rep., 1900, No. 4.

[4] Plehn, cited by Marchiafava and Bignani, Twentieth Cent. Practice, XXI, 807.

[5] Christophers and Stephens, Reports of the Malarial Commission of the Roy. Soc. (Eng.), 2nd Ser., 1900–03, 15.

[6] Thompson Yates' Lab. Rep., 1900, III, Pt. 2, 201.

[7] Deutsche med. Wchnschr., 1900, XXVI, 399, 642, 753, 769.

age were infected. In Panama Kendall[1] found 57 per cent infected of the natives of all ages examined in the village of Bahio, and 73 per cent of foreigners. While many of the latter were more or less sick, many were entirely well. Darling[2] in villages in the Panama Canal zone where there were no *Anopheles*, nevertheless found that 10 per cent of the laborers at work were infected though they were not at all sick. Among the families of the Spanish and the West Indians, the latent infection reached 30 per cent. It is this latent infection in the blood of the native population which is the cause of the malaria which so certainly attacks arrivals from non-malarial regions. The greater the distance that can be placed between the natives and the strangers the less the danger of the latter contracting the disease.

Sleeping Sickness. — African sleeping sickness has been shown to be due to a protozoan, *Trypanosoma gambiense.* This disease has been much studied of late, and it seems certain that it is transmitted by means of the tsetse fly (*Glossina palpalis*), though whether it is a purely accidental mechanical transference on the proboscis of the fly, or whether it passes through a part of its life history in the body of the fly, as the *Plasmodium* of malaria does in the mosquito, is still uncertain. In any event the parasite is frequently found in the blood of apparently healthy subjects, just as is the malarial parasite. According to Todd[3] it may remain in the blood for 15 years, causing no symptoms, and frequently remains for many months. The expedition from the Liverpool School of Tropical Medicine[4] found many natives infected, but who exhibited no symptoms, or only slight symptoms. The greater the prevalence of the disease the more common are these latent cases. In Gambia, where the disease is rare, not more

[1] Kendall, J. Am. M. Ass., Chicago, 1906, XLVI, 1151, 1266.

[2] Darling, J. Am. M. Ass., Chicago, 1909, LIII, 2051.

[3] Todd, Tr. Epidemiol. Soc., Lond., 1905–06, XXV, 1.

[4] Liverpool School Trop. Med. Memoirs, 1904, XIII; Med. News, N. Y., 1904, LXXXV, 526, 615.

than one native in 1000 examined showed the parasites, while in the Congo 46 in 100 were infected, and in Uganda the percentage was still higher. Whether the disease is always transferred from man to man, or whether some of the lower animals also harbor the parasites and thus serve as a " reservoir " from which the human disease is derived, is as yet uncertain.

Syphilis. — The spirochete of syphilis has in one instance been reported as remaining latent in a healed lesion of that disease.[1] According to Bosquenet[2] the spirochetes are commonly found in gumma, where they may apparently remain latent for a long time. The fact that gumma have not been considered infectious has been urged as an argument against the pathogenicity of the spirochetes. It is now, however, generally thought that the spirochetes in these tumors are infective.

Relapsing Fever. — There are several types of relapsing fever having more or less well marked geographical limitations. The disease is characterized by well defined febrile " relapses " with equally well defined afebrile intervals. The different forms of the disease are caused by slightly differing species of spirochetes, and, as will be referred to in the last chapter, these parasites are undoubtedly transmitted by insect carriers. According to Craig,[3] it has been demonstrated by Breinl and Kinghorn and by Dutton and Todd that though *Spirocheta duttoni* is not found in the blood during the afebrile period, the blood nevertheless is infectious. Mackie has shown the same for *S. carteri*, and Darling[4] has shown that the blood from the afebrile stage and from entirely recovered animals is still infectious. Darling's work was done in Panama.

[1] Pasini, cited by Rosenberger, New York M. J. [etc.], 1908, LXXXVII, 394.

[2] Bosquenet, Spirochætes, Phila., 1911, 51.

[3] Craig, The Malarial Fevers, New York, 1909, 447.

[4] Darling, Arch. Int. Med., Chicago, 1909, 150.

Vincent's Angina. — It seems highly probable that this disease is caused by the spirochetes which are found constantly in the lesions. That many mild missed cases, and perhaps true carriers occur is probable. Farley,[1] in reporting an institutional outbreak of this disease, says that a number of children were found without any constitutional symptoms, but with a slight exudation on the tonsils or with spongy gums, and that in these the spirochetes were found to be present. These cases were not discovered until a systematic examination was made of all the children and the outbreak ceased on their removal from the institution. Kerr[2] reports an outbreak in the Linden Lodge School in London, consisting of about 20 cases, and due apparently to unnoticed chronic and subacute cases which attracted no attention until they were sought for.

Yellow Fever. — The parasite which is the cause of yellow fever is still unknown, although fortunately for preventive medicine we have very accurate knowledge of the manner in which the disease is transmitted. As in scarlet fever, so in yellow fever lack of knowledge of the parasite renders difficult the recognition of carrier cases if they exist. But there is abundant clinical evidence that many very mild and atypical cases occur which it is impossible to recognize. It is in young children chiefly that this slight disturbance is produced by the infection. A similar phenomenon is noted in malarial disease, and young children are the chief source of infection in both yellow fever and malaria. The fact of the mildness of these cases, their frequency, and the impossibility of making a diagnosis, has been insisted upon by Finlay, Gorgas, Guiteras, Carter, Agramonte, Marchoux and others. Even in adults, walking cases, which it is impossible to discover by an ordinary examination, are not rare. Thus it was claimed that during an outbreak in Louisiana a single walking case carried the disease to three different communities.

[1] Farley, J. Am. M. Ass., Chicago, 1910, LIV, 1516.
[2] Rep. Med. Off. of Education, Lond., 1909, 63.

Amebic Dysentery. — A number of observers have reported finding *Entameba histolytica*, which is the cause of this disease, in the intestines of healthy persons. It is now believed that most of these reports are based on error due to confusing the pathogenic species named above with harmless saprophytes. This is the view of Vedder [1] and Craig.[2] Although the laboratory evidence of the existence of carriers of dysentery amebæ is uncertain or lacking, there is epidemiological evidence that these parasites are sometimes found in persons for a long time after recovery, and may also be found in the feces before the disease develops. Martini [3] reports a case in which the sickness lasted from the 15th of September to the 1st of December, 1907, but in which the amebæ persisted until the last of January, 1908. Vincent [4] reports several instances in which persons were carriers for five months after their return to France from Tonkin. Lemoine [5] had under observation a man who contracted the disease in China in 1897 and returned to France and transmitted the disease to another in 1908. Cameron [6] reports a soldier returned to Scotland from the Boer War, and apparently well for 6 years, but who then developed a liver abscess in which amebæ were found.

Poliomyelitis. — The disease known as acute anterior poliomyelitis, or infantile paralysis, has been, during the past fifteen years, occurring with increasing frequency. It usually appears in well-defined local outbreaks lasting from a few weeks to a few months. Except in the largest cities the outbreaks are not often of long duration. "Sporadic" or somewhat isolated cases also doubtless occur,

[1] Vedder, J. Am. M. Ass., Chicago, 1906, XLVI, 870.

[2] Craig, J. Infect. Dis., Chicago, 1908, V, 324; The Parasitic Amœbæ of Man, Phila., 1911.

[3] Martini, Arch. f. Schiffs- u. Tropen-Hyg., Cassel, 1908, XII, 588.

[4] Vincent, Bull. Soc. path. exot., Par., 1909, II, 78.

[5] Lemoine, Bull. et mém. Soc. méd. d. hôp. de Par., 1908, 3d Ser., XXV, 640.

[6] Cameron, Brit. M. J., Lond., 1911, I, 973.

though it is not unlikely that some which are reported under this name may be due to a totally different cause from that which gives rise to the "epidemic" form, just as cases of cerebro-spinal meningitis, closely resembling the disease caused by the Weichselbaum diplococcus, may be produced by several other infective agents. For many years epidemiologists have considered poliomyelitis as an infectious and contagious disease, though many have thought the evidence of communicability not to be entirely satisfactory. In fact, the epidemiological evidence of the contagiousness of this disease, and of cerebro-spinal meningitis, is almost on a par. The contagiousness of both diseases is certainly not very marked; that is, the chance of a frank case giving rise to another frank case, either in homes or in institutions, is very small. When an apparently contagious disease, yet one only slightly so, appears in well-marked outbreaks, it is pretty safe to assume the existence of large numbers of carriers or of mild atypical and unrecognized cases. The epidemiology of cerebro-spinal meningitis was inexplicable until the carriers of that disease were discovered. The explanation of its spread now involves no more difficulties than does that of scarlet fever or diphtheria. The epidemiological, and indeed clinical resemblance of cerebro-spinal meningitis and poliomyelitis led some, even before the work of Flexner and Clark, and Lucas and Osgood, to suspect the existence of carriers. The existence of numerous "abortive" cases, as they have been called, had long been considered probable.

Laboratory Studies. — To determine definitely the existence of either carriers or atypical cases of any infectious disease by means of epidemiological studies is extremely difficult, and to determine their number is entirely impossible. Fortunately experimental laboratory work, culminating in the investigations of Flexner and Lewis,[1] have

[1] Flexner and Lewis, J. Am. Med. Ass., Chicago, 1909, LIII, 1639, 1913.

shown, by repeated transfers of the virus through monkeys, that poliomyelitis is in all probability due to a living *contagium*. Subsequent studies have shown that the virus is filterable; that it is found in various fluids and organs of monkeys including the nasal and pharyngeal mucous membrane, and presumably also in the mucus; and that animals may be infected not only by injection into the central nervous system, but also by injection into the subcutaneous tissue, and by application of the virus to the scarified and healthy mucous surfaces. The spinal fluid very early shows quite characteristic changes, and "immunity principles" (capable of neutralizing the virus in the test tube) are found in the blood of animals, and human beings who have had the disease.[1]

Poliomyelitis Carriers. — By means of the experimental methods rendered possible by this work, it has been shown that in monkeys, at least, the virus of this disease remains in the nose and throat after the clinical symptoms have subsided. Thus Osgood and Lucas [2] found the virus in the naso-pharyngeal mucous membrane of two monkeys 6 weeks and 5½ months respectively after the acute symptoms of the disease had disappeared, and Flexner and Clark found the virulence to persist 4 weeks in a monkey studied by them. Thus the existence of chronic convalescent carriers in inoculated monkeys is definitely proved. As the virus has been shown by Flexner and Clark [3] to exist in the tonsillar tissue of human beings during the disease, just as it is found in the mucous membrane of monkeys, it seems reasonable to expect that it only needs further investigation to demonstrate the existence of human carriers of this disease. Occasionally observers have, for epidemiological reasons, suspected certain persons of being

[1] Flexner and Lewis, J. Am. Med. Ass., Chicago, 1910, LIV, 1780.

[2] Osgood and Lucas, J. Am. Med. Ass., Chicago, 1911, LV, 495.

[3] Flexner and Clark, J. Am. Med. Ass., Chicago, 1911, 1685.

carriers. Thus Lovett[1] states that he has a number of such cases in his records, and in 11 instances the disease followed intimate contact with persons who had previously suffered from it. Such cases have also been reported by Krause.[2] Anderson[3] in Nebraska notes a number of instances in which the disease seems to have been carried by well persons. Thus a girl who had visited in Stromberg, where the disease prevailed, returned to a farm many miles distant and a few days later a case of poliomyelitis developed, followed by others on that and a near-by farm. In another instance a thresher apparently carried it from his own family to the place where he worked. In two other instances peddlers seemed to be carriers. Similar observations have, in England, been made by Reece and Farrar.[4]

Poliomyelitis: Atypical Cases. — Ever since Wickman's studies in Sweden it has been believed that so-called "abortive" cases of this disease are quite common. These cases may show some slight symptoms referable to the nervous system, such as headache, pain, tenderness and rigidity of neck, hypersthesia and neuralgic pains; and some think that tonsillitis and gastro-intestinal irritation without nervous symptoms may be due to the same pathogenic agent. According to Frost,[5] Wickman found such abortive cases to equal in number 15 per cent of the frank cases. In Massachusetts in 1909 there were 49 possibly abortive cases observed in connection with 150 acknowledged cases. Frost himself in an outbreak in Hancock County, Ia., found 25 abortive cases and 5 frank cases. That some at least, and perhaps a large proportion, of these abortive cases are really poliomyelitis, is shown by the finding of

[1] Lovett, Rep. State Bd. of Health, Mass., 1909.

[2] Krause, Therapie der Gegenwart, 1911, LII, 145.

[3] Anderson, Pediatrics, N. Y. & Lond., 1910, XXII, 543.

[4] Reece and Farrar, Rep. to Local Gov. Bd. Lond., 1912, No. 61.

[5] Frost, U. S. Pub. Health and Mar. Hosp. Serv., Pub. Health Bull. No. 44, 1911.

"immunizing principles" in their blood. Anderson and Frost[1] state that Netter and Levaditi demonstrated a case in this way, and the authors themselves showed the presence of "immunizing principles" in the blood of 6 of 9 suspected abortive cases.

In view of the epidemiological facts, and the experimental data, it seems not unsafe to surmise that, with the perfection and extended application of laboratory methods of diagnosis, carriers and mild atypical cases of poliomyelitis will be shown to be common, and it is not unlikely that they may prove, as in cerebro-spinal meningitis, many times more numerous than are frank cases of the disease.

Latency a Common Phenomenon. — The laity and not a few physicians are still incredulous that there can be diphtheria infection unless the patient is sick in bed and the throat choked with exudation, or that there can be scarlet fever without high fever and an extensive eruption. Still less are they willing to admit that perfectly well persons can carry and reproduce in their bodies the virus of the infectious diseases. It is difficult for many to realize that the virus of disease may remain latent in the body, for long periods, without causing symptoms. The facts presented in the preceding pages have been gathered to show that latency is a common phenomenon, and for this purpose, besides many common human infections, a number of diseases have been referred to, not transmissible to human beings and of little interest to health officials, but which seem to illustrate this phenomenon. Infection without symptoms is no cause for surprise, but may be expected in any parasitic disease. There may be exceptions, as is said to be the case in relapsing fever and African East Coast cattle fever (caused by *Th. parva*). But these exceptions, rather than the existence of latency and atypical types, should be cause for surprise.

[1] Frost, J. Am. Med. Ass., Chicago, 1911, LVI, 663.

Laboratory Evidence of Carriers. — Definite knowledge as to the existence and number of carriers must rest almost entirely upon evidence furnished by the finding in the body of the causative agents of disease, bacteria or protozoa, or the demonstration in the blood or tissues of an unknown infective principle, as in the case of poliomyelitis. Actually, almost all such evidence depends upon the finding of disease-producing bacteria or protozoa in the bodies of healthy persons or animals. Those persons who do not believe that the causative relation between these minute forms of life and disease has been established with a reasonable degree of certainty will of course attach little weight to the bacteriological evidence of the existence of carriers. With such I cannot agree. On the contrary, the causation of certain diseases by bacteria seems to me to be one of the best-established truths of medical science, and it is consequently entirely legitimate to make use of bacteriological evidence in developing the theory and practice of preventive medicine. Many, while admitting that we have satisfactory evidence that some diseases are caused by specific bacteria or protozoa, are unwilling to admit that the evidence is conclusive as to the causative relation of certain other alleged pathogens and the diseases said to be due to them. Indeed, almost everyone takes this attitude towards some disease. It happens, however, that in the opinion of the majority of the most competent observers the evidence is especially strong as regards the causative agent of cholera, typhoid fever, diphtheria, cerebro-spinal meningitis, sleeping sickness and malaria. And it is particularly for these diseases that we have abundant evidence as regards the numbers and importance of carriers.

Laboratory Evidence of Atypical Cases. — While acute clinical observers have at all times recognized many atypical cases which would have been overlooked by the average man, it was from the nature of things impossible to know how far or how often a disease could deviate from the normal when the only criterion for the determination of the disease was the symptom complex of the normal type. It is only the discovery of the germ, and the ability to recognize it, which enables us to take a wider view of an infectious disease, and to see that it includes far more types and cases than was at first suspected. It is only the work of the laboratory that makes it possible to recognize the mild atypical cases of diphtheria, typhoid fever and malaria. The clinicians have been willing to accept, though, it must be confessed, with a little hesitancy, the teachings of the laboratory men in regard to prevalence of atypical cases. Some are even emboldened to proceed along lines where the laboratory men cannot as yet go, and to recognize atypical scarlet fever which they would formerly have passed by, and to postulate the "abortive" type of poliomyelitis. Yet when the laboratory man points out the true carrier and suggests danger from him as well as from the atypical case, many a clinician, and not a few epidemiologists as well, hesitate to follow.

Carriers Vary in Numbers. — One of the important facts noticeable in the study of this subject is the great variation in the number of carriers in different diseases. It ought to be determined by a sufficient number of observations just how many carriers there are in different diseases among the general public and among contacts at different ages, at different seasons, and in different places. Unfortunately the observations have not as yet been extensive enough to warrant any definite conclusions, though some quite striking differences are apparent. Probably the number of carriers is on the whole greater in pneumonia than in any other disease, including at times half the total population. In certain protozoan diseases the percentage of carriers may be even higher within limited groups, as among children in intensely malarious districts. So, too, carriers of the trypanosomes of sleeping sickness are at times very numerous. In the case of animal diseases, as

Texas cattle fever, the proportion of infected animals is very large. Among human diseases it would appear that influenza carriers are very numerous, though the identity of the causative agent has not been so well determined, and the number of observations is not as large as for many other diseases. It is certain that cerebro-spinal meningitis carriers are many times more numerous than the cases—in the opinion of many, from ten times to twenty times as numerous. Under ordinary conditions, with a moderate prevalence of the disease, diphtheria carriers equal about one per cent of the population, and during outbreaks the percentage, particularly among children, is many times as great. Probably typhoid carriers are not so numerous as are diphtheria carriers, but there are not many data as to the numbers among either the general public or among contacts. In neither human nor rat plague do carriers appear to be either numerous or important. There is even less evidence of the existence of carriers, certainly of chronic carriers, of smallpox; and for measles the clinical evidence that there are no carriers is very strong.

Relation between Number of Carriers and Infectivity. — Here again data are too few to warrant more than a suggestion, but one cannot but be struck by the fact that the most infectious diseases show the fewest carriers, while some of the diseases which are only slightly contagious show very many more carriers than cases. Thus smallpox and measles, considered perhaps the most contagious of diseases, are not certainly known to give rise to the carrier condition. Diphtheria is not so infectious as measles; that is, a case, brought in contact with susceptibles, does not so surely give rise to other cases; and carriers of diphtheria are quite numerous. Cerebro-spinal meningitis exhibits many carriers, and its ineffectivity, as measured by contagion in the family and institution, is small. Pneumonia has the most carriers of all and is the least contagious.

Virulence of Germs in Carriers. — The question of the infecting power of carriers is the crucial one of the whole subject. One way of testing this is by testing by animal experiment the virulence of the germs which the carrier is producing. Unfortunately, owing to insusceptibility of the lower animals, or the difficulties of the technique, or the cost of susceptible animals, like the apes, renders numerous observations out of the question. In one disease, diphtheria, in which experimentation is comparatively easy, it has been shown that in a varying percentage of carriers the bacilli are virulent, often exceedingly virulent, though there is a large number of carriers in which they are not virulent. The actual number of carriers of virulent germs is nevertheless shown to be very large. The pneumococcus found in well persons is virulent for rabbits, though less so than are cocci from cases of pneumonia. Tests on the lower animals for the virulence of typhoid bacilli are of little value, but it is worthy of note that a case of typhoid fever in a human being has recently resulted from drawing into the mouth a culture of a typhoid bacillus derived from a carrier.

In some of the diseases of the lower animals direct experiment has demonstrated the virulence of disease germs from healthy individuals. This has been abundantly proved in Texas cattle fever and in certain trypanosome infections.

Carriers as a Source of Protozoan Disease. — There seems to be little disposition in any quarter to question the importance of carriers of the malarial plasmodium in the extension of malarial disease. Yet so far as I know there are no experiments which demonstrate such transmission, and few if any clinical observations which would indicate such transmission. It is simply assumed that the numerous well persons carrying plasmodium must be a source from which oftentimes the mosquitoes get the infection which they transmit to others. Probably the reason why this view is so readily accepted without any demand for rigid experimental or epidemiological proof is that the mode of transmission of this disease is established on such convincing evidence. It seems certain that it is only transmitted by mosquitoes, and that mosquitoes obtain the parasites only by previously biting infected human beings. So, too, because the mode of transmission of sleeping sickness is definitely determined, no one looks for the origin of this disease outside the bodies of living beings, and as many human beings are shown to be "carriers" of the trypanosome, such persons are believed to be a principal source of the disease.

Carriers as a Cause of Bacterial Diseases. — In at least one bacterial disease, namely "white diarrhea of chicks," due to *B. pullorum*, it has been definitely shown that adult carrier hens infect their eggs and are thus the principal factor in the spread of the disease. In no other animal disease due to bacteria does the carrier question appear to have been so well worked out.

While the existence of numerous carriers has been amply demonstrated in such diseases as cholera, typhoid fever, dysentery, diphtheria and cerebro-spinal meningitis, their importance in the spread of these and similar diseases has been questioned by many who never question the importance of carriers in the spread of malarial disease. The reason for this, doubtless, is that the mode of transmission of these diseases is not so well understood because they do not readily permit the use of experimental methods. Everyone feels sure how every case of malaria is caused. On the other hand, we are often, perhaps usually, in doubt in cases of typhoid fever, cholera and diphtheria as to the mode of transmission of the infection and the source from which it comes. When there are many possible sources and modes of infection it is not easy to determine the right one.

Evidence of Contagion the Same as for Cases. — It is fair to claim that the evidence of the infectivity of carriers is the same as the evidence of the infectivity of cases. We believe that frank cases of diphtheria are contagious because it very generally happens that persons exposed to them develop the disease, and, conversely, because a certain proportion of the recognized cases have been in relation to other cases. We believe that typhoid fever is contagious because a certain number of persons exposed to cases of the disease contract it, even though the proportion is smaller than in diphtheria. It is considered a further proof that many cases of typhoid can be shown to have had some connection with previous cases. When a considerable number of cases of typhoid fever are caused by the consumption of milk, and the milk is known to have been handled by a typhoid patient, or even to have come from premises occupied by such a patient, it is generally assumed that the contagion was derived from the patient.

In precisely the same way it has been shown in the preceding pages, and much more additional proof of the same kind is obtainable, that persons in contact with diphtheria carriers, and indeed the carriers themselves, not rarely develop the disease. It has also been shown that persons with diphtheria have often been in relation to carriers. The number, it is true, is not very great, and it cannot be so great as for cases; for while it is comparatively easy to recognize any frank case in the environment of any given patient, it is not possible to recognize any carrier there may be, except by cultures from every one with whom the patient has come in contact.

In typhoid fever it is easier to find carriers because typhoid fever, more than any other disease, is spread through milk, water or food; and outbreaks so caused are often traced to some definite locality, often to a single house, so that the search for carriers becomes easier. Hence we have more definite proof that typhoid fever is caused by carriers than we have that any other human bacterial disease is so caused. The outbreaks of typhoid fever which have been shown to have a definite relation to carriers afford as good evidence that carriers are the cause of this disease as there is that cases give rise to other cases.

Lack of Statistical Evidence Alleged. — Hamer[1] has urged that the mere association of a carrier and a case is no proof of a causative relation, and he says that the finding of carriers in connection with certain outbreaks of typhoid fever is of little importance unless we have some idea of the number of carriers in the general population. He does well to call attention to the lack of satisfactory data, but when only 1 carrier is found among 250 persons and 3 among nearly 1000, it is fair to assume that carriers are not very common.

Carriers Often Appear not Dangerous. — It is certainly a fact that carriers often appear to be non-infectious. Many carriers of typhoid bacilli and of diphtheria bacilli have been known to remain such for long periods of time without apparently infecting members of their families or others brought in close contact with them. As shown on page 84, diphtheria carriers have been followed in schools in Boston and Providence and no infection from them has been discovered. Diphtheria carriers have been discharged from hospitals and no cases have developed in their homes. These and similar facts certainly demonstrate that all carriers do not at all times cause disease in those with whom they are brought in contact. Why this is so may be due to a variety of causes. Thus the excretion of bacteria is in many cases notoriously intermittent. There is also good reason for believing that the bacteria have in many cases lost their virulence. Perhaps sometimes they are produced in relatively small numbers. Again, many of the persons exposed are doubtless immune. Furthermore, we must bear in mind, as will be referred to in the following chapter, that the infecting power of even frank cases of disease is very much less than has generally been supposed. Such cases may often remain in close association with susceptible per-

[1] Hamer, Proc. Roy. Soc. Med., 1911, IV, Epidemiol. Sect., 105.

sons without the conditions being present for a transfer of an effective amount of infective material. One would expect this to happen still more often with carriers.

On the other hand, there is much evidence which shows that carriers at times do cause disease. To most persons the evidence of this is conclusive. The question at issue merely is, How often does this occur? To what extent are carriers a factor in the maintenance of the infectious diseases? To the writer it appears that many things strongly point to carriers as a factor of great moment. The probability of this is, I believe, sufficient to warrant our modifying our restrictive measures accordingly. I nevertheless freely admit that we are greatly in need of more statistical evidence.

There are still many problems concerning the relation of carriers to disease which need further careful study, and it is not for a moment claimed that the "carrier theory," so called, satisfactorily explains every epidemiological phenomenon. There are many which it does not explain at all. On the other hand, some of the most important phenomena of the extension of the contagious diseases are far better explained by the newly discovered facts concerning carriers than by any of the theories of former years. We still have much to learn, but we are not on that account justified in neglecting the facts which have already been learned and in basing our practice on disproved theories of the sources of infection.

No Sharp Separation between Varieties of Carriers. — That typical cases of disease are the source of similar cases follows necessarily from the very definition of contagiousness. That mild cases, even very mild and atypical cases, may give rise to typical as well as to other mild cases is recognized by everyone. Both clinicians and epidemiologists have always believed that perfectly well persons may be the bearers of infection from the sick to others. It was believed by most, and is now by many, that such persons carry the infection in the hair or clothing or on the hands. The discovery that the germs of disease may grow in the body without causing symptoms has forced most rational persons to the belief that when well persons carry infection it is because they are "carriers," that is, are growers, of germs.

It is probably true that all carriers are not dangerous, certainly not at all times, even when they are excreting bacilli. We know that in some diphtheria carriers the bacilli are not virulent for test animals and probably not for human beings. Certain observers of high standing have assumed that it is only the convalescent carriers and the carriers who are in immediate contact with the sick who are dangerous; that is, it is these only who carry virulent germs. If these can be controlled the carrier problem is solved, they think. I am willing to admit that the severe case is potentially more dangerous than the mild case, that the mild case may be more dangerous than the carrier, and that the convalescent carrier may be more dangerous than the chance carrier found among the public at large. There is some evidence of this, and it is not improbable that bacteria may tend to lose their virulence in passing through a succession of immune persons (as it is not improbable that they may increase in virulence by passing through susceptible persons); but I can see no ground at present for the assumption that virulent bacilli derived from a sick person may be carried by one well person but that when they pass to another well person they cease to be dangerous. There seems to be no ground for assuming that a virulent germ cannot pass from carrier to carrier.

Conclusions. — We are justified from the evidence presented in coming to the following conclusions:

1. Mild atypical and unrecognized cases of the infectious diseases are often extremely common. In many diseases they may be more numerous than the recognized cases.

2. Disease-producing micro-organisms, whether bacteria

or protozoa, frequently persist in the body without causing symptoms.

3. Sometimes the germs remain only a few weeks or months after convalescence, and sometimes they may persist for years, perhaps for life. Sometimes these carriers give no history of ever having been sick.

4. While the bacteria found in carriers are sometimes lacking in virulence, many times they show the highest degree of virulence.

5. There is ample epidemiological evidence that healthy carriers as well as mild unrecognized cases are the source of well-marked outbreaks.

6. The number of carriers varies greatly in different diseases. From 20 to 50 per cent of the population are carriers of pneumococci. It seems probable that the influenza bacillus is as widely distributed. During outbreaks of cerebrospinal meningitis the number of carriers may be from 10 to 30 times as numerous as the number of cases. Even when diphtheria is not prevalent 1 per cent of the population may be carrying the bacilli, and during outbreaks the number may be several times greater. Probably 25 per cent of all typhoid fever cases excrete bacilli for some weeks after convalescence, and it is estimated that from 1 in 500 to 1 in 250 of the population are chronic carriers. What little evidence there is indicates that carriers are as numerous in dysentery and cholera as they are in typhoid fever. In yellow fever, sleeping sickness, and particularly in malaria, carriers are very numerous. There is evidence that there are not many carriers of measles or smallpox.

7. Any scheme of prevention which fails to take into account carriers and missed cases is doomed to partial and perhaps complete failure.

CHAPTER III.

LIMITATIONS TO THE VALUE OF ISOLATION.

Number of Mild Cases and Carriers. — In the first chapter the attempt was made to show that pathogenic organisms do not usually develop outside of the body. Except for a few diseases, or under unusual circumstances, the saprophytic existence of disease germs is not to be looked for. Such sources of infection are much rarer than is generally assumed, and for most diseases may be entirely neglected. In the second chapter, evidence was presented that certain other sources of infection are very much more numerous than is generally believed, and it is here contended that no scheme of sanitation can have a scientific basis, or can have any possibility of success, which does not take full cognizance of them.

It must be admitted by all that mild atypical cases of contagious diseases are very numerous. Every one who has had any experience with the last epidemic of smallpox in the United States and England must have had many unpleasant reminders of this. Health officers' reports are full of instances of the introduction of the disease into a community by persons unsuspected by any one of having the disease, and who often give rise to a whole series of cases. Similar experiences with scarlet fever are often reported. The most critical investigation, such as that of our surgeons in the Spanish War, indicates that mild unrecognized cases of typhoid fever fully equal, if they do not exceed, the number of cases which are recognized and reported. Even with every facility for diagnosis, the amount of sore throat due to the diphtheria bacillus, but not so suspected, is fully equal to the amount of recognized diphtheria; and in many other infectious diseases these mild cases occur with varying degrees of frequency.

Usually not Recognized. — The extent to which these mild atypical cases escape recognition varies with the disease, the social condition of the people affected, the intelligence and conscientiousness of the physician, and the attitude of the health officer. That the majority of people will not consult a physician unless they are decidedly sick, is certain. That they will refrain from doing so if they expect to be reported to the health officer and to be placed under various restrictions, is but in accord with human nature. A slight sore throat, or a fleeting rash, little suggestive of danger, will be lightly passed over, no physician will be called and no precautions taken, and often there will be no thought of danger to others. It has always been known that a certain number of mild cases, difficult to recognize, could be expected in almost all infectious diseases, but it remained for the laboratory worker to show how numerous they are in such diseases as typhoid fever, diphtheria, plague and malaria. The microscopic demonstration of the frequency with which clinically unrecognizable attacks of the above named and other diseases occur, had called the attention of clinicians and epidemiologists to their probable occurrence in such other diseases as scarlet fever, smallpox, and yellow fever, the specific organisms of which have not as yet been discovered. So that at the present time the most careful epidemiologists, clinicians and laboratory workers begin to realize that very large numbers of mild atypical and unrecognizable cases are bound to occur in most infectious diseases. But as yet few text-books on sanitation, clinical medicine, or even on bacteriology, lay sufficient emphasis on this fact. Nothing is more common than to find the young man just from the medical school, as well as the old practitioner, quick to deny the presence of scarlet fever, diphtheria, or typhoid fever because the symptoms are not severe enough or because they deviate too much from the text-book description. But the large number of the mild and aberrant cases, which usually remain "missed cases," and their importance in the extension of the infectious diseases, must now be admitted.

Carriers Exceedingly Numerous. — Still more numerous are the pure carriers, those persons in whose bodies the pathogenic bacteria and protozoa develop without causing symptoms. The recognition of this element of danger is due entirely to laboratory investigation, but, strange to say, most workers on bacteriology lay no more stress on this epidemiological factor than do the writers of treatises on hygiene or of text-books of medicine. In the preceding chapter sufficient evidence was presented to demonstrate the very great frequency with which these carrier cases occur. Their existence and the virulence of the germs which they carry are now established facts. Numerous instances were given where such carriers appeared to have transmitted the disease to others. Indeed it is almost inconceivable that it should be otherwise. It is hardly possible that virulent typhoid bacilli or diphtheria bacilli produced in large numbers, as they frequently are in carriers, should not be equally as dangerous as those which develop in the bodies of the sick. That is, they are equally dangerous potentially; actually the well person moving freely about may be more dangerous to the community than the sick person who is confined to the house.

Approaching the subject from another standpoint, it is interesting to see how the discovery of these missed and carrier cases has explained so much which we formerly did not understand.

Effort to " Stamp Out " Disease. — Twenty-five or thirty years ago we heard a great deal about "stamping out" the contagious diseases. That was the era of the building of hospitals for these diseases, of the organization of the sanitary service, of the discovery of pathogenic bacteria. The wonderful decrease in smallpox, the successful fight against cholera, the almost total disappearance of typhus fever, and the complete disappearance of plague, only foreshadowed, it was said, the extermination of typhoid fever, diphtheria, scarlet fever and measles. It was claimed that in those diseases which are exclusively contagious, if every case can be isolated until it is free from infection, the disease will be exterminated. It was believed that if people, and especially physicians, would take only a little more care, practically all cases of these diseases could be recognized and isolated. It was also thought to be not very difficult to control them until infection had disappeared. This confidence in the efficacy of isolation was in the then existing state of knowledge not unreasonable.

Isolation and its Results in Providence. — Previous to 1884 there had been in Providence no isolation to speak of in any of the contagious diseases except smallpox. In fact very many physicians did not consider that scarlet fever and diphtheria were very contagious, if contagious at all, but were inclined to look upon them as filth diseases. Restrictive measures, including isolation at home and fumigation, began to be applied in 1884 and were quite steadily strengthened during the next sixteen or seventeen years. I hoped, as did most health officers, that if scarlet fever and diphtheria could not be stamped out, they could be reduced to an insignificant remnant. But they were not stamped out in Providence, as they have not been in other cities. On the contrary, we had twice as many deaths in 1887 from scarlet fever as we had had during any year for seven years. Diphtheria from 1886 to 1890 also caused nearly double the number of deaths that it had in the preceding four years. Of course we talked about epidemic waves, and noted that the mortality from the last wave was very much lower than from many that had preceded it, and congratulated ourselves that the outbreak was not so severe as in former years. But I began to ask myself what there was about epidemic waves that made restrictive measures of little use, and also to inquire if there was anything wrong about the restrictive measures. If we were limiting these diseases at all, it was certainly in a very moderate way.

Infection by Air and Fomites Thought Most Important. — It was fully appreciated that in cities at least most cases of contagious disease cannot be traced to their source. Two theories have from antiquity been advanced in explanation. One is that most contagious diseases are easily carried by the atmosphere. Thus a person going by a house where there is scarlet fever, or passing an infected person in the street, might contract the disease. Such unconscious exposure might be quite common. But the principal source of the untraced cases of contagious disease was believed to be fomites. Walls and furniture were thought to become infected with the virus, and for weeks and months persons entering the room might contract disease through the breath. Books, toys, clothing and, in fact, every material thing, might readily become a source of infection and retain its virulence for months and years. These were perhaps not unreasonable *a priori* hypotheses, and they had some apparent backing of facts. At any rate they were the best theories we had. So health officers everywhere, including Providence, set about improving methods of disinfection. Sulphur fumigation was abandoned and the use of formaldehyde gas adopted in its place. Many cities set up a steam disinfecting plant, in Providence as early as 1887, and carpets, bedding and clothing were disinfected by steam. Some cities, particularly on the continent of Europe, sent a band of uniformed disinfectors to wash and scrub everything in the infected house. Scarlet fever and diphtheria refused to be exterminated, though in Providence we did have rather less during the early nineties than we had had before. But I was not satisfied. It seemed to me that we were having too much of these diseases, that there must be a leak somewhere.

Cultures Expected to Discover Much Diphtheria. — Then for one disease a new weapon was put into our hands. Many had long recognized that the diagnosis of diphtheria was difficult. It was suspected that many cases, because of this difficulty, escaped isolation entirely. When the culture method of diagnosis was devised I became enthusiastic and hopeful. We adopted it in Providence in January, 1895, and soon after required a negative culture before the patient was released from isolation. Hill has shown that without cultures the chance of error in the diagnosis of diphtheria is 50 per cent, which corresponds entirely with my frequently expressed opinion before the advent of the culture method. It is evident, then, that the general use of cultures ought to bring to light great numbers of cases of diphtheria which were formerly unrecognized, and this it certainly does. If such an improvement in diagnosis, and consequently in isolation, is brought about by the use of cultures, and if by the same means isolation can be maintained until the patient is certainly free from infection, there ought to follow a marked reduction in this disease. But it was quite otherwise. The deaths in Providence, which in 1894 had numbered 45, rose to 79 in 1895 and 125 in 1896, nearly twice as many in proportion to the population as there were in 1883, when there was no isolation, no disinfection and no antitoxin. The cases rose from 166 in 1894 to 386 in 1895 and 890 in 1896. The apparent reduction in the fatality rate from 27.71 to 14.07 indicates very plainly that the culture method of diagnosis had discovered a very large number of mild cases that would have previously been unrecognized, for antitoxin was only a minor factor in reducing the fatality, as it had been used in only a little over one-third of the cases. Isolation, disinfection, the use of cultures, and the opening of the contagious hospital had been accompanied by the greatest prevalence of the disease for ten years. I do not mean to say that the adoption of the measures described had no effect upon the amount of diphtheria in Providence. I am sure that they had, and that this disease on the whole has been lessened, cases prevented and lives saved. But better results were expected. I was disappointed, and I think other health officers have been disappointed also. It seemed that the measures, carried out as they were, ought to have given better results.

It seemed that there was something which we did not understand.

Failure of Hospital Isolation. — One of the most effectual means of isolating cases of contagious diseases is by removal to the hospital. Certainly while in the hospital they can do no harm, and with reasonable care there is not much danger of their carrying infection back to their homes. Return cases do not occur in scarlet fever and diphtheria in more than about one to three per cent of discharges, and are not a factor of moment in the extension of these diseases. The idea that such hospitals would be a powerful factor in the extermination of these diseases was not unreasonable. Smallpox hospitals have been in general use for a very long time, but they are not here under consideration, though it is questionable whether the hospital isolation of smallpox can ever accomplish much alone and unaided by vaccination. But it is the hospitalization of scarlet fever and diphtheria that is particularly instructive.

English Hospitals. — The use of hospitals for contagious diseases has been carried farther in England than elsewhere. Fifteen or twenty years ago the larger municipalities began building them on a considerable scale, and at present most of the English towns are provided with large hospitals for scarlet fever, and to a less extent for diphtheria. At the time when their construction was first strongly urged it was believed that their use would result in the eradication of the diseases for which they were provided. The result has certainly been disappointing, and there has recently been an active discussion as to whether they do an amount of good in restricting disease at all commensurate with their cost.[1] There is no doubt that the mortality from scarlet fever, both in

[1] O'Connor, Geo. Wilson, Waddy and others, Brit. M. J., Lond., 1905, II, 630; Millard, Biss, Fraser, etc., Med. Press & Circ., Lond., 1904, LXXVIII, 215, 218, 241, 327, 377; Newsholme, Tr. Epidem. Soc. Lond., n. s., 1900–01, XX, 48; J. Hyg., 1901, I, 145; Millard, Pub. Health, 1901, XIII; J. T. Wilson, Pub. Health, 1896–97, IX, Sup., p. 21.

England and the United States, has greatly diminished during recent years, but whether this has been due to restrictive measures or to lowered virulence has been disputed. The small death rate would indicate that the disease is really milder. This is also indicated by the fact that plural deaths, that is, more than one death in a family, are less frequent now than formerly. Again, local outbreaks of the old-time severe type occasionally appear. There was such an outbreak in Providence in 1906–07, during which the case fatality ran up to 12.85 per cent. Similar outbreaks have been noted in Keene, N. H., Haverhill, Worcester and Montreal. The relatively lowered fatality in recent years has rendered it difficult to determine from the number of deaths just what influence restrictive measures, like hospital isolation, have had on the prevalence of scarlet fever, and increasing accuracy and care in reporting cases render it difficult to draw conclusions from the number of cases. But after all has been said it is clear that hospital isolation in scarlet fever has checked the disease very much less than was expected, and sometimes appears to have had little effect. In Huddersfield, a city of nearly one hundred thousand people, from 1890 to 1899 the percentage of removals to the hospital was 90, yet the mean attack rate for the period was 4.3 per thousand. From 1900 to 1908 the removals to the hospital were 92.4 per cent and the attack rate 2.96. This is certainly a surprisingly high morbidity rate for a city where practically all reported cases have for twenty years been subjected to most excellent isolation. A similar state of things is noted in other cities. Some cities with a high per cent of removals to the hospital have more of the disease than do cities with no hospitals. The same is noted in rural communities. O'Connor,[1] medical officer of health of Leicestershire and Rutland combined sanitary districts, reported that in five parishes where the percentage of hospital isolation had for ten years reached 66 per cent, the attack rate was 6.2 per thou-

[1] O'Connor, Brit. M. J., Lond., 1905, II, 630.

sand, while in five other parishes where hospital isolation was applied to only 14 per cent of the cases, the attack rate was 2.8. In another district, one parish which sent 60 per cent of its scarlet fever to the hospital, had three times as many cases as contiguous parishes which had little hospital isolation. Neech[1] says that in Cornwall from 1898 to 1907 there was practically no difference in the incidence of scarlet fever, in both urban and rural districts, connected with the use or failure to use isolation hospitals. Again, a city after it builds a hospital may have more of the disease than before. The abandonment of hospital isolation may do no harm. In Leicester[2] the hospital was closed temporarily, and all the scarlet fever cases sent to their homes, with an actual decrease in number of reported cases. The hospital in other cities also has been closed without harm. I have thought it possible that at times hospital isolation might actually favor the spread of disease. When a case is removed to the hospital, comparatively little restraint is placed upon other members of the family, and if some of them are carriers, as they certainly usually are in diphtheria, much harm may result. If, however, the case is kept at home, the rest of the family, particularly the children, are under considerable restraint for several weeks. Observations in Providence demonstrate that the retention of the case at home very rarely leads to the extension of the disease to other families in the house, and presumably to still less extension outside of the house.

Why the Failure? — It may be admitted, and is doubtless true, that hospitals have prevented very many cases of disease, and they may have been somewhat of a factor in its lessened prevalence. Nevertheless it must also be admitted that, notwithstanding the complete and excellent isolation secured in some cities like Huddersfield, scarlet fever has still prevailed to an alarming extent. When eighty to ninety per cent of the cases are removed to the hospital it is certain

[1] Neech, Pub. Health, Lond., 1908–09, XXII, 296.
[2] Rep. on Health of Leicester, 1902, 36.

that the remainder will be so situated that home isolation will quite effectually prevent extension from them. In such cities almost all of the reported cases are thus effectively isolated, either in hospital or home. Yet the disease continues to prevail. There is evidently some source which escapes control. Newsholme has very clearly shown this. While admitting that isolation does prevent much sickness, he says that the disease still prevails and outbreaks still occur owing to some "epidemic influence." Now our purpose is to determine, if possible, what this "epidemic influence" is. What is the factor which is so powerful and continuous in its action that 90 to 95 per cent of perfection in the isolation of a contagious disease is unable to prevent a continued high prevalence and repeated epidemic waves?

American Hospital Experience. — It is not merely English hospital experience which has shown the inefficiency of isolation. We have numerous instances in our own country. I have already referred to the experience of Providence, where increasing stringency in isolation was not followed by a decrease in contagious diseases. There has been much difference between American cities as regards the strictness of enforced isolation. Some have been notoriously lax, while others have for years endeavored to secure a complete registration of scarlet fever and diphtheria, and have adopted rigorous measures of isolation and disinfection, though in no American city has hospitalization been carried so far as it has in many English towns. But no one would be able, by studying mortality rates, to pick out the cities which pursue a rigorous policy of isolation. I collected data relating to the prevalence of scarlet fever and diphtheria in American cities for the decade 1890–1899,[1] and it is surprising to note that the cities with the best sanitary administration frequently have a comparatively large amount of scarlet fever and diphtheria. During the period mentioned, Boston, in my opinion, had the best sanitary administration of any of the large cities,

[1] Chapin, Municipal Sanitation, Providence, 1901, Table op. 480.

though New York stood high. The death rate from diphtheria in both cities was 84 per 100,000 living, from scarlet fever 25 for Boston, and 33 for New York. Certainly neither Chicago nor Cincinnati enforced such rigorous measures, yet the rates in these two cities were 72 and 71 for diphtheria and 17 and 7 for scarlet fever. Among the smaller Massachusetts cities Fall River has usually had a rather inefficient health service and little hospitalization, yet the death rate from diphtheria was 21 and from scarlet fever 15 per 100,000 living, while in Worcester the figures were 48 and 8, and this notwithstanding the fact that in Fall River the proportion of children is much greater than in most American cities, and that the population is exceptionally ignorant as measured by illiteracy. Worcester has had a contagious-disease hospital since 1897, and has removed to it in some years as high as 63 per cent of its diphtheria cases. In general, Worcester secures an excellent registration of cases, and consequent isolation. Nevertheless Worcester has recently had, notwithstanding its increasing hospitalization and good home isolation, a severe outbreak of the disease. It seems a fair assumption that some factor much more important than the recognized cases of the disease has been at work in Worcester. If it were not so, the reported cases of the disease should not have risen from 132 in 1905 to 1178 in 1907.

Diphtheria Isolation at Home. — In Providence for some years previous to March, 1902, isolation in diphtheria was terminated only when a negative culture had been obtained from the patient. At that date a change was made, terminating isolation ten days after the disappearance of exudation. This certainly liberated many cases still infectious, but this factor was of so little moment that the disease continued to decrease until on a certain day in August the city was entirely free from reported cases, a condition again nearly reached in 1907.

Isolation in Institutions. — It is by no means uncommon to see outbreaks in institutions lasting many months, although every case is promptly isolated and all persons in the institution are repeatedly examined by cultures from throat and nose. I have records of several such in Providence, and most health officers and managers of institutions have been through such unpleasant experiences. Here again we are forced to look for sources other than the recognizable cases.

At a school in Owatonna, Minnesota,[1] there had been more or less diphtheria for years until a sharp outbreak in 1896 caused a very energetic effort to be made to stamp it out. Cultures were taken from everybody, and all persons in whom diphtheria bacilli were found were isolated, at first in a common ward, but later each person in a separate room. Isolation was maintained until three successive negative cultures were obtained from throat and nose, and efficient disinfection was practiced. Still the disease persisted month after month, and some of the carriers, after release, were found to be still harboring the bacilli. One boy carried the bacilli for nineteen months. The attempt at the isolation of carriers was abandoned, and several years later there was still more or less diphtheria in the institution.

A still more notable failure of the isolation of diphtheria was at the Willard State Hospital for the insane in New York.[2] In this institution practically the same methods were adopted as at Owatonna, but nevertheless the disease persisted several years. Patients and carriers released from isolation after several negative cultures were still found to be carriers. If in an institution of this kind, where the strictest discipline is maintained, and where carriers can be isolated indefinitely, the most stringent measures of isolation and disinfection fail to stamp out the disease, what is to be expected of any such measures which can be adopted in an ordinary community?

An outbreak in a hospital in California was managed in

[1] St. Paul M. J., 1900, II, 223; Brit. M. J., Lond., 1898, I, 1008; Rep. St. Bd. Health, Minnesota, 1897–98, 465; Rep. Am. Pub. Health Ass., 1899, XXV, 546.

[2] Rep. State Commission in Lunacy, N. Y., 1904, XVI.

the same way.[1] At first no effect seemed to be produced, and the outbreak lasted from April to August, but was assumed to have been finally checked by the same measures which failed at Owatonna and Willard. But as many outbreaks last even a shorter time, though no attention is paid to carriers, it is uncertain whether the outbreak was stamped out or died out. Sidney Davies[2] reports that at the Bostall-lane School in Woolwich diphtheria prevailed for three years notwithstanding repeated closures and bacterial examinations of the pupils. There is little doubt that at times a careful search for carriers and missed cases in schools and institutions and their isolation until two successive negative cultures from throat and nose are obtained, prove successful in checking outbreaks; there is no doubt, too, that outbreaks frequently die out of themselves; and it is shown by the examples given above that it is at times impossible by any degree of isolation to stamp out an outbreak. How to manage such institutional epidemics cannot be determined until the control of carriers is more carefully studied than it has been.

Isolation a Failure in Measles. — Measles is a disease which in cities it seems to be impossible to check to any appreciable extent by isolation. In Aberdeen[3] this was faithfully tried for twenty years, 1883 to 1902, but no apparent effect was produced on the prevalence of the disease. Similar failures have been noted elsewhere. During the last half of this period in Aberdeen, when there was far more accurate registration and better control than before, the number of cases rose to 24,254, about fifty per cent more than in the first half of the period. A census of the children in certain schools indicated that from ninety to ninety-three per cent of children over ten years of age had had the disease. Restrictive measures which protected only seven to ten per cent of the population from attack were then wisely abandoned. The very

1 Rep. State Bd. of Health, California, 1906–08, 201.

2 Rep. Med. Off. Health, Lond., 1908, 36.

3 Aberdeen, Report of Med. Off. of Health, 1904, 41.

excellent report of the medical officer of health of Aberdeen discusses the subject very fully. In New York measles was first isolated in 1896, but not until 1902 were the regulations very rigorously enforced. The average death rate from 1895 to 1904 was 2.40, and the highest death rate since 1896 was reached in 1906, when it was 2.69. There is no evidence that the measures adopted in New York have had any more influence on the prevalence of the disease than did isolation and disinfection in Aberdeen. It seems in the highest degree probable that the disease prevails because of the unrecognized but infectious prodromal stage. No amount of isolation after the disease is recognized can atone for the harm done before the diagnosis is made.

Isolation a Failure in Meningitis. — Within a recent period the city of New York suffered from an exceptionally long and severe outbreak of cerebro-spinal meningitis. The attack rate was higher than in any of the other large American cities, and the outbreak lasted longer; and it lasted longer than it has in most of the German cities. On April 19, 1905, after the epidemic had continued for about two years, very stringent restrictive measures of isolation and disinfection were adopted. The outbreak was then declining, and that it would afterwards decline still more was to have been expected. But it was not "stamped out," for in 1907 there were reported 642 deaths and in 1908, 351. In Leith[1] great efforts were made to isolate all suspects and carriers, and the outbreak appeared to be checked, but in Edinburgh also it died out, though without such energetic measures. The experience in Germany seems to be that if in the beginning diligent search is made for carriers, and strict isolation is maintained, the outbreak may sometimes be checked, but after the disease has become established, and carriers are numerous, isolation is of little avail. These appear to be the views of Lingelsheim, Ostermann, Selter, Flatten and others.

[1] Ker. Practitioner, Lond., 1908, LXXX, 66.

Isolation often a Failure in Smallpox. — Smallpox is less likely to escape detection than is any other disease. Yet epidemics grow in the face of the most rigid isolation. Unrecognized cases, even in this disease, are so numerous that the isolation of the recognized cases often seems to be a complete failure. The State Board of Health of Minnesota, realizing this,[1] has had the boldness to advise that no attempt be made to isolate, and that entire reliance be placed on vaccination. It was hoped that this would lead to more complete vaccination. There has been no alarming increase in smallpox in Minnesota, and Montana[2] is now following the lead of the former state.

Why Does Isolation Fail? — The epidemiological evidence is conclusive that the isolation of recognized cases of contagious diseases often fails to check outbreaks which grow in spite of it; that it does not stamp out disease, and that it only reduces in a moderate degree the prevalence of the disease. We are forced to conclude that there is some defect in our procedures, or some other source of infection more important than the recognized cases. The error cannot be that isolation is too brief, for return cases and recurrences are not important factors. It is not that isolation is imperfect, for isolation in the hospital is well-nigh complete, and careful observations in Providence indicate that the danger of extension outside the family from cases at home is very slight.

Importance of Carriers and Missed Cases. — As has been previously stated, two theories have been advanced to account for the appearance of untraced cases of contagious diseases: that of distant aerial infection, and that of the persistence of infection on things, i.e., fomites. In other chapters of this book it is shown that both of these modes of infection are of little moment, and in the first chapter it was shown to be

[1] Resolution adopted July, 1906, to go into effect January, 1908, Am. J. Pub. Hyg., 1907, III, 227.

[2] Am. J. Pub. Hyg., 1909, V, 815.

unlikely that the specific organisms of our common diseases grow outside of the body. In the second chapter it was shown that they may grow in the body and yet produce few or no symptoms. It appears, then, highly probable that by far the most important factor in the causation of the contagious diseases are the "carrier" and "missed" cases.

It is not for a moment suggested that the existence of carriers explains all epidemiological problems. There are, for instance, quite a number of contagious diseases which exhibit a varying degree of periodicity. We have as yet only the vaguest notions as to the causes of the variations in the prevalence of disease, its seasonal irregularities, and the rise and fall of epidemics. There is no reason to believe that these phenomena depend on the extra-corporal growth of pathogenic organisms, and it is probable that the seasonal distribution of such diseases as smallpox and scarlet fever is only in the most indirect manner dependent upon temperature, rainfall, etc. It is not unlikely that the factors affecting the extension of these diseases are so numerous that their prevalence is really to a large extent a matter of chance. But whatever the factors may be, we must believe that they affect carriers as well as clinical cases. Why we have more carriers and more cases at one time than another, we cannot at present say. But it appears to be in the highest degree probable that in times of outbreaks, as well as in inter-epidemic periods, the chief factor in the extension of the disease is the existence of unrecognized infection in human beings or, in some diseases, in the lower animals.

Need of Further Study. — I would be the last person to assert that the views here set forth are unassailable and unalterable. They doubtless will be modified; it may be that they are entirely erroneous. What is needed is further investigation along the lines indicated, and a great deal of it. Unfortunately sanitary science is far from exact. We have few established truths, but many theories of greater or less probability, on which to base our practice. The probability of each theory must be carefully weighed. Which is the most probable source of infection, the cesspool in the yard, the fomites that escaped disinfection, the patient who was released too soon, or the unknown carrier ? The chances are greatly in favor of the last, and yet to-day sanitary practice almost completely ignores the carrier. It is not surprising that many health officers fail to appreciate the importance of the question which is here discussed. It is remarkable, however, that bacteriologists as a rule minimize the danger to be apprehended from carriers.

Carriers not to be Ignored. — It may be admitted that only 1 per cent of the population are diphtheria carriers, though as a matter of fact it must often be more than that; also that only 15 per cent of these carry virulent germs, though it is really often much greater. It may also be admitted that these bacilli are not usually so numerous as in the sick, though it is known that they sometimes appear in pure culture; yet even admitting all this, there will be in inter-epidemic periods in a city of 100,000 people at least 150 well persons carrying virulent diphtheria bacilli. Why should the bacteriologist ignore these 150 sources of infection and insist on two throat and nose negative cultures from every reported patient ? Or why should he, as he occasionally does, recommend isolating the carriers in the family but ignore all other carriers ? Why neglect this whole question of carriers, and spend endless time in devising methods of liberating formaldehyde to kill the few bacilli that may remain about the house ? Why worry about the saliva that may have gotten onto a book, a coat, or the wall of a room, and neglect the reader of the book, the wearer of the coat and the dweller in the room, who is probably growing the germs in his throat and nose ? It is not easy to answer these questions, and so the bacteriologist withdraws to his laboratory and ingores them. But the health officer *must* answer them in one way or another.

Principles of Diphtheria Isolation. — To confine the discussion for the moment to diphtheria, concerning which we have more accurate knowledge than we have for any other disease, there appear to be only two logical positions which the health officer can take in regard to its management. There is the possible policy of non-regulation. This the public would certainly not permit, and I think with very good reason. Or we can go to the other extreme and attempt to isolate every person carrying diphtheria bacilli, until they disappear from throat and nose, or until they are shown to be non-virulent. That is, of course, entirely impracticable except in small isolated communities or institutions, and it is often very difficult, and sometimes impossible then. In every large city there are hundreds of carriers who can never be detected, and who could not be controlled if they were. Virulent bacilli may remain for months, and the attempt to isolate for a prolonged period prominent lawyers, business men, or physicians, would result in a breakdown of the whole system. As a matter of fact, such carriers escape from isolation while still infected. If cultures are taken daily, or every few days, it is usually not very long before the two negatives required by rule are secured and the patient is released, though subsequent cultures not infrequently reveal the bacillus. The ideal of health officers has been to keep up isolation until every spark of infection has died out, — a very reasonable ideal, until it was learned that there are many hidden sparks scattered about the community, some of which are sure sooner or later to burst into flame. As it is impossible to attain the ideal of stamping out all infection, and as it is certain that many infected persons cannot be restrained at all, it is unreasonable to require restraint to the uttermost limit, of the recognized cases. It is often argued that the fact that all infected persons cannot be isolated, is no reason for not isolating all that can be found, any more than the fact that many thieves escape is no reason for not imprisoning those thieves who are caught. But there is no true parallel here. The thief is a criminal, and his imprisonment is a punishment. The bacillus carrier is not a criminal, and he is isolated, not as a punishment, but to protect the community. If the protection secured is not commensurate with the hardship inflicted, the procedure is unjust, and unwise from a sociological standpoint.

A Compromise Necessary. — But just as soon as we depart from the orthodox ideal, absolute isolation, we have to adopt some sort of compromise, a compromise which has no strictly logical defense. We are thus forced to follow one of three policies, — either do nothing, which is unwise and would not be permitted, or attempt absolute isolation of all sources of infection, which is manifestly impossible, or employ a moderate degree of restriction, which, though not strictly logical, is nevertheless practicable, reasonable and to a considerable degree effective.

Isolation of Real Value. — While the most rigorous isolation does not stamp out diphtheria, we know that restriction does some good. The removal of a case to the hospital is shown by statistical evidence to prevent to some extent the development of secondary cases in the family. So too does good isolation at home. The warning sign on the house keeps out many people, some of whom would otherwise certainly contract the disease. The regulation of school attendance prevents some school outbreaks, and others are checked by the prompt removal of the infecting child. The evidence points to an appreciable reduction in diphtheria prevalence in recent times, which I believe it is fair to consider as due, in part at least, to deliberate separation of the sick from the well under the direction of the sanitary authority or otherwise. Why more has not been accomplished by isolation is explained by the facts set forth in the preceding chapter. If because of the existence of so many unrecognized sources of infection, isolation can effect only a limited degree of prevention, could not substantially as much be accomplished by more moderate methods than are usually employed? Why keep the patient indoors for six weeks when other members of the family with infected throats are going about?

Why keep from work the wage earners in an infected family when scores of other carriers are attending to their business without restraint?

Typhoid Carriers cannot be Isolated. — The isolation of typhoid carriers is no more possible, just, or effectual in checking disease, than is the isolation of diphtheria carriers. As was shown in the preceding chapter, the number of carriers and convalescents excreting bacilli is probably much larger than the number of cases confined indoors. It seems to me useless to attempt to confine convalescents two or three months after their recovery. There certainly would be most energetic opposition on the part of the public, which probably would ultimately be sustained by the courts. The health officer who attempted to isolate convalescents until bacilli were no longer to be found in their urine, would be in an awkward position if he allowed chronic carriers to go at large, and he would be in a still more awkward position if he attempted to isolate all chronic carriers indefinitely. There are probably 200,000 cases of typhoid fever in the United States each year, and 3 per cent of these would be 6,000. To attempt to isolate 6,000 carriers would of course be futile. Not one-tenth of them could even be discovered. To isolate the small fraction of carriers who can be discovered is practically useless, and therefore unjust. It may be, and probably is, wise to regulate the life of such carriers as may be discovered, and at times to forbid their engaging in certain occupations, such as those of cook, waitress and milk dealer, but to attempt their isolation under present conditions seems to me most unwise.

Isolation too Rigorous. — I believe that, on the whole, isolation in our prevailing contagious diseases is carried farther than is necessary; that less rigorous measures would accomplish practically as much good, and that there would be less temptation to conceal cases and to interpret doubtful symptoms in line with the patient's desires. It is impossible here to lay down in detail a scheme for the proper isolation of contagious diseases. What are the best methods of dealing with these diseases is a matter for free discussion, and also for experiment. It is to call attention to the new facts, and to elicit discussion from the new viewpoints, that these pages are written.

Degree of Contagiousness. — Before considering some of the principles which should guide the application of measures of isolation, we should consider what are, under the ordinary conditions of life, the chances of infection from a single individual. Until recently it has been believed to be very great. That smallpox hospitals are placed a mile or more from inhabited districts, that physicians clothe themselves with gowns and caps and rubber boots on their visits to infectious cases, and that it is insisted that the ceiling of a room occupied by such a case be disinfected, indicate a belief that the virus of the contagious diseases is exceedingly diffusive and exceedingly virulent. Why such a belief is not well founded will be shown in succeeding chapters, and it will suffice here to call attention to the fact that the chance of an infected person transmitting the infection to another is not nearly so great as is generally supposed. This is a mathematical necessity. We now know that the number of infected persons is very much greater than was formerly believed, and that they often remain infected for much longer periods than was suspected. It necessarily follows that the danger to be apprehended from any one person at any one time is much less than was once thought.

Factors Involved. — The chance of an infected person giving rise to the disease, or of transmitting the infection to others, varies greatly with the intensity of the infection, or the number of disease germs in the secretions or excretions, their virulence, the volume of the excretions, the care exercised, the occupation, and the surroundings generally. Conditions in the home and in institutions are usually much more favorable than elsewhere for the transmission of infection. Yet in the home the chance of such extension of disease is not as great as has been supposed. In Providence,[1] the chance of persons contracting diphtheria from another member of the family who has the disease is only about 1 in 15. The chance of a child between two and six years contracting it is 1 in 5; of an adult, 1 in 40. The chance of a woman contracting the disease in the family is about three times as great as that of a man. For scarlet fever the figures are not very different. Every one must have noted repeated instances where only one of a family of children is attacked by scarlet fever or diphtheria, the rest of the family remaining well, though isolation may have been far from satisfactory.

Danger Less outside Family. — Outside of the family, in school, in factory and in ordinary social relations, except perhaps in the play of young children, the chance of transmitting the disease must be very much less. Instances are not rare where children, presumably in the infectious stage of scarlet fever, have mingled freely with others for many days, or perhaps weeks, with little or no extension of the disease. I have notes of an instance where a boy with scarlet fever in the sore-throat stage attended a Sunday-school festival, and no other case developed among the large number of children present. At an infant asylum a child was sick with mild scarlet fever for 17 days, mingling freely with about 75 children, mostly under 5 years of age, and only 3 other cases resulted. At a large school a girl returned at the end of the first week of an attack of scarlet fever, and continued her attendance for 20 days. Only 3 or 4 cases developed in that school. Similar and even more marked instances of apparently feeble infectivity are reported by others. I have made no attempt to collect such cases, but I happen to have before me three reported by Butler.[2] One child, taken sick November 5, attended school from November 11 to November 19. Two other children, attacked December 26 and 27 respectively, attended different schools up to January 16. In only

[1] Rep. Supt. of Health, Providence, 1909.
[2] Butler, Proc. Roy. Soc. Med., Lond., 1908, I, Epidemiol. Sec., 225.

one of the three schools did even a single case occur. I have known of a teacher with virulent diphtheria bacilli in her throat from the first of January to the middle of April, who taught in a kindergarten all that time, but who did not transmit the disease to any one. Many of the instances of typhoid carriers which have been referred to, show that such persons may for long periods of time fail to infect any one, even though employed as cooks or handlers of milk. I have known of cases of smallpox remaining for several days in lodging houses or hospital wards, or traveling on railroads, without any one contracting the disease. Failure to infect may be due sometimes, perhaps, to intermittency in the excretion of germs, sometimes to lack of contact, and sometimes to lack of susceptibility on the part of the receiver of the infection. Whatever the cause may be, we must recognize that an infected person often mingles freely with the public without transmitting the infection to another.

Carriers less Infective than the Sick. — As has been stated, it is not improbable that the infectivity of a well carrier may for several reasons be less than that of a person sick with the disease. It may then be argued that the danger from carriers has in the preceding pages been very much exaggerated. It is not to be denied that the probable danger from a *single carrier* is small. Their number, however, is large, so that the danger from *all carriers* is large, and is, I believe, a very considerable factor in the maintenance of the contagious diseases.

Isolation should Vary. — In applying isolation to the prevention of disease it must be kept in mind that different conditions require different procedures. Thus when an ordinary contagious disease first appears, after a considerable absence, in a small community, or in an institution, very rigorous measures of isolation are usually desirable, as experience has shown that very often an outbreak is thus effectively checked in its beginning.

Isolation in Villages. — The efficacy of isolation under such circumstances is well illustrated by the history of outbreaks of the common contagious diseases in the smaller cities, townships and villages of Michigan. The data given in the annual reports of the board of health of that state are of great epidemiological interest, and my discussion of the subject on another occasion is here given.[1]

" Only those places are considered which have remained free from the disease for at least sixty days, and this unfortunately is never true of a city of any considerable size. The outbreaks reported are arranged in groups, one in which isolation and disinfection were both enforced, one in which they were both neglected, and one in which the reports did not state with sufficient exactness what restrictive measures were carried out. The following is a summary of some of the tables in the report:

	Number of Cases per Outbreak.			Number of Cases per Outbreak.	
	Restrictive Measures not Enforced.	Restrictive Measures Enforced.		Restrictive Measures not Enforced.	Restrictive Measures Enforced.
Typhoid fever, 10 years..	5.82	3.13	1900	6.72	2.22
Diphtheria, 14 years.....	11.12	2.11	"	4.85	1.71
Scarlet fever, 14 years....	11.95	2.32	"	10.43	2.53
Measles, 11 years........	48.30	3.03	"	27.60	4.67
Smallpox...............	....	.....	"	32.00	3.80

Isolation Effective. — " Several things are to be noted in connection with these figures. In the first place, isolation and disinfection accomplish very much in preventing the extension of all these diseases. The number of facts is so great, the outbreaks of each disease running into the hundreds, and the difference between good and bad sanitation is so manifest in each one of the years for each one of the

[1] J. Mass. Ass. Bds. Health, Bost., 1904, XIV, 226.

diseases, that the success achieved must be a very real one. It appears certain that isolation and disinfection as practiced in the smaller communities of Michigan reduce the cases of contagious disease in round numbers from forty-five to ninety-five per cent. In scarlet fever, diphtheria, measles and smallpox, isolation appears from the reports, as one would expect, to have very much more restrictive effect than disinfection.

"As will be shown later, disinfection probably has little influence in restricting contagious diseases, but in view of existing ideas and practices it is probable that isolation and disinfection were not so distinctly separable as is indicated by the reports of the local health officers. One of the things which appeared most remarkable to the writer in these reports is the apparently great restriction of measles. It has certainly been the experience in all our larger cities that restrictive measures, no matter how energetic, have had very little effect in reducing the mortality from this disease. But in the smaller communities in Michigan it appears that where isolation and disinfection are well carried out there is nearly ninety-four per cent less cases per outbreak than where precautions are neglected.

Cause of Success. — "But if one examines the original returns of the health officers it appears plain why such good results are obtained. If the first case of the disease coming to a community is early recognized and isolated the chances are good that the outbreak will be at once checked. The chances that such a case will be so recognized in a village are very much greater than in a city. If, however, the outbreak is not checked at its very outset, the chances are, even in the country, that its extension will be very considerable. As a matter of fact, a great many of the first cases coming to small communities are promptly recognized and isolated, and as a result an outbreak is prevented. It is because outbreaks are in rural communities so often nipped in the bud that the application of restrictive measures in such communities makes such a good showing. What is true of measles is true also of other diseases, particularly of scarlet fever and diphtheria. It is success in applying restrictive measures to the first case that is the principal cause of the apparent efficiency of these methods. If every appearance of contagious disease in these rural communities had gained some headway before restrictive measures were applied, the showing would not be nearly so favorable. In fact, in the large cities in Michigan, where these diseases are always epidemic, restrictive measures, even of a very rigorous type, have not enabled the health officers to 'stamp them out.' Thus in Detroit it was the custom for many years to 'quarantine' absolutely every house where there was scarlet fever or diphtheria. No one was allowed to go out, and the inspectors visited the house twice a day and furnished provisions for the poor at an expense of thousands of dollars annually. Yet these diseases were no more 'stamped out' in Detroit than they have been in Chicago or other cities where milder methods have prevailed."

Isolation in Common Diseases. — When measles, diphtheria or scarlet fever appears in a town or institution which has for some time been free from the disease, the patient ought to be isolated until it is as certain as medical science can determine that he is free from infection. At least this should be attempted. If it should happen, as it sometimes does, that the diphtheria patient retains virulent bacilli for many months, or that the scarlet-fever patient has a discharging ear for a similar period, isolation will probably have to be abandoned. But isolation is worth trying, for in the majority of instances safety is secured in a few weeks. Contacts also should be carefully examined and isolated, or otherwise restricted as to their relations with the community. If after a reasonable time the disease is "stamped out" the health officer is to be congratulated. If it is not stamped out he may well temper the rigor of his restrictive measures.

When a rare disease, as plague, leprosy, or cholera, appears in Europe or North America, equally stringent measures should be employed. At present smallpox belongs rather to this class of rare diseases, and strict isolation of the first case and careful examination and supervision of contacts is desirable and useful.

Many Carriers make Isolation Useless. — The effectiveness of isolation, and the consequent reason for its practice, varies inversely as the number of carriers and missed cases. With the enormous number of carriers of pneumococci, it is entirely useless to enforce isolation of cases of pneumonia. Influenza belongs to the same class as pneumonia, in which compulsory isolation is useless. It is probable also that nothing which the health officer can do in the way of isolation will have any effect on the extent of outbreaks of cerebrospinal meningitis. The enforced isolation of typhoid fever, owing to the number of carriers, will usually prove of little value. While it is probable that there are few carriers of measles, yet the long prodromal but extremely infectious stage renders ineffectual measures of restriction. If isolation of measles is attempted, little can be hoped for other than a slight postponement of the age of attack, and no measures should be adopted which inflict any great hardship. No one advocates the isolation, in the ordinary meaning of the term, of pulmonary tuberculosis. It is not attempted in this disease simply because infected persons are so numerous that it is impossible. If tuberculosis were as rarc as leprosy, strict isolation would be, and should be, demanded. On the other hand, there are so few carriers of smallpox that, even with the mild type of the disease prevailing, strict isolation is often advisable.

To discover the proportion of carriers to recognized cases, for each disease, is a matter of the greatest practical importance. We must have a fairly clear idea of how many unrecognized human foci of infection there are before we can determine upon what methods of isolation, if any, are likely to prove effective. Yet the investigation of carriers has received comparatively little attention at the hands of bacteriologists.

Value of Hospitals. — Hospitals are useful for protecting the family, for checking outbreaks in institutions, for receiving cases from lodging houses and hotels, for furnishing better medical service, and for relieving the overworked housewife in the families of the poor. It is an unnecessary expense to provide hospital accommodations for all cases of scarlet fever and diphtheria, or for ninety per cent or even eighty per cent. That half or two-thirds of the cases of these diseases can, for all practical purposes, be equally well cared for at home, is not unlikely.

Home Isolation. — In home isolation of scarlet fever, diphtheria and measles, the patient should, for the benefit of the public, be kept in the house. It does not seem reasonable to prolong isolation until all possible chance of infection has ceased. Exactly what the period should be in each disease should now be a topic for renewed discussion.

Isolation in Providence. — In Providence at present the period of isolation for scarlet fever is four weeks from the beginning of the case. Up to 1902 the period was five weeks. Since the reduction in the period of isolation, the attack rate has been about 33 per 100,000 living, although one of our largest epidemic waves occurred during this period, and registration is certainly far better than formerly. From 1884 to 1901 the attack rate was about 34 per 100,000. In diphtheria, isolation is maintained for ten days after the disappearance of the membrane. The decrease in the prevalence of the disease which followed the adoption of less rigorous isolation has been previously alluded to.

Family. — When the attempt is made to isolate the patient in the family from the family, in order to protect other members, the duration of isolation may well be left to the discretion of the family. It is the duty of the health officer to explain that the longer the separation of sick from well is maintained, the more likely it is to be effective. In scarlet fever there is no means of determining when the patient is free from infection. I am in the habit of recommending separation from the family for six weeks, perhaps a somewhat shorter time if the case is a mild one, and longer if there is aural or nasal discharge. In Providence, scarlet-fever cases are usually sent home from the hospital in four or five weeks, if free from nose and ear discharge. No regard need be paid to desquamation, as the experience of English hospitals has shown that no danger is to be feared from that source.[1] It is absurd to isolate with strictness a diphtheria patient from the rest of the family unless cultures have shown that the rest of the family are free from the bacilli. If such home isolation is to be undertaken at all, it should be continued, if possible, until two or three successive negative cultures have been obtained.

Hospital. — Diphtheria cases in Providence are usually in the hospital until two, three or four successive negative cultures from the throat have been secured, the greater precaution being taken when the child is to return to an institution. Sometimes the patient is sent out while still harboring bacilli. The duration of isolation of the living cases is 19.65 days, and the percentage of return cases has been 1.9. In London [2] the period of detention of 6866 cases was 57.5 days, and the percentage of return cases was 1.2, about 0.5 per cent less than in Providence, although the period of detention was almost three times as long. The duration of stay in the Providence hospital for scarlet fever, surviving cases, is 45.67 days, and the percentage of return cases is 3.4. In the London hospitals the period of detention is 64.9 days,[3] and the percentage of return cases, 1902–04, was 3.22.

[1] Metropolitan Asylums Board Report on Return Cases of Scarlet Fever and Diphtheria, 1902–04, 6. See also my discussion of this subject in Fiske Fund Essay LII, published by R. I. Medical Society, Providence, 1909.

[2] Metropolitan Asylums Board Report on Return Cases of Scarlet Fever and Diphtheria, 1901-02, 59, 62.

[3] Metropolitan Asylums Board Report on Return Cases of Scarlet Fever and Diphtheria, 1902–04, 5, 23.

School. — School children in infected families should be excluded from school for a liberal period, for this works little hardship, and the state should make special effort to keep its schools free from disease. Yet school exclusion may be, and often is, carried to excess. In Providence children living in a family where there is scarlet fever are excluded from school for four weeks from the beginning of the last case. In all except the poorer class of houses children living in other families in the house are permitted to attend school. In diphtheria, children in the infected family are not allowed in school for four weeks, provided that if all the school children in the family yield two throat and nose negative cultures, they may attend school after the warning sign has been removed (which is ten days after the disappearance of the exudation). Children in other families in the better class of houses are admitted to school if one negative culture is obtained from throat and nose. After the expiration of a month, all children in families where there has been diphtheria are usually admitted to school whether or not they are carrying morphologically typical bacilli, and of course quite a number do go to school while infected. Doubtless these carriers may at times infect others in school, but even if two negative cultures were required before readmission, some children would probably still prove infectious. Absolute security is impossible, and the rule should be so framed as to accomplish a maximum amount of good with a minimum amount of annoyance.

Wage Earners. — There is little reason for excluding wage earners from their work except in a few occupations. Most of the carriers we cannot restrain, and therefore why penalize those who have the additional misfortune of sickness in their families?

The most dangerous carriers are those who handle milk; hence milk producers and dealers living in infected families should be excluded from work. Judging from the number of reported outbreaks, the danger is probably greater for typhoid fever than for any other disease. It is probably wise to regulate the occupation of all typhoid contacts who handle any kind of food that is eaten raw. Perhaps the same should be done with diphtheria contacts. Teachers and nurses may very properly be prevented from following their usual vocations if they live in infected families. It has been my custom also to exclude from work car conductors, postmen, barbers and department-store clerks. I doubt, however, whether this is always advisable. I am very sure that laborers, mill operatives and office clerks need not, under ordinary circumstances, be kept from their business.

Summary.—As regards the employment of isolation for the prevention of the spread of infectious disease we may fairly conclude:

1. The danger to be apprehended from a single infected person is much less than has been supposed.

2. Isolation is of far less value than was believed a few years ago.

3. The fewer the infected persons in any community or institution the more likely is isolation to be successful. Isolation in an extensive outbreak rarely accomplishes much.

4. The effectiveness of isolation varies inversely as the number of missed cases and carriers.

5. Hospitalization in such diseases as scarlet fever and diphtheria cannot be expected to exterminate them, and the majority of patients can be as well cared for in their homes.

6. In diphtheria, scarlet fever and measles there is rarely, and only in certain occupations, any necessity for interfering with the freedom of the wage earners of the family.

7. The isolation of school children should be more strict than that of adults, for less hardship results, and there is more danger in the mingling of children than in the intercourse of adults.

CHAPTER IV.

INFECTION BY CONTACT.

Most Obvious Mode. — Contact infection is the most obvious mode of transmission of the infectious diseases. For the sick to touch the well, and thus infect them, seems to be the most natural way of accounting for the spread of these diseases. If contact infection can explain epidemiological phenomena, there is no occasion for assuming the growth of pathogenic germs outside of the body, or of infection by fomites or infection by air, or any other similar theory, and no such theory should be adopted as a working hypothesis unless pretty strong evidence can be brought to its support.

Venereal Diseases. — Gonorrhea and syphilis are universally believed to be transmitted exclusively by contact, and almost invariably by a special kind of contact. This idea is so firmly fixed in the minds of medical men and the laity, that no matter how many cases occur which it is impossible to trace to their source, no one ever suggests that these diseases are air-borne, or that their germs maintain a saprophytic life. No matter how much the patient may protest, it will still be held that the infection is due to contact, and in the vast majority of cases to contact involved in the sexual act. Gonorrhea, particularly, is believed to be almost never transmitted except by the most direct contact; yet there is at times as much reason for assuming that the gonococcus is air-borne, or clings to the walls of rooms and thence infects their occupants, as there is to assume the same for scarlet fever. Yet so firmly are we held by tradition that if any of us should suggest such an origin for gonorrhea it would provoke only a smile, while such sources of scarlet fever are accepted as well established.

Gonorrhea in Babies' Hospital. — The spread of gonococcus infection in institutions for children is very suggestive of the ways in which other infections are transmitted.

A very interesting account of institutional infection is given by Holt.[1] At the Babies' Hospital in New York, from 1894 to 1898 inclusive, 64 cases of gonococcus vaginitis were admitted, and 16 cases developed in the hospital. In the summer of 1899, three children suffering from gonococcus vaginitis were inadvertently admitted to the country branch of the hospital, and though the danger was realized, and every effort was made to prevent the extension of the disease, by providing separate nurses for the infected cases, by washing the napkins separately, and boiling and disinfecting them, nevertheless 15 girls contracted vaginitis. In 1901 similar trouble was experienced, and notwithstanding the most vigorous measures of isolation and napkin disinfection, 22 cases developed in the one cottage to which the three original cases were admitted. The physicians were inclined to look upon general house infection as the only explanation of the origin of the cases. In November, 1902, a new hospital building was occupied for the first time, and it was hoped that it could be kept free from the disease, but 5 cases were unwittingly admitted during the first six months, and 29 cases of vaginitis and 8 of gonococcus arthritis developed in the institution. During the year, 13 cases were admitted, and 66 were contracted in the hospital. Although the infected cases were all strictly isolated, on two occasions a child, even in another part of the hospital, developed the disease. For a time napkins were discarded and pads used, which could be burned; separate thermometers, baths and supplies were required for each child; wash cloths were burned, and tub baths forbidden. Bed clothing was disinfected with the greatest care. There was thought to be absolutely no opportunity for direct contact between child and child. When diphtheria or scarlet fever persists in an institution in

[1] Holt, N. York M. J. [etc.], 1905, LXXXI, 521.

such a manner, it is at once attributed to persistent infection of the building itself, and it is suggested by Holt as a possibility in this instance also.

Carried by Nurses. — But the gonococcus is an exceptionally frail organism, and it is impossible to believe that persistent infection of a building or its contents can occur. Actually, in the Babies' Hospital, it was found that the nurse was the carrier of the germs from child to child, and the two cases which developed in distant wards, and which were supposed to be perfectly isolated and under the care of different nurses, were attended by the same night nurse who looked after the infected cases. Finally, when the strictest disinfection had failed to check the disease, it was at last controlled by requiring that the nurses should practice a strict medical asepsis, and disinfect the hands in every instance immediately after bathing or changing the napkins of each child. Here was a disease which continued to spread after the erratic and persistent manner of scarlet fever and diphtheria, and which was shown to depend exclusively upon contact infection. Air-borne infection and fomites infection can have no part in institutional gonococcus infections, for the gonococcus dies so quickly that such modes of transference are impossible. Yet this infection is most persistent and troublesome in many institutions for the care of young children.

Contact not always Direct. — Gonorrheal infection is not only quite common in institutions, but it is often found in infants and young children in their homes. It is believed to result usually from the child sleeping with its parents, or to direct contact with the hands of the mother while washing or dressing the child. I have also known of cases of the direct transfer of the disease on instruments in a physician's office.

It has thus been necessary to modify our conception of the mode of transmission of gonorrhea, and although it is still conceived of as due exclusively to contact infection, it is now recognized that the contact need not always be direct between the sick and the well, but some infected person or thing may act as intermediary. Yet from what is known of the weak resistance of the gonococcus, the interval of time must be brief. The term contact infection as now employed means just that kind of transference of rather fresh infecting material from one to another. It does not necessarily imply actual contact between sick and well, but it does imply that there are no long intervals of time in which the infective materials may become dry and inert. The transfer of gonorrheal pus from child to child on a syringe, or on the fingers of the nurse, are examples of contact infection. If the pillow used by an infected child were put away for a week or two, and when brought out caused ophthalmia in the infant who used it, it would be an example of fomites infection. The distinction between the two types of disease transference, though not sharply or accurately defined, is a reasonable and practical one. Thus every one admits that gonorrhea is frequently transferred by indirect contact infection, as it may be called, but it is never suggested that this disease is spread by fomites.

Syphilis spread solely by Contact. — While it appears to be pretty well determined that *Treponema pallida* is the cause of syphilis, we have as yet no data as to the cultivation of this organism or its persistence outside of the body. Its cultivation outside the body certainly is not easy, and it may be suspected that its life is short; but it is not impossible that the virus may retain its virulence for some days or weeks, as does that of rabies, variola and vaccinia. At present we have to rely solely on clinical evidence as to these points, and the universal opinion of this much studied disease is that the virus develops only in human beings (and some of the apes), that it is not very persistent, and that it is transmitted solely by contact. No one has ever suggested that syphilis is an air-borne disease in the ordinary sense, though one or two cases of droplet infection have been reported.[1]

[1] Buckley, Syphilis in the Innocent, N. Y., 1894, 176.

No matter how obscure may be the origin of cases, no one would attribute them to aerial infection, or to dwelling in an infected house. Infection during the sexual act is undoubtedly the cause of by far the larger proportion of the cases of this disease, yet in the aggregate a great number of cases are caused in other ways.

Non-sexual Contact. — Buckley in the work just quoted shows that probably ten per cent of the initial lesions are extragenital. Exceedingly infectious lesions at times are found in the mouth so that kissing is a not unusual mode of infection. At a party in Philadelphia, where there were kissing games, 8 persons were infected by a young man. One of these was a man who received his infection indirectly on the lips of a girl just previously kissed by the syphilitic.[1] Syphilis is often transmitted by nursing and the sucking of wounds. Mediate contact by all sorts of infected articles is common and Buckley has collected many hundreds of instances. Among the articles named are cups, glasses, spoons and other eating-utensils, pipes, toilet articles, underclothing, bathing suits, handkerchiefs, bedding, pins, string, wind instruments of all kinds, glass blowers' tubes, pencils, coins, nursing-bottles, sponges, syringes, surgeons' instruments, dentists' tools and barbers' utensils. Buckley's book is mainly taken up with an enumeration of these modes of infection. A perusal of these reports is extremely interesting, for though it is not claimed that every case narrated was caused in the manner assumed, yet it is evident that all such modes of transmission are possible, and one is greatly impressed by the vast number of ways in which fresh secretions may be passed from one to another. While the time during which the various articles retained their infection is unknown, or at least is not given in the reports of cases, it is apparent that almost none of the instances of mediate contact were the result of long persistent infection. Fomites infection is not an important

[1] Shamberg, J. Am. M. Ass., Chicago, 1911, LVII, 783.

factor in the spread of syphilis. Buckley[1] says that the danger from soiled clothing, rags, or second-hand garments "is infinitely less than is commonly supposed, and relatively few instances have been recorded, and none of these are very clear or satisfactory." In the few instances which he gives, the infective material might well have been very fresh.

Typhoid Fever by Contact. — Of late years a great deal has been written about the transmission of typhoid fever by contact from case to case, and this mode of infection appears to have attained greater prominence in connection with this than with any other of the common infectious diseases. My attention was first drawn to the importance of contact infection in typhoid fever by the vivid description given by Sedgwick of an outbreak which he investigated in 1892 in Bondville, Massachusetts. He says:[2] "Children abound; and, as there are no fences, and because it is the custom, they mingle freely, playing together and passing from house to house. The families are of that grade in which food always stands upon the table; meals are irregular except for those who must obey the factory bell. The children play awhile, then visit the privies, and with unwashed hands finger the food upon the table. Then they eat awhile and return to play. Or, changing the order of things, they play in the dirt and eat and run to the privy, then eat, play, and eat again, and this in various houses and in various privies. For them, so long as they are friendly, all things are common, — dirt, dinners and privies; and, to illustrate exactly how secondary infection may go on, I may describe in detail one case which I personally witnessed. A whole family (of six or more) was in one room. Four of them had the 'fever.' Two of these were children in the prodromal stage. A table stood by the window covered with food, prominent among which was a big piece of cake. It was early September, and a very warm day; but every window was shut and the odor sickening. Flies innumerable

[1] Buckley, Syphilis in the Innocent, New York, 1894, 156.
[2] Sedgwick, Rep. Bd. Health Mass., Bost., 1892, 736.

buzzed about, resting, now on the sick people, now on the food. A kind-hearted neighbor was tending the baby. By and by one of the children having the fever withdrew to the privy, probably suffering with diarrhea, but soon returning, slouched over to the food, drove away some of the flies, and fingered the cake listlessly, finally breaking off a piece, but not eating it. Stirred by this example, another child slid from his seat in a half-stupid way, moved to the table, and, taking the same cake in both hands, bit off a piece and swallowed it. The first boy had not washed his hands, and if the second boy suffered from secondary infection, I could not wonder at it.

"This was one case; but I have seen so often the table of food standing hours long in the kitchen, and serving as one station in the dirty round of lives like these, that it is easy for me to understand how dirt, diarrhea and dinner too often get sadly confused. The privies had been obviously in bad condition, and, from some, filthy streams ran down between them and the houses. In and around these streams the children played. Given any original imported case, the infection might easily have reached these trickling streams. Children's fingers might thence carry the germs to the food, and thus the journey of the germs from one living intestine to another be completed. Or, again, given in such a community an imported case and no disinfection, as was the condition here at first. The importer, while in the early stages, handles with unclean hands food for others; or the clothing of such a person gets infected and is handled; there need be, then, no difficulty in completing the history. It follows as a matter of course."

Contact Typhoid in Spanish War. — Probably the report of Reed, Vaughan and Shakespeare[1] did more than anything else to call attention to the importance of contact infection in the epidemiology of this disease. This commission found

[1] Abst. of Rep. on the Origin and Spread of Typhoid Fever in U. S. Military Camps during the Spanish War of 1898, Wash., 1900.

that infected water played little part in the development of typhoid fever in the camps. They also found that probably every regiment brought into camp one or more mild unrecognized cases or carriers, and that these were the starting points of outbreaks. It was shown that the fever was not evenly distributed through the regiments, but was more or less localized in companies or squads (p. 111 et seq.).

While they attributed a certain amount of the disease to carriage by flies and by dust, they considered contact infection from man to man the most important cause. Of 1608 cases especially studied, and which were accurately located as to place and time, 35.01 per cent were directly connectible and 27.79 per cent indirectly connectible attacks; total connectible attacks, 62.80 per cent (p. 184). Owing to the unsatisfactory methods, or lack of method, of excreta disposal, the shoes, clothing and hands of the men, as also the blankets and tentage, became more or less soiled with excreta, and infection of the men became easy, and in fact unavoidable. Men detailed as hospital orderlies were, after they had performed the duty of emptying bedpans, seen to go directly to their meals without washing their hands, and even to distribute food to their comrades.

In South Africa. — Similar conclusions were arrived at by the surgeons who studied typhoid fever, which proved equally disastrous to the English, in the Boer War, but on the whole, however, the English, while recognizing the importance of contact infection, did not place so much stress upon it as did the Americans.[1]

Contact Typhoid in Civil Life. — Outbreaks in civil life have of late frequently been attributed largely to contact infection. Winslow[2] reported an outbreak in Newport, R. I., which probably had its origin in an infected well, but which

[1] Col. Lane-Notter, Tr. Epidemiol. Soc., Lond., 1904, XXIII, 149; J. Roy. Army Med. Corps, Lond., 1905, IV, 587, 693; Tooth, Brit. M. J., Lond., 1901, I, 642.

[2] Winslow, Technology Quarterly, 1901, XIV.

was continued by contact infection. He coined the word "prosodemic" to describe this extension of the disease from case to case. Water-borne and milk-borne outbreaks of typhoid fever usually develop suddenly, a large number of cases being reported within a short time. That they do not end so suddenly but, even after the infected water and milk are eliminated, continue, decreasing gradually, is a phenomenon which becomes apparent from the examination of the charts of such outbreaks. This prolongation of the outbreak is due to the prosedemic infection of Winslow, and has been noted by Whipple[1] for water outbreaks, and by Trask[2] for milk outbreaks. During a water-borne outbreak at Lincoln, England, from 50 to 60 per cent of the cases were due to personal contact.[3]

Municipal Outbreaks. — Many local outbreaks have been believed to be due almost, if not quite, exclusively to contact infection. Such an outbreak was reported by Weston and Tarbett in Knoxville,[4] Jordan in Winnipeg,[5] Magrath in Springfield,[6] Noetel in Beuthen,[7] and Weil in Rathsweiler.[8] Freeman[9] states that the majority of the outbreaks in the smaller towns of Virginia appear to be due to contact infection. The authority of Koch has done much to direct attention to the importance of contact infection in the spread of typhoid fever in civil life. In a report on a village outbreak in Trier[10] he says that small country epidemics will usually

[1] Whipple, Typhoid Fever, 1908, 209.

[2] Trask, U. S. Pub. Health and Mar. Hosp. Serv. Hyg. Lab. Bull. No. 41, 38.

[3] Pub. Health, Lond., 1905, XVIII, 129.

[4] Weston and Tarbett, Am. Pub. Health Ass. Rep., 1907, XXXIII, Pt. 1, 63.

[5] Jordan, Abst. in J. Am. M. Ass., Chicago, 1905, XLIV, 563.

[6] Magrath, Am. J. Pub. Hyg., Bost., 1905, I, 467.

[7] Noetel, Ztschr. f. Hyg. u. Infectionskrankh., Leipz., 1904, XLVII, 211.

[8] Weil, Med. News, N. Y., 1904, LXXXIV, 467.

[9] Freeman, J. Am. M. Ass., Chicago, 1909, LIII, 1263.

[10] Koch, Die Bekämpfung des Typhus, Berlin, 1903.

be found to be due to this mode of infection. In the particular outbreak investigated all the cases were found to be due to contact, that is, to the direct transfer from person to person, and the source was in most instances unrecognized mild cases, often in children. He then describes conditions very much like those reported by Sedgwick. Fecal matter was observed in the dooryards where it could readily infect the children playing about, and would certainly be carried indoors on their shoes.

Fulton,[1] Egbert [2] and others have shown that typhoid fever prevails far more extensively in the country than in the city. Formerly, when less was known about the etiology of the disease, polluted well water was believed to be the chief factor in its causation, but it now appears that it is far more likely to depend on contact infection.

In Hospitals. — Typhoid fever frequently develops in hospitals and other institutions, presumably by contact infection. Occasionally explosive outbreaks due to infected milk or food are observed, but many institutional outbreaks are characterized by a slow and irregular development of cases. The disease chiefly attacks those who are brought in close contact with the sick, physicians and especially nurses. Fifty or sixty years ago few cases of hospital infection were recorded. It is suggested that this may have been due to the fact that nurses in those days were usually women well along in years, and therefore not so susceptible to the disease, and usually immune. During recent years typhoid fever among nurses and ward tenders has been quite common. It is stated that in 1902–6, of an annual average of 322 nurses in six hospitals, 26 contracted typhoid fever and 12 of an average of 94 ward tenders contracted typhoid fever while on duty. It is said that in the London hospitals typhoid fever is twenty times as common

[1] Fulton, J. Am. M. Ass., Chicago, 1904, XLII, 73.

[2] Egbert, Am. Med., Phila., 1905, IX, 649.

[3] Joslin and Overlander, Boston M. & S. J., 1907, CLVII, 428.

among nurses as among women of the same ages in other occupations.[1] Goodall[2] says that during the years 1892–1899 there were treated in the London hospitals 5913 typhoid patients, and 100 attendants contracted the disease. In four hospitals not admitting typhoid fever no cases developed. Schuder,[3] Neufeld,[4] McCrae,[5] Talayrach,[6] Edsall[7] and others have reported an excessive prevalence of typhoid fever among the attendants on cases of this disease in hospitals, and they have also noticed numerous instances in which it has developed among other patients. Nurses and others infect their hands while caring for typhoid patients, and then without washing the hands, or after careless washing, infect their own mouths directly, or by handling their food and drink. Through the same carelessness they also infect other patients. Neufeld refers to the transfer of the germs on a thermometer and in a bath. Edsall has seen a nurse given the double duty of emptying the bedpans of typhoid cases and preparing special diet, and a patient was observed to empty a bedpan and then proceed to his dinner without washing his hands. Nurses also wipe out the mouths of patients with a bit of gauze on the finger, a procedure which was believed by Holt to be one of the means of spreading gonorrheal infection in the Babies' Hospital. By introducing strict cleanliness Edsall was able to stop this transference of the disease.

In Other Institutions. — Sometimes quite marked outbreaks occur in institutions, due presumably to contact infection. Usually water, milk and other food as sources of infection can be excluded, and the irregular and slow development of the cases, and perhaps the discovery of carriers or

[1] Pub. Health, Lond., 1905, XVIII, 142.
[2] Goodall, Trans. Epidem. Soc., Lond., 1900.
[3] Schuder, Ztschr. f. Hyg. u. Infectionskrankh., Leipz., XXXVIII, 251.
[4] Neufeld, Kolle u. Wassermann, Handbuch [etc.], Jena, 1903, II, 296.
[5] McCrae, Mod. Med. [Osler], Phila. & N. Y., 1907, II, 82.
[6] Talayrach, Arch. d. méd. et de pharm. milit., Par., 1903, XLII, 393.
[7] Edsall, Am. J. M. Sc., Phila., 1908, n. s., CXXXV, 469.

missed cases, renders the extension of the disease by personal contact highly probable. In an almshouse in New Haven,[1] 37 cases occurred during a period of some months. Mild cases were concealed and worked in the kitchen, and it was impossible to teach the inmates cleanly habits. At a soldiers' home at Lafayette, Indiana, there were 65 cases due to contact infection, probably chiefly from the physician.[2] At the State Hospital for the Insane at Trenton there occurred between April 8 and August 13, 1907, 80 cases with 16 deaths, due in all probability to contact infection, largely in the kitchen and pantry.[3] Ravenel[4] reports an outbreak in a boarding house at the University of Wisconsin, where 41 cases developed, probably as the result of a patient working in the pantry during the prodromal period of his illness. Sedgwick[5] reports the case of a chambermaid, and also of a laundress, who contracted typhoid fever from handling soiled linen. A waitress, also, who ate bread cut by the other two, developed the disease. Wolcott tells of the matron of a hospital who caught the disease from handling infected bedding and neglecting to wash the hands. McCrae[6] reports an instance of infection from careless handling of typhoid cultures in the laboratory, and a similar case occurred in an insane asylum at Northampton, Mass.[7] Dr. Mann tells me that a number of nurses eating at the same table in the Homeopathic Hospital in Boston contracted typhoid fever, probably from a waitress whose sister was sick with the disease, and who herself was perhaps a carrier.

[1] Rep. Bd. Health, New Haven, 1905, 6.

[2] Hurty, J. Am. M. Ass., Chicago, 1909, LIII, 1263.

[3] Rep. St. Bd. Health, New Jersey, 1907, 149.

[4] Ravenel and Smith, K. W., J. Am. M. Ass., Chicago, 1909, LII, 1635.

[5] Sedgwick, J. Mass. Ass. Bds. Health, Bost., 1900, X, 148.

[6] McCrae, Mod. Med. [Osler], Phila. & N. Y., 1907, II, 82.

[7] Rep. Bd. Health, Mass., Bost., 1899, 762.

Contact on Shipboard. — Many of the instances of infection by carriers referred to in Chapter II were almost certainly the result of contact infection, and many more could be easily collected. Occasionally small outbreaks occur on shipboard, where it is possible to exclude all modes of infection but contact. Thus, 9 cases on an Atlantic liner were traced to a saloon steward.[1] On the United States ship *Connecticut* there were three outbreaks in 1907, almost certainly due to contact infection.[2]

In the Family. — During 1908 I noted three small outbreaks of typhoid fever in Providence, due apparently to contact infection. In one instance there were 10 cases in three closely related families, in another 8 cases in three such families, and in the third outbreak there were 7 cases in two families. Such family outbreaks are noticed in Providence nearly every year, and they are referred to so often in current medical literature that it does not seem necessary to give additional references. Contact outbreaks in hotels and boarding houses, as well as in various public institutions, are also frequently reported. Hill in Birmingham, in 1898, traced 10 per cent of the typhoid-fever cases to contact with other cases. In Manchester in the same year about 13 per cent were traced in the same way, and in 1906, 36.8 per cent. Edsall attributed 27 per cent of 250 cases to contact, and Forster 117 of 386 cases, and McCrae 68 of 500 cases. It would be easy to prolong the discussion and show that medical men are everywhere attributing more and more importance to contact infection in this disease. It is to be noted that in few of the reported instances of contact infection is there any direct and conclusive proof that the disease was caused in the manner alleged. The evidence is by no means so convincing as to mode of infection as it is in so many water-borne and milk-borne outbreaks, and from the nature of things it rarely can be so.

[1] Rep. Med. Off. Health, Glasgow, 1907, 147.
[2] McDonnold, Mil. Surgeon, Carlisle, Pa., 1908, XXIII, 29.

Evidence of Contact Infection. — But when water and food as vehicles of infection are excluded, when the disease develops in persons who are in contact with the sick or with carriers, and when the fingers, possibly or perhaps evidently soiled with excreta, are seen to touch food, eating-utensils, and sometimes the lips, the probability of the development of the disease in this manner is so evident that observers are constantly seeing in contact infection the cause of family, institutional and community outbreaks of this disease. The importance now attributed to contact infection is the result of a careful estimate of probabilities.

Amount of Contact Infection. — In 1908 there were 11,375 deaths from typhoid fever in the registration area of the United States, which doubtless means considerably over 100,000 cases. The registration area includes about one-half the population of the country. While a certain amount of typhoid fever is caused by milk, it must be a very small fraction of the great total. As will be shown, milk outbreaks are usually well marked, and probably not a very great deal of milk-borne infection escapes notice. Again, while in some cities the larger part of the typhoid fever is due to infected water, it is not so in most cities, and certainly only a small part of the total typhoid fever in the country can be traced to such a source. It is not likely in my own city for instance that more than 20 per cent of the 4300 cases of typhoid fever during the past twenty-five years have been due to infected water or milk; and infected oysters, celery, etc., certainly play a very unimportant part in the causation of the disease. As we shall see, it is improbable that air-borne infection or dust infection is of any moment in civil life. The only other important source of typhoid fever which has been suggested is fly-borne infection. It will be shown also that infection by means of flies probably accounts for only a small part of our typhoid fever. By exclusion, then, we are led to the conclusion that contact infection is the chief source of our typhoid fever.

Why should we not, in the absence of direct evidence as to other modes of infection, assume at once that contact, that is, the more or less direct transfer of infective material from person to person, is the principal source of contagious disease? Why neglect the most obvious and direct mode of transfer in favor of more circuitous paths? There are several reasons why contact infection in this disease has been neglected.

Why Contact Infection has been Neglected. — One reason has been the undue emphasis laid upon other modes of transmission. Formerly air infection was considered of great moment, and as this fell into disrepute, undue weight was attached to water and milk infection, partly, no doubt, because of the dramatic character of so many outbreaks. Another reason for doubting the importance of contact infection is the prevalent notion that typhoid fever is essentially an intestinal disease, and that it must be caused by infected food. It now appears that typhoid fever is not an intestinal disease, and in some cases the intestines are not involved and the feces are free from bacilli during the whole sickness. But the bacilli are found in the blood stream in the earliest stages, and it seems to be more likely that they enter the circulation through the upper part of the alimentary tract than through the intestines after running the gauntlet of the gastric secretions. Even if it be denied that the tonsils and stomach are the portals of entry of the typhoid bacilli, it is highly probable that bacilli taken into the mouth in small masses find their way to the lower part of the alimentary tract by means of the small quantities of saliva which are constantly swallowed. It has certainly been demonstrated that tubercle bacilli are swallowed and thus reach the intestines.

People are not Cleanly. — Then, too, contact infection in typhoid fever supposes an intimacy with the most offensive substances, which most persons would vehemently deny. Nevertheless it appears that the fingers of human beings, and secondarily everything that the fingers touch, are frequently contaminated with excremental matter. The colon bacillus is for all practical purposes a good test for the presence of excrement, and it is somewhat of a shock to learn that it is found on the hands of five to ten per cent of ordinarily cleanly people. Winslow[1] and Hall,[2] while studying the dissemination of typhoid fever by carriers, recovered fecal bacteria from the finger nails and hands after the usual procedures following the use of the closet and toilet. An inspection of the privies or water-closets in railway stations, factories, shops and tenement houses shows that they usually present evidence of contamination with feces and urine, and in many instances are constantly in a horribly filthy condition. It is only in the better class of hotels and residences that these apartments are kept in even an apparently cleanly condition, and this is only by dint of constant vigilance and frequent cleansing. There can be no doubt that even very careful people frequently infect the seat, their fingers, the pull, the door, etc., and that in a large proportion of privies and water-closets the users almost certainly infect their fingers with at least traces of their own or others' excremental matter. Yet how many persons are there who invariably wash the hands after the use of a closet? How many make it a rule never to put the fingers in the mouth? Yesterday I saw a workman carrying a can of beer to his friends. His thumb was immersed a couple of inches in the beverage. Had he washed his hands after leaving the barroom water-closet? At a recent sanitary convention I noticed the colored waiter stick his finger into a glass which he, however, did not remove, and which the speaker soon drank from. What was the recent history of that finger? Does the fruit peddler wash his hands after using the tenement privy before he ventures to sort his fruit? Do the waitress, the milk peddler, the candy seller, the Pullman porter, the soda-water clerk, the baker's boy, the delicatessen man *always* wash the hands before taking

[1] Winslow, J. Mass. Ass. Bds. Health, Bost., 1903, XIII, 144.
[2] Hall, Rep. Med. Off. Health, Bristol, Eng.. 1908, 27.

up their work? Are the toilets in their places of business so cleanly that such a precaution is not necessary? However shocking it may seem, it is certain that it requires only a little observation to demonstrate that the path from intestines to mouth is not always a circuitous one.

Contact with Carriers. — Until recently it would have been argued that contact infection is not an important factor in typhoid fever because only a small proportion of the cases can be shown to have been in contact with this disease, and because the large proportion of cases of this fever are more or less isolated in their homes because of the sickness. But we now know that there are vast numbers of mild unrecognized cases, and most important of all, that the number of carriers is very great. There are doubtless 200,000 cases of this disease in the United States each year. If only 3 per cent of these become chronic carriers, and if a carrier remains such only three years, we should have a carrier population of 18,000 persons, practically all unknown and taking no precautions against infecting others. If we add to these the 25 per cent of convalescents, who for some weeks are excreting the bacilli in their urine, it appears that there is a very respectable army of unrecognized sources of typhoid infection.

At present we have no definite knowledge of the origin of the larger number of our cases of typhoid fever. In view of the almost universal careless habits of the people, and the great number of carriers, why not adopt as a working hypothesis the most obvious source of infection, infection by contact?

Danger from Privies. — This view that contact infection is the most important factor in the causation of this disease, is borne out by the observation that the more promptly and effectively human excrement is disposed of, the less chance there is for contact infection and the less the disease prevails. When the disposal is exceptionally bad, as in army camps, lumber, mining and railroad camps, then this disease is almost always very common. In thoroughly sewered and clean cities, provided the water and milk are not contaminated, typhoid fever is comparatively rare. The privy vault stores up fecal matter on the premises and is rarely kept as clean as a water-closet, and the area around privies is often filthy also. It has often been noted that the removal of privy vaults has been followed by a decrease in typhoid fever. In Providence the disease fell off forty per cent after most of the privy vaults were abolished. Many other American cities in which typhoid fever is not maintained by a polluted water supply, show a steadily decreasing prevalence of this disease as privy vaults are gotten rid of. In England Pringle[1] has shown that in fourteen towns with middens the typhoid rate was 0.25 per 1000, while in fourteen water-closet towns it was 0.19. In Ipswich there was a marked decrease in typhoid fever following the removal of the middens.[2] A similar decrease was noted in Oldham, Leicester[3] and other cities. On the other hand more "pail closets" remain in Nottingham than in most English cities, and to this Boobbyer[4] attributes the fact that typhoid fever has decreased less in that town than in the other great towns of England. Like reports of a decrease in the disease following removal of privies come from such widely separated places as Winnipeg[5] and Melbourne.[6]

There are also numerous reports to the effect that in the same town typhoid fever is much more common in houses without water-closets than in those with them. This may be due in part to the storing of fecal matter on the premises of the former, and it may be due also to the fact that houses with privies are usually of a poorer class, and the inhabitants less cleanly in their personal habits, or to other reasons; but

[1] Pringle, Pub. Health, Lond., 1902–03, XV, 630.
[2] Pub. Health, Lond., 1908–09, XXII, 414.
[3] Rep. Med. Off. Health, Leicester, Eng., 1908, 29.
[4] Boobbyer, Rep. Health of Nottingham, 1908, 53.
[5] Rep. Dept. Pub. Health, Winnipeg, 1908, 4.
[6] Jamieson, J., Australas. M. Gaz., Sydney, 1903, XXII, 56.

these facts of typhoid distribution accord with the view that the disease is largely spread by contact from person to person. In Birmingham,[1] the incidence of typhoid fever in "pail" and water-closet houses was as 65 to 43, and there has been a steady decrease in the disease as the "pail closets" have been abolished. In Nottingham there was (in ten years) 1 case in each 37 houses with privies, and 1 in each 558 water-closet houses; in Salford it was 1 to 20 and 1 to 42 respectively,[2] and in Gorton the cases were two or three times as numerous in privy houses as in water-closet houses.[3] At Leigh,[4] typhoid fever was four times as prevalent among colliery workers as among the rest of the population, owing, in the opinion of the inspector, to the filthy mode of excreta disposal in the mines. In Glasgow[5] secondary cases of the disease developed in 23 per cent of the cases in houses with privies and in 6 per cent of the cases in houses with water-closets.

Every one who has had practical experience in sanitary inspection work knows that privy vaults not only serve as storehouses for excrement, but their presence encourages its careless disposal in the yards and on ash heaps. The filthy condition of the ground about the houses, leading to contamination of feet and hands of children, as reported by Sedgwick and by Koch, is rarely noticed on premises provided with water-closets. It may be urged that the excess of typhoid fever in privy towns is due to infection by flies rather than infection by contact, and this may be true to some extent; but if flies were the chief factor we should scarcely expect a great difference between water-closet and privy houses in the same town. So also the infection of miners, as noticed

[1] Rep. Health of Birmingham, 1906, 49, and 1908, 49.

[2] Pringle, Pub. Health, Lond., 1902–03, XV, 630.

[3] Martin, Pub. Health, Lond., 1904–05, XVII, 709.

[4] Sweeting, Rep. Med. Off. Local Gov. Bd., Lond., 1907–08, XXXVII, 57.

[5] Rep. Med. Off. Health, Glasgow, 1902, 97.

by Sweeting, cannot be due to flies. In Providence after the removal of privies the decrease in typhoid fever was as great in winter, when there were no flies, as during the fly season.

Amebic Dysentery. — There is no reason why amebic dysentery may not be transmitted by personal contact, but if, as is generally believed, the ameba is quite widely distributed in the soil, it is likely that in countries where the disease is endemic, man is the least common source of infection. Nevertheless cases do develop from contact with other cases. Lemoine[1] has reported such infections in France, in one instance at least, probably due to the use of the same bedpan, douche, etc. The infecting case was a carrier of ten years' standing. Allan[2] writes that in Charlotte, N. C., he observed four cases of amebic dysentery which he believed were due to contact with chronic carriers.

Bacillary Dysentery. — Bacillary dysentery, like typhoid fever, is a great scourge of military life, and outbreaks of a serious character are not rare in institutions such as hospitals for the insane. The bacillus is found in the feces of the patients and also in convalescents. There is every reason for believing that this disease, like typhoid fever, is frequently spread by more or less direct contact.[3] Conradi[4] described a village outbreak near Metz where 70 cases occurred during a period of three months. Several carriers were found in infected families, and conditions favoring contact infection were noted, very similar to those observed in the outbreaks of typhoid fever studied by Koch in Trier. Dodge[5] reports the case of a laboratory worker who got some of a culture of the dysentery bacillus in his eye; the tears ran profusely and were swallowed, and in twenty-four hours an attack of

[1] Lemoine, Bull. et mém. Soc. méd. de hôp. de Par., 1908, 3 s., XXV, 640.

[2] Allan, Med. Rec., N. Y., 1910, LXXVII, 63.

[3] Shiga, Mod. Med. [Osler], Phila. & N. Y., 1907, II, 781; Scheube, Diseases of Warm Climates, 2d Ed., Phila., 466.

[4] Festschrift von Robert Koch, 1903, 555.

[5] Dodge, Am. Pub. Health Ass. Rep., 1905, XXX, 310.

dysentery developed. An outbreak of 49 cases, developing in the characteristic slow irregular manner of contact outbreaks, was reported in the Connecticut Hospital for the Insane.[1] Kruse[2] reports a similar outbreak in Germany, and two in Holland. Epidemic dysentery is quite common in hospitals for the insane, and its prevalence is explained as due chiefly to contact infection, for the carelessness of many patients and the impossibility of controlling their habits offer every opportunity for this sort of diffusion.[3]

Cholera and Contact. — If typhoid fever and dysentery are spread by means of contact infection, we should expect that cholera would be. That less is written about it is due probably to the fact that in recent years less attention has been paid to cholera than to the more common diseases. The literature relating to typhoid fever has of late been many times more voluminous than that relating to cholera. Nevertheless most writers attribute some importance to contact infection in this disease, and some consider it an etiological factor of very great importance. The filthy conditions of village life described by Sedgwick in America and Koch in Germany as giving rise to typhoid fever, are far surpassed in danger by the habits of vast numbers of the poorer people who dwell in cholera-infested countries. The opportunities for the direct transference of fecal matter from person to person are far greater in Asiatic countries than they are with us, and a number of writers have emphasized the part played by personal contagion in this disease. Gotschlich [4] refers to

[1] Rep. St. Bd. Health, Connect., 1903, 234.

[2] Kruse, Deutsche med. Wchnschr., 1901, XXVII, 370, 386.

[3] See Reports of Commissioners in Lunacy (Eng.) since 1903; also Heuser, Deutsche med. Wchnschr., 1909, XXXV, 1694; Ryder, Boston M. & S. J., 1909, CLXI, 681; Haenisch, Ztschr. f. Hyg. u. Infectionskrankh., Leipz., 1908, LX, 245; Mott, Tr. Epidem. Soc., Lond., 1901–02, and Arch. Neurol. Path. Lab., Lond. Co. Asyl., Lond., 1903, II, 735; Prior, Australas. M. Cong. Tr., Victoria, 1909, III, 383.

[4] Gotschlich, Kolle and Wassermann, Handbuch [etc.], Jena, 1904, IV, 108.

this factor, and a number of our officers in the Philippines have dwelt upon its importance. Woodruff [1] says that while infected water played some part in the great epidemic in Manila, the filthy habits of the people were the chief cause of the extension of the disease. He speaks of an outbreak of eighty cases in a provincial town due to food prepared in Manila by a caterer who soon died of cholera. Heiser [2] considers that the handling of foodstuffs and of the leaves in which the betel nut is wrapped, by dealers and prospective purchasers, is one of the chief ways in which cholera is spread, and McLaughlin [3] considers the "carrier" with filthy habits the greatest source of danger. He says that contact infection of visitors in the houses of the sick is a common means of disseminating the disease. Schumburg [4] reported several small outbreaks of cholera near Hamburg caused by contact infection. Shakespeare [5] reports several instances in which cholera was apparently caused by handling soiled linen, some of which might perhaps be considered rather as examples of fomites infection. Macrae [6] reports the infection of hospital nurses with cholera in a manner similar to the infection of nurses with typhoid fever. Heiser [7] says that in the Philippines, physicians and nurses who had been trained to aseptic methods did not contract cholera but untrained attendants frequently did through contact with patients.

Diarrhea. — Newsholme [8] believes that much infantile diarrhea is due to direct contact infection in the home, and he suggests that it is brought about by "sucking infective

[1] Woodruff, J. Am. M. Ass., Chicago, 1905, XLV, 1160.

[2] Heiser, J. Am. M. Ass., Chicago, 1907, XLVIII, 856.

[3] McLaughlin, J. Am. M. Ass., Chicago, 1909, LII, 1153.

[4] Schumburg, Ztschr. f. ärztl. Fortbild., Jena, 1905, II, 567.

[5] Shakespeare, Rep. on Cholera in Europe and India, U. S. Gov. Printing Office, 1890, 81.

[6] Macrae, Indian M. Gaz., 1909, XLIV, 361.

[7] Heiser, Bull. State Bd. Health, N. Y., Sept., 1911.

[8] Newsholme, J. Hyg., Cambridge, 1906, VI, 139.

matter from dirty fingers, from dummy teats and in other ways." Naish[1] and Niven[2] are largely in accord with this view. Sandilands,[3] in an extended article, cites others as reporting hospital and laboratory infection as well as evidence from house and neighborhood outbreaks. From his own study of multiple cases in houses, and of local distribution, he is convinced that contact plays an important part in the causation of this disease. Doubtless the most complete epidemiological study of summer diarrhea has been made by Peters,[4] and it should be read by every one interested in the subject. Flies are considered as possible carriers of infection, and while no evidence against this theory is found, much positive evidence is presented to show that contact infection is an important factor in the causation of this disease.

Hook Worm Disease. — The European type of the disease is caused by *Anchylostoma duodenalis*, while the American type is due to a slightly different species, *Uncinaria americana*.[5] The symptoms are caused by the growth of the worms, which are about half an inch long, in the intestine, where they fasten themselves to the intestinal wall, and not only suck blood themselves, but also cause considerable free bleeding from the wounds which they make. The eggs, which are laid in the intestine, do not there develop, owing to lack of oxygen, but hatch soon after the feces are voided, and the young worms then pass through several stages of growth in moist earth or mud.

Until recently it was believed that human infection resulted from drinking water containing the young worms, or by get-

[1] Naish, Pub. Health, Lond., 1909–10, XXIII, 168.

[2] Niven, Proc. Roy. Soc. Med., Lond., 1909–10, III, Epidemiol. Sect., 131.

[3] Sandilands, Proc. Roy. Soc. Med., Lond., 1909–10, III, Epidemiol. Sect., 95.

[4] Peters, J. Hyg., Cambridge, 1910, X, 602.

[5] Stiles, U. S. Pub. Health and Mar. Hosp. Serv. Hyg. Lab. Bull. No. 10, 1903.

ting them onto fingers or into food, and so into the mouth. It was first suggested by Looss in 1898 that infection might take place through the skin, and he believed that he had himself become infected in that way. In 1901 he proved the correctness of his surmises by experiments. Later Grassi, Pieri and Noe placed a few drops of water containing worms upon the skin, but only one of the three became infected. In 1902 Looss successfully repeated his experiments. It had meantime been noticed by Bentley and Boycott and Haldane that dermatitis was apt to be found in regions where the disease prevailed, and it was suspected that it might be due to the passage of the worms through the skin. Smith[1] showed that by placing infected earth on the arm, not only was infection caused, but there resulted a dermatitis at the site of the application. Ashford, whose careful study of the disease in Porto Rico, and whose brilliant success in curing its victims give his opinion great weight, believes that the skin is by far the most important avenue by which the worms infect the body.[2] Uncinariasis is, then, *par excellence*, a disease due to contact infection.

Fortunately the disease is usually easily curable under medical treatment, and the freeing of individuals from worms by this treatment is necessarily an important part of the prevention of the disease. It is evident from the mode of infection that the pollution of the soil with human feces is the principal factor in the spread of the disease. Properly constructed privies or water-closets, with the ultimate disposal of the fecal matter by deep burial, or some other means to prevent the pollution of the upper layers of the soil, are the essentials of prophylaxis.

Contact Infection less Easy in Some Diseases than in Others. — Gonorrhea is a disease in which the infecting secretion is not likely to be much handled, and when it occurs

[1] Smith, C. A., J. Am. M. Ass., Chicago, 1905, XLV, 1142.

[2] Ashford, Rep. of Commission on Study and Treatment of "Anemia" in Porto Rico, 1904, 37.

in young children the secretion is often received on a diaper. Yet it has been shown in the preceding pages that infantile gonorrhea is spread exclusively by contact infection. Although the children themselves take little part in the spread of the disease in hospitals where they are isolated from one another, and although nurses and physicians have been shown the danger of carrying the disease, and have been instructed to take the greatest precautions, yet this disease may be maintained for months in an institution solely by means of infection borne on thermometers, syringes, etc., but particularly on the hands of attendants.

In typhoid fever the bacilli are contained in the feces and urine, which even careless people are supposed to avoid touching. Nevertheless it appears that the fingers of careful people, and even of trained nurses, are infected in this manner, and that transfer to the mouth with the subsequent development of typhoid fever results. There is much evidence that this mode of transference is an important, if not the most important, factor in the spread of this disease.

Contact with Saliva. — If contact infection is important in such diseases as gonorrhea, typhoid fever, dysentery and cholera, in which the infecting material is not constantly at hand, and is usually strenuously avoided, how much more important must this mode of transference be in diseases in which the specific germs are found in the secretions of the nose and mouth or in the sputum.

Danger from Fingers. — Probably the chief vehicle for the conveyance of nasal and oral secretion from one to another is the fingers. If one takes the trouble to watch for a short time his neighbors, or even himself, unless he has been particularly trained in such matters, he will be surprised to note the number of times that the fingers go to the mouth and the nose. Not only is the saliva made use of for a great variety of purposes, and numberless articles are for one reason or another placed in the mouth, but for no reason whatever, and all unconsciously, the fingers are with great frequency raised to the lips or the nose. Who can doubt that if the salivary glands secreted indigo the fingers would continually be stained a deep blue, and who can doubt that if the nasal and oral secretions contain the germs of disease these germs will be almost as constantly found upon the fingers? All successful commerce is reciprocal, and in this universal trade in human saliva the fingers not only bring foreign secretions to the mouth of their owner, but there exchanging them for his own, distribute the latter to everything that the hand touches. This happens not once but scores and hundreds of times during the day's round of the individual. The cook spreads his saliva on the muffins and rolls, the waitress infects the glasses and spoons, the moistened fingers of the peddler arrange his fruit, the thumb of the milkman is in his measure, the reader moistens the pages of his book, the conductor his transfer tickets, the "lady" the fingers of her glove. Every one is busily engaged in this distribution of saliva, so that the end of each day finds this secretion freely distributed on the doors, window sills, furniture and playthings in the home, the straps of trolley cars, the rails and counter and desks of shops and public buildings, and indeed upon everything that the hands of man touch. What avails it if the pathogens do die quickly? A fresh supply is furnished each day.

Drinking Cups. — Another important vehicle of transfer must be the common drinking cup. Davison[1] estimated that there were as many as 20,000 epithelial cells on a drinking glass that had been in use in a school for nine days, which well illustrates the amount of infection which may be thus carried. Cars, steamboats, hotels, schools, offices, factories, theaters, churches, all provide a common vessel from which large numbers of persons drink, thus furnishing an almost ideal method by which perfectly fresh saliva may be transferred from one to another. Hundreds of thousands of persons must be each day in this manner exchanging the

[1] Davison, Tech. World Mag., Chicago, 1908, IX, 623.

secretions of the mouth. When traveling in the steam cars I have noted the shocked expression on the face of passengers as a fashionably dressed woman was seen to allow her pug dog to drink from the common glass, — not a pleasant thing, of course, but infinitely less dangerous than for the woman to drink from it. She might have tuberculosis, or carry diphtheria bacilli, or perhaps even have mucous patches on her lips.

Other Kinds of Contact. — Besides the moistening of the fingers with saliva and the use of the common drinking cup, the mouth is put to numberless improper uses which may result in the spread of infection. It is used to hold pins, string, pencils, paper and money. The lips are used to moisten the pencil, to point the thread for the needle, to wet postage stamps and envelopes. Children "swap" apples, cake and lollipops, while men exchange their pipes and women hatpins. Sometimes the mother is seen "cleansing" the face of her child with her saliva-moistened handkerchief, and perhaps the visitor is shortly after invited to kiss the little one.

Children have no instinct of cleanliness, and their faces, hands, toys, clothing and everything that they touch must of necessity be continually daubed with the secretions of the nose and mouth. It is well known that between the ages of two and eight years children are more susceptible to scarlet fever, diphtheria, measles and whooping cough than at other ages, and it may be that one reason for this is the great opportunity that is afforded by their habits at these ages for the transfer of the secretions. Infants do not of course mingle freely with one another, and older children do not come in such close contact in their play, and they also begin to have a little idea of cleanliness.

Contact Dangerous because of Missed Cases. — A little observation and reflection will show that the ways are numberless in which fresh secretion of nose and mouth is passed from person to person. Enough has been written to demonstrate that the opportunities for contact infection are sufficiently numerous to account for the spread of the contagious diseases without invoking any other mechanism. The chief objection to this view is that while it is true that there is much interchange of secretions, it is between well persons, and not between the sick and the well. That this objection is untenable is amply demonstrated by the evidence presented in Chapter II. There can no longer be the slightest doubt that there are large numbers of mild and unrecognized cases of infectious disease mingling freely with the public, and that in some diseases, and perhaps in most, there are also larger numbers of perfectly well carriers who also are unknown. These unrecognized foci are clearly numerous enough to cause, by their contact with others, the recognized *cases.* The transfer of the disease by fairly direct means is so obvious and easy that there is no necessity for invoking the agency of other and more circuitous modes of dissemination. Indeed it is sometimes said that the arguments here presented prove too much, and that if carriers were as numerous, and contact with them as frequent, as is here alleged, none could escape. But, as was stated in Chapter II and on page 153, infection does not take place so readily as is generally believed. This is demonstrated clinically, and the reasons are apparent. There are often long intervals in which carriers are not eliminating the pathogenic organism, and the saliva may not contain the germs, even when they are in the throat and nose. Germs are not evenly distributed through saliva, sputum or feces, and the particle transferred may be free from them. The infective material is often small in amount and spread in a thin layer, and the contained organisms very speedily die. Lastly, small numbers of pathogens are often, perhaps usually, destroyed by the body. We must believe that *usually* continued or somewhat massive infection is necessary to cause disease, but that nevertheless *sometimes* a single infection with a very small number of germs suffices. The number of unrecognized foci of infection in human beings, the opportunities for contact infection, and the natural obstacles to successful infection, appear admirably to explain many otherwise inexplicable phenomena of epidemiology.

Bacteria on the Hands. — Reference has already been made to this on page 179. Neumann,[1] by finding fecal bacilli on water-closet fixtures, showed how the hands are infected, and he also showed[2] how by another transfer on the hands they may infect bread, rolls, fruit, butter and milk. Colon bacilli have also been found on 3 of 12 roller towels.[3] Pus-forming organisms have their natural habitat on the skin, and the work of the surgeons has shown the tremendous importance of contact infection, which they have now learned most successfully to avoid.

Danger from the Shuttle. — As weavers habitually thread the shuttle by sucking the yarn through the eye, mouth bacteria may in this way be transferred from one to another. This has been alleged as a mode of infection in tuberculosis, and indeed Brown[4] claims to have traced three cases to this.

Bacteria on Cups, Pencils. — Vincenzi found diphtheria bacilli in the holy water in a church font. Kinyoun[6] found them in 2 of 85 swabbings from the woodwork and drinking glass of a railway car. They have also been found on glasses and cups by Albert and Boyd,[7] Perrow,[8] and in Chicago.[9] Forbes, in Rochester, found them upon a drinking glass which was believed to have been the cause of an outbreak. This has been frequently referred to, and though I

[1] Arch. f. Hyg., München. u. Leipz., LIX, 174.

[2] Neumann, Deutsche med. Wchnschr., Leipz. u. Berl., 1910, XXXVI, 2046.

[3] Bull. Mass. State Bd. Health, Nov., 1911.

[4] Brown, Med. Officer, 1911, IV, 27.

[5] Vincenzi, Semaine méd., 1898.

[6] Kinyoun, Med. News, N. Y., 1905, LXXXVII, 193.

[7] Albert and Boyd, Bull. State Bd. Health, Ia., Oct.–Dec., 1911, 37.

[8] Perrow, Rep. Health Dept., Lynchburg, Va., Sept., 1911.

[9] Bull. Dept. Health, Chicago, April 22, 1911.

have not been able to find Forbes' original article, Dr. Goler, the present health officer of Rochester, informs me that the facts are as reported. Williams[1] recovered diphtheria bacilli from pencils moistened by the lips of children sick with the disease. The observations referred to in the chapter on fomites show that the germs of this disease are rarely found on fomites and then only on objects that have been recently and grossly infected.

Tubercle Bacilli in Mouth.—Not only are tubercle bacilli found in enormous masses in the true sputum, but they are often present in the saliva as well. Neild and Dunkley[2] found them in saliva from the tip of the tongue in 29 of 50 cases of pulmonary tuberculosis. Park found them in the saliva of 10 of 15 cases,[3] and refers to Möller recovering them in 3 of 20 cases. Le Noir and Camus[4] found virulent tubercle bacilli in the nose as well as from the mouth of tuberculous cases.

Pathogenic Bacteria on the Hands.—With the present habits of human beings these germs must be constantly transferred to the fingers, and to a lesser degree to everything that the fingers touch. Graziani[5] found tubercle bacilli on the hands of 4 of 8 tuberculous patients, and on 3 of them 3 hours after washing with soap and water. He also obtained the bacilli from the hands of 4 out of 6 non-tuberculous patients. After shaking hands with tuberculous patients he was able several times to recover the bacilli from his own hands. Baldwin[6] found bacilli on the hands of patients in the Adirondack Sanatorium. They did not use handkerchiefs. Of 10 patients seen in private practice 8 had tubercle

1 Williams, Scientific Bull. 2, 1895, Health Dept., N. Y. City, 14.

2 Neild and Dunkley, Lancet, Lond., 1909, I, 1096.

3 Park, Sixth Internat. Cong. on Tuberc., Wash., 1908, I, 157.

4 Le Noir and Camus, Comp. rend. Soc. de biol., Par., 1908, LXV, 464.

5 Graziani, Ann d' Ig. Sper., XV, 709, referred to by Rosenau, Sixth Internat. Cong. on Tuberc., Wash., 1908, I, 28.

6 Baldwin, Tr. Am. Climat. Ass., 1898, XIV, 202.

bacilli on their hands. The other two were exceptionally careful. Preisich and Schütz [1] found tubercle bacilli on the hands of children in a children's hospital at Budapest. Of 66 examinations of the dirt from under the finger nails 14 were positive under the microscope, but owing to the death of the animals from sepsis their virulence was not demonstrated. Of the 14 positive cases, 11 had tuberculosis, or were associated with it, while of the 52 negative cases only 5 were associated with tuberculosis. Dieudonné[2] by inoculation demonstrated tubercle bacilli on the hands of 2 of 15 children. In this connection may be mentioned the experiment of Schumburg,[3] in which he rubbed an *öse* of a culture of bacteria on his hands, and recovered the germs after 15 and 16 handshakes. Ostermann,[4] on the other hand, does not consider contact infection of much importance in tuberculosis. While he recovered tubercle bacilli from the hands of 7 of 14 phthisical patients and from 1 attendant, he obtained them only 4 times from 42 children living in tuberculous families and 2 times from the floors occupied by these families. He does not find that bacteria are transferred from hand to hand as readily as have other observers. He also made a few cage experiments with guinea pigs to show that infection by contact is less effective than infection by air.

It scarcely needed the experiments of Annett at Liverpool[5] and Higgins[6] at Birmingham to show that virulent tubercle bacilli may be found in the sputum on sidewalks, or those of Dixon[7] to demonstrate that they may be swept up on the skirts of ladies' dresses.

[1] Preisich and Schütz, Berl. klin. Wchnschr., 1902, XXXIX, 466.

[2] Dieudonné, Münch. med. Wchnschr., 1901, XLVIII, 1439.

[3] Schumburg, Ztschr. f. ärztl. Fortbild., Jena, 1905, II, 567.

[4] Ostermann, Ztschr. f. Hyg. u. Infectionskrankh., Leipz., 1908, LX, 375.

[5] Annett, Thompson Yates Laboratory Rep., 1901–02, IV, Pt. 2, 359.

[6] Higgins, Pub. Health, Lond., 1909–1910, XXIII, 100.

[7] Letter from Dr. Samuel A. Dixon to author.

In Communion Cups. — Anders[1] found tubercle bacilli in the dregs from communion cups in a Philadelphia church, and Möller[2] from the communion cup of a sanatorium chapel. Davison[3] found them on a glass used for some weeks in a high school. He also demonstrated pneumococci. Klein[4] obtained a positive tuberculous reaction once after inoculation of the swabbings of six telephones, although on twelve telephones on another occasion[5] he was unable to find either diphtheria or tubercle bacilli, and Rickards[6] was unable to find either bacillus on twenty-four mouthpieces of lung-testing machines in Boston. Huhs[7] found tubercle bacilli on napkin rings in the sanatorium at Stadtwald, but did not find them on the spirometer which was in daily use. Price[8] used some water in which sanatorium dishes had been washed to inoculate eight guinea pigs, all of which died of tuberculosis. Washings from dishes which had been first washed in the ordinary way showed no bacilli.

Contact Chief Mode of Infection. — Since it is true that pathogenic organisms begin to die or lose their virulence when thrown off from the body, we are forced to conclude that the closer the relationship in time and space with the bearers of the germs, the greater the chance of infection. Now that the number of unknown foci of infection and the opportunities for direct transfer of secretions have been demonstrated, the deduction is certainly permissible that contact infection is more important than the more indirect infection by fomites or by air.

We are also compelled by inductive methods to place the greatest emphasis upon contact infection. In the chapter on

[1] Anders, J. Am. M. Ass., Chicago, 1897, XXIX, 789.
[2] Möller, Deutsche med. Wchnschr., 1905, XXXI, 548.
[3] Davison, Tech. World Mag., Chicago, 1908, IX, 623.
[4] Klein, Lancet, Lond., 1908, I, 1862.
[5] Ref. J. Am. M. Ass., 1905, XLIV, 1866.
[6] Rickards, Rep. Bd. Health, Boston, 1906, 91.
[7] Huhs, Ztschr. f. Tuberk. u. Heilstättenw., Leipz., 1906, IX, 396.
[8] Price, Sixth Internat. Cong. on Tuberc., Wash., 1908, I, 167.

infection by fomites, and particularly in that on infection by air, much evidence is presented to show that infection usually does not take place unless contact is fairly close. The views here presented as to the great importance of contact infection, and the comparatively slight importance of air infection and fomites infection, gradually developed after consideration of much experimental and epidemiological evidence. The two facts which more than all others have contributed to these views have been the restriction of scarlet fever and diphtheria to single families in the same house, and the success of certain hospitals in preventing cross infection, when contact infection is strictly guarded against.

Disease Spreads in Dwellings only by Contact. — The rarity with which scarlet fever and diphtheria pass from one family to another in the same house has already been alluded to, but it is worth considering again. Of 4306 other families in Providence living in the same house with a case of scarlet fever, only 295, or 6.8 per cent, were later invaded by the disease. This includes all families, whether careful or careless, and whether or not the initial case was removed to the hospital; but as less than 10 per cent of the cases have been removed to the hospital during the 23 years covered by the figures, hospital isolation can have been of little moment. This amount of infection is surprisingly small, and of itself indicates very strongly that close and intimate contact is usually necessary for the extension of this disease. A further study of the facts indicates this still more clearly. During the last 5 years, scarlet fever has extended to 118 of 1888 other families, or 6.3 per cent. In 54, or 22 per cent, of the cases infection occurred during the first two weeks, of which 37 were during the first week. Most of these cases during the first two weeks probably derived their infection from the first family before the disease was recognized. Only 24 second families developed their infection after the end of the second week and while the warning sign was on the house. This is the time when the patients are desquamating and when the disease is popularly believed to be most infectious. These 24 cases are 1.3 per cent of the 1888 other families in the infected houses. As in a number of these cases there was known to be considerable communication between the families, it seems to be certain that in an ordinary tenement house scarlet fever is not readily carried from one family to another, and that effective isolation is comparatively easy. In fact, everything goes to show that two or more families may live in the same house, using hallways, doors, and even water-closets in common, without scarlet fever extending from one to the other. All that is necessary is that there shall be absolutely no visiting between the families, and that the children shall never meet in play. I do not know that similar data have been collected elsewhere, but Cameron[1] has shown by his study of "return" cases of this disease that in many instances the infecting case may remain in the family for some time, providing there is no direct contact with the well persons.

Diphtheria is as little likely to extend from family to family without direct contact as is scarlet fever. During the last twenty-one years, in Providence, of 3667 other families living in a house with diphtheria, only 263, or 7.2 per cent, were invaded by the disease. During the five years 1904 to 1908, of 1648 other families, 114, or 6.9 per cent, have acquired the disease. Of these, only 38, or 2.3 per cent, were attacked after the first week of the initial sickness and before the warning sign was removed. As was shown above, many of these infections are due to the fact that the first case is not recognized and hence the different families in the house continue to visit one another; or in some instances to the fact that persons in the second family carry the bacilli for a time without being sick. Probably a large part of the infections during the first week take place before the disease is recognized, so that it seems very probable that less than 2 and perhaps less than

[1] Cameron, Rep. on Return Cases of Scarlet Fever and Diphtheria, Lond., 1901–02, 98.

1 per cent of families living in a house with a case of diphtheria contract the disease while the warning sign is on the house. I have given particular attention to the cases of diphtheria arising in other families in the house while the warning sign remained on the apartment where the disease first appeared, and almost always there is known to be direct intercourse between the families. Contact infection, then, seems to be necessary for the transfer of diphtheria from one family to another living in different apartments of the same house.

Disease spreads in Hospitals only by Contact. — Another strong reason for this view that contact infection is the chief mode of extension for the common contagious diseases is the success of certain hospitals in preventing cross infection by minimizing in every way the opportunities for infection by contact. The Parisian hospitals, particularly the Pasteur Hospital, have been leaders in demonstrating the success of this method. In most hospitals for contagious diseases great effort is made to prevent cross infection by separating the different diseases to a considerable distance, since the theory prevails that air-borne infection is the chief mode of spread. This view so dominates hospital practice that numberless ways escape notice by which disease is spread by very direct contact, with the result that in most hospitals cases of cross infection are continually developing.

French Hospitals. — The French seem to have been the first to appreciate the importance of guarding against contact infection, and an interesting account of the efforts made is given by Grancher,[1] who was one of the pioneers. Strict methods of "antisepsie médicale," as Grancher calls it, were introduced, and it was found possible to care for patients with different diseases even in a common ward with far less danger of transfer than before. He employed wire screens around the beds to impress upon the nurses the necessity for guarding against infection by contact. During the years

[1] Grancher, Cong. Internat. de med., XIII., C.-r. Par., 1900, Sec. de méd. de l'enfance, 478.

1890 to 1900, 6541 patients were treated in Grancher's wards, and diphtheria was introduced 43 times, but only once did a case develop in the wards. Scarlet fever was introduced 19 times, and 7 cases developed in the wards. Less success was obtained in isolating measles, but infections were reduced two-thirds. Grancher was satisfied that even this disease was spread by contact. He believed that in clean wards infection is rarely air-borne; it is "objective," not "atmospheric." In several other French hospitals the importance of preventing contact infection has been realized. In some of them isolation is made easier by placing the patients in separate rooms or cubicles; in some, partitions are placed between the beds. These partitions may be full height, or may stop short of the floor, and reach only just above the head. Sometimes screens only are used. In 1897 the Minturn Hospital in New York, a small private hospital, was built to provide isolation in separate rooms for cases of scarlet fever and diphtheria. But the most notable example of the new method is the Pasteur Hospital in Paris, opened in 1900. The success of these various hospitals in preventing cross infection is correlated, not with the amount of isolation as ordinarily understood, but with the care with which aseptic measures are carried out by the attendants. The cubicles, partitions and screens certainly cannot prevent infection if the nurses without taking proper precautions pass from one case to another. This is shown by the constant development of cross infection in the ordinary hospital. It was in the Pasteur Hospital that the principles of medical asepsis were first fully appreciated and carried out in a practical manner. The hospital consists of two pavilions with about fifty beds each, designed ostensibly, one pavilion for scarlet fever and one for diphtheria; but, as is shown below, all sorts of cases are admitted. For the care of all these "other diseases" and mixed and doubtful cases, twelve single rooms are provided in each ward, all opening into a common corridor, the doors of which are usually left open. The same nurses look after different diseases, often in adjoining rooms. The discipline of the hospital attempts to secure an entire avoidance of contact infection, and is remarkably successful. Yet the procedures are all very simple. The nurse always sterilizes her hands after waiting on the patient; she wears a gown, which is kept in the room, when anything is done which would be likely to infect her clothing. Nothing goes into the room except what is sterile, and nothing comes out without being at once sterilized. To train nurses sufficiently to take charge of a ward, two years are necessary, but the nurses whom I saw there were carrying out these details with the same precision and unconsciousness which are shown by the bacteriologist in his laboratory.

English Hospitals. — The principles of aseptic nursing as applied to contagious diseases have been employed in a number of places in England, as, for instance, in the North Eastern, South Western and London Fever hospitals in London, at Walthamstow and Manchester, and doubtless in other places. The methods adopted in the Monsall Hospital at Manchester, and described by Gordon,[1] are as follows:

"The patient's bed in the general ward is surrounded with a screen covered with sheets, which are kept constantly wet with a weak solution of some disinfectant. The main purpose of this screen is to serve as a label, and to remind the nurses that certain precautions must be taken for the patient behind it. At the same time, I think the wet sheets may possibly arrest infective particles that are projected against them in the acts of coughing and sneezing. The only other requisites are two glass shelves fixed on the wall behind the bed, and a locker or portable cupboard made of metal, with an enameled surface, which can easily be disinfected and kept clean.

" The precautions to be taken by the nurses in attending patients behind this screen or 'barrier' are printed on a card fixed to the screen, and are as follows:

[1] Gordon, Rep. on Health of Manchester, 1908, 154

Rules in Manchester. — " Precautions to be Observed in the Nursing of Barriered Cases.

"(1) Rubber gloves are to be worn by the Nurse for all manipulations connected with the case, including the handling of clothes. The gloves are to stand in a bowl of 1 in 400 Izal solution.

"(2) The following utensils are to be marked and kept on the glass shelves or in the locker provided:

Spatula Nozzles Clinical Thermometer	To be kept completely immersed in a 1 to 400 Izal solution.

At least two bowls.
All feeding utensils (plates, spoons, forks, etc.).

"(3) A plentiful supply of wet swabs, with a bowl containing Izal solution to receive these when used, is to be kept on the locker. Handkerchiefs or muslin squares are not to be employed.

"(4) No toys or books that have once been used inside the barrier are to be taken outside it except to be destroyed.

"(5) In every case a square of jaconette is to be placed on the pillow slip, and over this a piece of muslin; the latter is to be renewed whenever soiled.

"(6) An overall is to be worn by the Nurse whenever either the patient or the clothes are handled. This is to be kept inside the barrier."

The success of the methods described in the preceding pages is well shown by the published figures. At the Pasteur Hospital from October 1, 1900, to April 19, 1903, the following cases were received:

Diphtheria	443	Scarlet fever	92
Sore throat	166	Erysipelas	163
Smallpox	524	Phlegmon of tonsil	20
Chicken pox	55	Other diseases	219
Measles	126	Mothers with infants	192

Such a combination furnishes a remarkably fertile field for cross infections. During the next year about 750 cases were admitted.[1]

During this whole period the only cases which developed in the hospital were 5 of smallpox, 2 of erysipelas and 1 of diphtheria. Dr. Loiseau writes me that since 1904 the percentage of cross infections has been less than 0.1 per cent. At the Minturn Hospital in New York there has been no instance of infection in the hospital. At the Monsall Hospital in Manchester in 1908 a large number of persons admitted with mistaken diagnosis were cared for in the wards by the methods described without contracting the disease, and a number of cases of mixed infection were cared for in the open wards without infecting others, except in one instance when, owing to a mistake in orders, "barrier" isolation was not promptly instituted. A letter just received from Dr. Arnold, who has succeeded Dr. Gordon at Monsall, states that in order that the patient may see and be seen, and to avoid the dampness of the wet sheet, he has substituted a tape which as effectually prevents the mythical aerial flight of the germs, or, to speak literally, equally well reminds the nurse that she must be clean.

Is Tuberculosis Air-borne? — It is assumed that tuberculosis, as it occurs in human beings, is usually an air-borne disease, and as will be shown on another page, there is more reason for such an assumption concerning this than concerning most diseases. Yet there is in certain quarters a growing tendency to attribute to contact infection more importance than formerly. Yet it must be confessed that most writers on this disease lay no emphasis on contact infection, and some scarcely mention it. Cornet,[2] in speaking of kissing, the most direct means of contact infection, says that it is incredible that tuberculosis should be transmitted in this way, for the saliva is ordinarily germ free, and the germs if

[1] Martin, Bull. méd., Par., 1904, XVIII, 251.

[2] Cornet, Nothnagel's Encyclopedia, Tuberculosis, 187.

present would not be carried to the lungs. Cornet's first contention is certainly not correct, for Neild and Dunkley, as before mentioned, found tubercle bacilli on the tip of the tongue of phthisical patients examined during intervals of freedom from cough. They also report cases of lupus, due in all probability to inoculation with saliva, and refer to others reported by Wild.[1]

There has been little experimental work to determine the part played by contact infection in tuberculosis. The work of Bartel and Spieler[2] indicates that guinea pigs exposed under natural conditions to contact with the members of a tuberculous family more often develop the disease than do animals exposed merely to the air of the room, while the experiments of Packard, though inconclusive, indicate little difference.

Infection by Alimentary Tract. — There seems to be evidence that the tonsils may be the seat of infection in many cases of tuberculosis. Harbitz[3] has very forcibly called attention to the probability that tubercle bacilli frequently gain access to the body through the tonsils. He examined the tonsils and lymphatic glands of a large number of children, and found latent tuberculosis in many of the tonsils, and latent bacilli in the cervical glands in 17 instances, much more often than in the mesenteric glands. He thinks that a more careful study of the tonsils and lymph nodes would reveal much latent tuberculous infection, and he thinks that a considerable amount of infection takes place through the tonsils. Harbitz mentions Grawitz,[4] Aufrecht[5] and Beckmann as supporting this view. Ravenel and Reichel[6] review much literature, and refer to Wood's experimental infection of swine

[1] Wild, Brit. M. J., 1899, II, 1353.

[2] Referred to in the chapter on infection by air.

[3] Harbitz, J. Infect. Dis., Chicago, 1905, II, 143, and especially 198.

[4] Grawitz, Deutsche med. Wchnschr., 1901, XXVII, 711.

[5] Aufrecht, Verhandl. d. deutsch. path. Gesellsch., Berl., 1901–02, IV, 65.

[6] Ravenel and Reichel, J. Med. Research, Bost., 1908, XVIII, 1.

through the tonsils, the course of the bacilli being apparently through the submaxillary and cervical glands. Benome [1] caused infection in animals through the mouth and pharynx. Bandelier[2] finds primary tuberculosis of the tonsils not so rare as is generally believed, but he does not consider the tonsils as a frequent starting point of phthisis. Mohler and Ravenel from experiments and observations consider the mouth as a frequent site of infection in the tuberculosis of hogs.

Contact Infection in Tuberculosis. — The nose also may be the seat of infection. Cornet,[3] by applying infective material by means of a feather to the nasal mucous membrane of guinea pigs, was able to produce disease of the nose and submaxillary glands. Renshaw [4] was able in the same way to infect seven of eight animals. As tubercle bacilli are numerous upon the hands of consumptives and upon various articles used by them, it is evident that fresh bacilli must be frequently carried to the mouth and nose of persons near by, and may either infect directly through the mouth, nose and pharynx, or may be swallowed and enter the circulation through the lower part of the alimentary canal. The only question is, How frequently does this happen? As was stated above, it is the opinion of many that it is a very common mode of infection. Moore[5] is of the opinion that in cattle tuberculosis is spread chiefly by the animals licking one another, and by their eating and drinking from the same vessels. Bartel[6] believes that infection by pharynx, stomach and intestines is more common than has been supposed, in which view he supports Weichselbaum,[7] Volland,[8]

[1] Benome, Ref. J. Am. M. Ass., Chicago, 1907, XLIX, 888.
[2] Bandelier, Beit. z. Klin. d. Tuberk., Würzb., 1906, VI, 1.
[3] Cornet, Nothnagel's Encyclopedia, Tuberculosis, 154.
[4] Renshaw, J. Path. and Bacteriol., Lond., 1901, VII, 142.
[5] Moore, Conference of Sanitary Officials, N. Y., 1907, 37.
[6] Bartel, Sixth Internat. Cong. on Tuberc., Wash., 1908, I, 95.
[7] Weichselbaum, Festsch. VI Konf. Internat. Tuberk., Wien u. Leipz., 1907.
[8] Volland, Berl. klin. Wchnschr., 1899, XXXVI, 1031.

Kavacs[1] and Preisich and Schütz.[2] Among others who attribute much importance to contact infection may be mentioned Wassermann,[3] Calmette and Landouzy.[4]

Certainly the opportunities for the direct transfer of fresh moist infective material in the home of a phthisical patient must be very great, while the chance of the infective material becoming dried, pulverized and, while still virulent, being carried to the pulmonary alveoli, must be comparatively small. Unless there is some good reason to think otherwise, one would naturally attribute to contact infection the chief rôle in the extension of this disease, at least in the family. The only objection is offered by the pathologists, many if not most of whom affirm that the evidence points to direct infection of the lungs by the inspired air. There are, however, many able experimenters who think otherwise, and who maintain that tubercle bacilli may enter the body at various points and reach the lungs through the lymph channels. It is impossible for the writer properly to weigh pathological evidence, but that the question is still *sub judice* must be admitted. Under the circumstances it seems to be wise to assume as a working hypothesis that contact infection is a factor of great importance in the causation of human tuberculosis. It is certainly essential to guard against such infection in every way, and from a person who does thus conduct himself in a cleanly manner at all times, diffusion of the disease through the air would be impossible. Undue emphasis laid upon the invisible and therefore terrifying infection in the air has done more than anything else to develop the unfortunate phthisiphobia which so often renders miserable the life of the tuberculous, and seriously interferes with rational measures for the restriction of the disease.

[1] Kavacs, Zeiglers Beitrage zur. Path. Anat., 1906, XL.

[2] Preisich and Schütz, Berl. klin. Wschnschr., 1902, XXXIX, 466.

[3] Wassermann, Berl. klin. Wchnschr., 1908, Nr. 48.

[4] Calmette and Landouzy, Sixth Internat. Cong. on Tuberc., Wash., 1908, I, 110.

Importance of Contact Infection. — I have sometimes been told that I lay too much emphasis on contact infection, but if it is the principal way in which disease spreads, too much emphasis cannot be placed upon it, and it seems to me that the evidence is that it is the chief mode of infection. Even if it is not so important as is here alleged, every one must admit that it is of considerable importance, yet until recently very little attention has been paid to it. If contact infection is the chief mode of extension of the contagious diseases, then defense against them becomes more largely a personal affair than we have been taught. We do not have to rely exclusively on the municipality for our protection, awaiting forced isolation, hospital construction, disinfection and the like, but can largely protect ourselves by keeping our fingers out of our mouths, and also everything else except what belongs there. It may not be possible to prevent all contagious sickness in this way, but some can be avoided, and perhaps most of it. Contact infection is avoided by personal cleanliness, and personal cleanliness is demanded by decency, good manners and refinement, as well as by hygiene. It is not much trouble to be decently clean, and it is not very expensive. It is a serious mistake to build an expensive isolation hospital that does not check disease, or to construct a filter when it is not needed; but no harm would be done if the views here presented should be found to be erroneous and people should learn to wash their hands and keep their fingers out of their mouths to no purpose so far as disease prevention is concerned. It seems certain that much can be done to prevent the spread of disease in the family and in hospitals, schools and institutions, if only personal cleanliness be insisted upon. Yet such cleanliness or medical asepsis is sadly neglected by physicians as well as by nurses. Rather strong preaching is needed when, as was referred to on another page, a typhoid nurse is detailed for the double duty of washing bedpans and preparing food. It is certainly necessary to insist somewhat strenuously on reform when such occurrences as the following take place.

Disregard of Contact Infection.— Thus, at one of the finest hospitals in this country, with separate wards for scarlet fever and diphtheria, a considerable number of cases have arisen in the general wards. The germs were supposed to be airborne, as it was said there was no other possible avenue of infection. When I saw the head nurse lick her finger to facilitate turning the bedside charts of diphtheria patients, I suspected that the principles of medical asepsis had not been entirely mastered. Called to see a case of scarlet fever in a well-to-do family, I found the door of the sick-room carefully hung with a sheet to keep the infection from the other children. After examining the throat with a spatula I handed the latter to the mother. She took it into the hall and put it on an upholstered sofa, and with her saliva-infected hands opened the door of an adjoining room. The attending physician meanwhile sat on the bed and handled the patient, an entirely unnecessary proceeding at that time, and except for the example set him, would have forgotten to wash his hands before leaving. A certain hospital determined to copy in one of its wards the cubicle system of the French, but had so missed its essential features that I found doctors and nurses going from cubicle to cubicle feeling the pulse, smoothing the bedclothes, and handling dishes without even stopping to wash their hands. Meanwhile the screen was supposed to prevent the microbes from passing from bed to bed, and we all carefully wore gowns and caps so that the wicked little germ might not jump into our hair and then jump off again onto the next patient. In another fine hospital for contagious diseases, where great stress is laid upon ample space between different diseases so as to prevent cross infection, the superintendent was observed freely to touch articles about the ward, and handle the patients, and then go to the public office without even washing his hands. Such incidents could be multiplied indefinitely. The superintendent of another hospital invited another visitor and myself to eat ice cream from the same spoon as himself, which spoon was then replaced in the freezer which was to supply the wards. I was most of all impressed with the fact that at the International Congress on Tuberculosis in 1908 a large number of the readers of papers moistened their fingers with their tongue when turning the pages, and in each of the sections only one drinking glass was provided for all the speakers; and this continued without protest for a day or two. If the most distinguished investigators and health officials of the world, gathered to study the most important contagious disease, show no appreciation whatever of the importance of contact infection, it is certainly time for some one to be emphatic.

Personal Prophylaxis. — The discovery that disease germs are rarely able to maintain themselves outside of the body clouded the hopes of those who expected by municipal house cleaning to "stamp out the zymotic diseases," and the later discovery of numerous missed cases and carriers has shown that isolation of the sick controls infection far less than was believed. These somewhat discouraging facts are to a large degree offset by what has been learned of the modes of infection. Formerly air infection was chiefly feared; now it appears that contact infection is of prime importance. Formerly dependence was placed upon the state to isolate and disinfect; now it appears that the individual can protect himself, and as easily protect others if he chance to be infected. It is usually comparatively simple so to live as not to allow the secretions of others to come in contact with one's own mucous surfaces, and it is easy, and should be considered immoral, to allow one's own secretions to be so placed that they may infect another. Personal cleanliness is less expensive than municipal cleanliness, and is within the reach of all.

Need of Education. — When one notes the utter disregard of medical asepsis shown in our hospitals and medical congresses, one is apt to feel that the education of the public in habits of personal cleanliness will take a very long time; but some encouragement is felt when it is remembered that it is not so very long ago that excrement was commonly thrown into the street and garbage was tossed under the tables of the great. It is only a few years since our sidewalks were flecked with saliva, but now nineteen persons out of twenty are ashamed to be caught spitting on the pavement. Perhaps we may all soon learn to stop distributing our secretions so freely among our friends.

Education in School. — As the avoidance of contact infection is chiefly a personal matter, the present need is for education. First of all, the teachers in the medical schools and the staffs of hospitals must learn to appreciate the importance of this mode of infection. It is not unreasonable to hope that in a few years the schools and the hospitals will place as much emphasis on medical asepsis as they now do on surgical asepsis, and it is to these centers that we must look for the education of physicians, health officers and nurses. To educate the general public is a more difficult matter. Some years ago Dr. Theobald Smith called my attention to the desirability of teaching school children something about the requirements of personal cleanliness, and since then I have each year distributed to each school child the following " dont's "

REMEMBER THESE THINGS.

Do not spit if you can help it. Never spit on a slate, floor, or sidewalk.

Do not put the fingers into the mouth.

Do not pick the nose or wipe the nose on the hand or sleeve.

Do not wet the finger in the mouth when turning the leaves of books.

Do not put pencils into the mouth or wet them with the lips.

Do not put money into the mouth.

Do not put pins into the mouth.

Do not put anything into the mouth except food and drink.

Do not swap apple cores, candy, chewing gum, half-eaten food, whistles or bean blowers, or anything that is put into the mouth.

Never cough or sneeze in a person's face. Turn your face to one side.

Keep your face and hands clean; wash the hands with soap and water before each meal.

PROVIDENCE, May, 1901.

An explanatory circular is sent to the teachers, and of late a short account of the sanitary reasons for personal cleanliness has been distributed to children above the primary grade. Large printed copies of the "don'ts" have been framed and hung in the schoolhouses.

Much kindergarten work is of such a nature as to inculcate rather than discourage cleanly habits. Children work in common in moist clay and sand, use the same "gifts" and toys and are brought into close contact in the games. Miss Bessie M. Scholfield, late supervisor of these schools in Providence, succeeded, without any undue expense or violent change of methods, in employing kindergarten work as a means of teaching some of the principles of personal hygiene.

Municipality should encourage Cleanliness. — Besides efforts that are directly educational the municipality can do much indirectly to encourage habits of personal cleanliness and to prevent the distribution of the secretions and excretions of the body. The common drinking cup is a most efficient means of such distribution, and it should be abolished in all schools and other public institutions. This has been done in many places, and individual cups or specially designed drinking fountains substituted. The example is now being followed by some railways, factories and shops. The states of Kansas, Michigan and Mississippi were the first to forbid the use of a common drinking glass on railways, and the Lackawanna and some other roads, and the Pullman Company advertise as an attraction free cups of paraffin paper for each passenger.[1] Since the above was

[1] J. of Outdoor Life, 1909, VI, 371.

written a dozen other states have forbidden the use of the common glass. Hundreds of churches have adopted the individual communion cup. In the first edition, I said that "the roller towel should go the way of the common drinking cup." Since then Massachusetts and Connecticut and the cities of New York and Chicago have enacted statutes or adopted rules forbidding the use of a common towel in public places.

People are more likely to keep clean if it is easy to do so. Hence the establishment of public baths may be considered a real sanitary measure. While compulsion can have little share in the campaign for cleanliness, certain prohibitions are entirely reasonable and feasible. Thus ordinances against spitting on the sidewalks and the floors of public places have done much to teach people to take proper care of their secretions. Reference has already been made to evidence that the abolition of privy vaults results in a decrease in typhoid fever. Privy vaults certainly encourage the improper disposal of excreta and general uncleanly habits. A good sewage system and the removal of vaults and cesspools do much to prevent contact infection, at least in the fecal-borne diseases.

CHAPTER V.

INFECTION BY FOMITES.

Definition of Term. — As was shown in the preceding chapter, it seems very probable that contagious disease may often be caused by the quite direct transference of the germs from one person to another on such objects as cups, pencils, pipes, the fingers, etc. This mode of transference should properly be considered a form of contact infection. The term contact infection, as commonly used at the present time, does not necessarily imply the immediate touching of two persons, but it does imply the comparatively direct transference of quite fresh material from one to another. Although almost any object may in this manner be the bearer of infection, it would not ordinarily be considered as fomites. By fomites are usually meant infected objects which retain the infection for some time. A toy used by a diphtheria patient and sent to a distant town and there giving rise to the disease, the dress of a scarlet-fever patient put away for weeks or months and brought out only to cause another case, a library book carrying the infection of smallpox from one household to another, blankets loaded with typhoid bacilli in South Africa transferring infection to England, infected hides from Asia causing anthrax in Philadelphia, blank cartridges as the bearers of tetanus germs, and the various objects in a room lately occupied by a case of any contagious disease giving rise to the same affection in newcomers, would all be recognized as fomites. The cup which carries the moist saliva from one school child to another, the borrowed pencil which transfers the fresh syphilitic virus from lip to lip, and the urine-moistened closet seat which infects the fingers and then the mouth of the next user, are not thought of as fomites but as the necessary media for that intimate mode of disease transference which is coming to be called contact infection. This distinction between the two classes of bearers of infection is somewhat arbitrary, and not very definite, but is eminently practical. In this book, by infection by fomites is meant a transference of infecting material on objects under such conditions that considerable time elapses, days at least, usually weeks, sometimes months.

Yellow Fever and Fomites. — If one takes up the older text-books on yellow fever it will be found that fomites were considered the most important means in the extension of this disease. The invasion of cities and countries was usually attributed to this mode of carriage. This was the general view up to, and indeed after, the discovery of the rôle played by the mosquito, and numerous instances of such transference are given. Thus the federal inspectors[1] attributed the outbreak at Brunswick, Ga., to ballast brought from Cuba. The disease was supposed to have been carried from New Orleans to Havana by means of second-hand oyster buckets.[2] Liceaga[3] gives instances of the transmission of yellow fever by a shipload of grain from New Orleans, by cloth spread out on the grass to dry, by general merchandise, by bagging, by clothing, and by ballast. Horlbeck[4] says that two persons at Key West contracted yellow fever from sleeping on a mattress that was brought from Cuba.

Never so Transmitted. — In all these instances the evidence is the same: a locality has long been free from yellow fever, something is imported from an infected place and the disease develops. What could be clearer? The proofs that it is a fomites-borne disease were far more numerous and stronger for yellow fever than for almost any other disease.

[1] Rep. Surg. Gen. U. S. Mar. Hosp. Serv., 1893, II, 33.

[2] Report on Shipment of Merchandise, U. S. Mar. Hosp. Serv., Special Report, 1899, 9.

[3] Liceaga, Am. Pub. Health Ass. Rep., 1898, XXIV, 122.

[4] Horlbeck, Am. Pub. Health Ass. Rep., 1897, XXIII, 436.

Yet we now know that yellow fever never was, nor could be, transmitted in any such way. Such a mistake, a mistake which cost millions upon millions because of the needless interruption of commerce, and disinfection, should make us careful how on similar, but weaker, evidence we attribute importance to fomites as a means of infection in other diseases, and should lead us to inquire what proof there is that the long persistence of infection on things is a weighty factor in the transmission of disease.

Smallpox. — It does not require much search in medical literature to find numerous instances of the alleged transmission of disease by fomites. Recent text-books and journals are full of them. Welch and Schamberg[1] state that smallpox was brought to Philadelphia on cotton from the South, but the only reasons for thinking so were that there was much smallpox in the cotton region and none in Philadelphia, and that the patient handled cotton. Not long since the health officer of a western city reported that the principal source of smallpox in that city was lumber, his assumption being based on the facts that there was much of the disease in the lumber camps, that the rough lumber was well fitted to carry contagion, and that in most families the first person attacked was engaged in some sort of woodworking. The above are fair samples of the kind of evidence on which the theory of fomites infection rests. Smith[2] reports that a man from Paris died in London of what was probably malignant smallpox. Two people who afterwards slept in the same bed, on different days, developed the disease, as did the girl who sorted at the laundry the soiled linen from this hotel.

Scarlet Fever. — A recent writer in *Public Health*[3] reports six instances of house infection giving rise to scarlet fever, in one case nine months after the first patient was sick. The

[1] Welch and Schamberg, The Acute Infectious Diseases, Phila., 1905, 160.

[2] Smith, Pub. Health, Lond., 1901–02, XIV, 211.

[3] Trotter, Pub. Health, Lond., 1906–07, XIX, 745.

only evidence was the recurrence of the disease in the house. Welch and Schamberg[1] quote from others reports of fomites infection in this disease. Boeck states that the hair of a scarlet-fever patient caused the disease twenty years after. Another physician caught the disease from a coat which he wore while attending a case a year and a half before. The health officer of Detroit[2] reports two cases due to infection from books which had been used by a patient some months before. Wende[3] states that quilts used by scarlet-fever patients in August, and put away without disinfection, caused the disease in November. The reports of the state board of health of Michigan[4] give instances of the persistence of the scarlet-fever virus for years in houses, letters, books, etc.

Diphtheria. — Buckley[5] quoted from the Newton, Victoria, Health Report an instance where a cornet used by a diphtheria patient was put away for four years, and was then found by some children, who contracted the disease from it. He gives another instance where the disease recurred in the house after a period of two years. At a time when Manila was absolutely free from diphtheria, an American child who had been there over a year received some Christmas presents from St. Louis, and was taken sick a few days later. Christian[6] writes of the transmission of diphtheria on carpenters' tools which were sent from one shop to another.

Cholera. — A number of instances of the transmission of cholera by soiled clothing are given in the Report of the Marine Hospital Service for 1893.[7] In nearly every instance the clothing was brought from foreign countries. Because

[1] Welch and Schamberg, The Acute Infectious Diseases, Phila., 1905, 344.

[2] Rep. Bd. of Health, Detroit, for year ending June 30, 1903, 11.

[3] Buffalo San. Bull., Nov. 30, 1908.

[4] Rep. St. Bd. Health, Mich., 1906, 134; 1907, 133.

[5] Pub. Health, Lond., 1906–07, XIX, 296.

[6] Bull. N. Y. St. Board of Health, June, 1907, 5.

[7] Rep. Surg. Gen. U. S. Mar. Hosp. Serv., 1893, Vol. II, 353.

a company of soldiers had suffered from typhoid fever for two years, and the disease ceased on disinfecting the barracks, the outbreak was believed to have been due to room infection.[1]

Before weighing the value of this evidence it is perhaps worth while to consider some of the things which are most often alleged to serve as fomites.

Infected Clothing. — From the time when the priest was directed how to detect leprosy in woolen and linen[2] to the present, clothing has been considered an important vehicle of infection. It is not to be doubted that disease germs may be carried on clothing. If clothing is soiled with a considerable quantity of infected saliva, feces, urine or pus, and if while fresh, say within a few hours or days, it is brought in contact with susceptible persons, disease may result. If it is folded and put away in the dark, especially if it be in a damp place, it may remain infectious perhaps for months. But as bacteria as a rule die rapidly, and as there must be a sequence of gross infection, favorable conditions for survival, and contact with susceptible persons, it does not seem likely that disease is often caused in this way.

Many instances are recorded, usually only of possible, rarely of probable, transference of disease by clothing. Of yellow fever more than of any other disease has this been alleged, yet we now know that such transmission of this disease is impossible. Many writers also report the spread of bubonic plague by means of clothing, but, as will be seen, the evidence is that plague is only under very exceptional circumstances carried by fomites.

Typhus not carried in Clothing. — When typhus fever appeared in New York in 1892, from sixty to seventy-five officers of the health department were, according to Doty,[3]

[1] Cited by Germano, Ztschr. f. Hyg. u. Infectionskrankh., Leipz., 1897, XXIV, 404.

[2] Leviticus, Chapter xiii, verses 47–59.

[3] Doty, Med. News, N. Y., 1905, LXXXVI, 730.

more or less in contact with the cases, often in intimate contact; gowns were not used, and the officials went freely between the patients and their own homes, and about their other business, yet no case of this disease could be traced to fomites infection.

Butler [1] speaks of a parlor maid in a contagious-disease hospital who for six months had been in daily contact with nurses coming directly from scarlet-fever cases without change of clothes, but she did not contract the disease until exposed to an incipient case in the person of a nurse, when she promptly developed scarlet fever. This is only one illustration of many of the failure of supposedly infected clothing to infect.

Physicians rarely carry Disease. — In scarlet fever and diphtheria physicians are constantly passing from the sick to the well. Some of them take great precautions to avoid carrying the disease in their clothes, but the majority take few or none, — or at least did not until very recently. Yet records of their transmitting disease are extremely rare. For many years I was on the lookout for this mode of transference, and only once or twice found any evidence that the physician was at fault. In such cases how much greater is the chance that the physician carries infection on his hands than in his clothes. Barlow [2] found that of 500 cases of scarlet fever in only 4 had the physician previously been treating the disease and these 4 cases were apparently traced to other sources.

Infection by Clothing is Rare. — If the gross infection of clothing is only in rare instances the cause of disease, how little must be attributed to slight infection! A few droplets of tuberculous saliva, a slight smear of moisture from the lips of a diphtheria patient, will soon lose their virulence after exposure to light and air. But usually the visitor in a sick-room will escape all infection except the hypothetical floating

[1] Butler, Proc. Roy. Soc. Med., Lond., 1908, I, Epidemiol. Sect., 225.

[2] Barlow, Med. Officer, 1910, III, 319.

particles. The danger from this floating matter will be shown in another chapter to be a negligible quantity. It is the common practice for physicians, nurses and visitors in a room occupied by a contagious case to wear a gown and cap. For physicians and nurses who are to move or lift the patient, or otherwise come into intimate contact with him, the gown is a reasonable protection against possible gross contamination. For the careless visitor too it may be useful. The cap is a useless frivolity. It is amusing to see how religiously it is worn, while no protection is given the feet, though Denny and Nyhen[1] have shown that infection by means of the shoes is bacteriologically possible, while the aerial infection of the hair has never been demonstrated and is highly improbable. More than once have I seen a physician don his cap to keep the germs from flying into his hair, and pass freely from one diphtheria patient to another, inspecting the throat, feeling the pulse or smoothing the bedclothes, and occasionally stroking his own chin or scratching his head, all without washing his hands. And physicians and nurses will continue to do such things as long as they fancy that air infection is all they have to fear, and forget that there is such a thing as contact infection. It has for some years been my custom not to wear a gown when called in consultation to cases of contagious disease, or when visiting hospital wards, unless I am to do much work about the patient. Under the conditions of a casual visit, even in smallpox, I do not wear a gown. It is not necessary to touch anything except with the hands, and these should be carefully washed before leaving. I have never carried infection to my home, or elsewhere so far as known, and I believe that there is no chance of my doing so.

Laundries and Disease. — If clothing can carry infection, sickness ought to make its appearance in laundries, to which enormous quantities of clothing go even while the infecting material is still fresh. Attempts have been made to show

[1] J. Mass. Ass. Bds. of Health, Bost., 1904, XIV, 109.

that disease is carried to laundry workers in this way, and it is probable that some of the alleged instances are true. Thus Sedgwick, and also Walcott,[1] report cases of typhoid fever where the evidence was very strong that the disease was contracted by handling soiled linen. Thorne-Thorne[2] also reports an interesting case of probable transmission of typhoid fever by clothing. That such accidents are common has never been shown. Certainly in Providence there is no excess of scarlet fever, diphtheria or typhoid fever among laundry workers. This cannot be due to the disinfection of the clothing, for much disinfection is not effective, and for six years there has been no disinfection after diphtheria, and moreover the linen from carriers and missed cases is nowhere subjected to disinfection.

It is true that Landouzy,[3] after examining 1590 laundry workers in Paris, states that tuberculosis is twice as prevalent among them as among other workers, and he attributes it to infection from soiled clothing. But certainly other occupations show an even greater excess of this disease, and there is no suggestion that it is due to infection from the materials handled. There may be many other reasons why laundry workers should show an excess of tuberculosis, such as age distribution, poverty and overwork.

Infection of Rooms. — It is generally believed that the room, or rooms, which have been occupied by a case of contagious disease are a fertile source of danger to others. The germs of diphtheria, scarlet fever and smallpox are supposed to become attached, not only to books, playthings, bedding and furniture, but also to the walls and ceilings. It is true that anything which can be reached by the patient or attendant may possibly receive infection, the chance increasing according to the frequency with which the thing is

[1] Sedgwick and Walcott, J. Mass. Ass. Bds. Health, Boston, 1900, IX, 145.

[2] Thorne-Thorne, Clin. Soc. Trans., Lond., 1892, XXV, Suppl., 67.

[3] Landouzy, Presse méd., Par., 1905, XIII, 633.

handled. That parts of the room or its contents not touched should be infected by floating particles, is highly improbable. The secretions and excretions which in various ways become attached to the contents of the room are usually small in amount and thinly smeared on the surface. Such material usually rapidly loses its virulence by drying, so that, as is shown in these pages, virulent germs are recovered from the sick-room in only a small proportion of tests. Nevertheless if people should, after the termination of the sickness, crowd into the room, rub their moistened fingers over the various objects and put the fingers in the mouth, infection might sometimes result. But as the germs die rapidly, as probably not many persons enter the room, as even visitors would usually run little chance of taking up whatever pathogenic organisms might be there, we are, I think, justified in assuming that infection from the room or its contents is not very likely to take place.

"Lung Blocks." — The celebrated "lung block" in New York, bounded by Cherry, Catherine, Market and Hamilton streets, has had enormous influence on modern views concerning the transmission of tuberculosis. The great excess of tuberculosis in certain tenement houses has given rise to a strong belief in its causation by infection which remains attached to the interior of the dwelling. We even hear much loose talk about the germs of the disease developing in the filth and dampness of these dark houses. What an important factor house infection is believed to be in the causation of this disease is well illustrated by the exceedingly prominent place which is given to room disinfection. To judge from the attention, time and money bestowed on room disinfection after the removal or death of a consumptive, this practice is considered of equal importance with hospitals, sanatoriums, dispensaries or district nursing as a preventive measure. Let us see what is the evidence on which house infection is supposed to rest. It is apparently that cases continue to occur in the same house during successive years. This judgment is based on the spot map. Thus in New York[1] during five years, 42 per cent of the deaths from tuberculosis occurred in 23 of the total houses infected, or in 5.25 per cent of all the houses in the city. In Ward IV, 55.8 per cent of the cases occurred in 10.5 per cent of the houses in the ward and in 28 per cent of the infected houses. In Ward VI, 44.7 per cent of the cases were in 7 per cent of the total houses and in 19 per cent of the infected houses. Many in other cities have noted the same phenomenon, but it has been especially well recorded by the New York Department of Health. But to say that these facts are to be largely explained by the persistence of the tubercle bacilli in the houses is no more reasonable than it would be to explain the recurrence of an excess of murders in certain areas to the persistence of a hypothetical microbe of homicide. It is true that the advocates of the importance of house infection point to numerous instances in which an apparently healthy family moving into a house recently occupied by a consumptive later develop the disease. That such should quite often happen merely as a coincidence is necessitated by the great prevalence of the disease. That in "lung blocks" exposure to living cases in the other tenements is a much more likely source of the disease than exposure to bacilli on the walls, is probable. To demonstrate the relation of the disease to house infection it would be necessary to go fully into the history of at least a large proportion of the cases, and that, particularly as we really know nothing about the latent period of the disease, is at present impossible. The excessive incidence of tuberculosis on certain houses is no proof of house infection, and we are obliged to appeal to the facts of bacteriology and the general principles of infection to estimate the probable danger from this source. When we consider the number of persons who are continually throwing off great numbers of tubercle bacilli, and the numberless chances there are, particularly in the crowded tenement districts, of coming in contact

[1] Rep. Dept. Health, City of New York, 1896, 244.

with fresh infective material, there seems to be no necessity of assuming that infection must be traced to the more or less feeble and scattered germs that may be clinging to the walls of a vacated apartment. What necessity or excuse is there for assuming that such infection plays more than an inappreciably minute part in the causation of this disease?

Rags and Disease. — Rags have often been considered an important vehicle of disease. At one time much attention was given to this subject in the United States, and great danger was apprehended from the importation of foreign rags, and stringent measures were taken to secure their disinfection. Lengthy discussions of the matter, and references to a great volume of literature, may be found in a report for the New York City Board of Health by Smith in 1886, and in the Marine Hospital Report for 1893.[1] Numerous references are given of the alleged transmission of various diseases by means of rags. Among the diseases mentioned are smallpox (126 outbreaks), influenza, scarlet fever, erysipelas, typhoid fever, septicemia, cholera, and a disease peculiar to rag dust, called "flock cough."

Rags and Smallpox. — It has been believed that smallpox is frequently introduced among the workers in paper mills by the rags which they handle. Numerous instances have been reported from Maine, Massachusetts and Wisconsin, as well as from foreign countries. Most of the evidence is very inconclusive, as no effort is made to exclude other sources of infection, and the disease is usually prevailing generally at the time. The most suggestive outbreaks are a series reported by the Massachusetts State Board of Health.[2] Here from one to three cases occurred in six mills in different localities at a time when there was no smallpox in the town. Dr. Abbott, who personally studied these outbreaks, was convinced that they were due to handling rags. Yet it is curious that almost nothing has been heard of this sort of infection

[1] Rep. Surg. Gen. U. S. Mar. Hosp. Serv., 1893, II, 330.
[2] Rep. St. Bd. Mass., 1888, xvi.

during the last twenty years, and this at a time when smallpox was of a remarkably mild type and great quantities of clothing worn by patients must have escaped disinfection. Abbott was also convinced that, owing to the length of time between the collection of the rags and the opening of the bales, no danger was to be apprehended from foreign rags. Doty[1] says "that the most careful investigation has failed to present satisfactory evidence that either foreign or domestic rags act as a medium of infection." He has personally carefully studied the question in Egypt, where many rags are collected for the American market, and he says that there is no evidence of the infection of the handlers of even the fresh rags.

Rugs and Plague. — Remlinger[2] has recently called attention to the supposed danger to be apprehended from draperies, and particularly also rugs, from the Orient. He rightly says that many of the rugs are very filthy, and must have been infected during their use or manufacture. Yet during all the prevalence of cholera and bubonic plague in Asia during recent years not a single case of these diseases has been brought into Europe or America in this way, though great quantities of rugs, draperies and rags have been imported without disinfection or with very imperfect disinfection.

Money and Disease. — Money is popularly believed to be a common means of spreading disease. Indeed there are few things which at first sight seem more likely to do so than paper money. Germs readily become attached to its surface, it passes rapidly from one person to another, it is kept in intimate contact with the person, held closely in the hand and often put to the lips. Nevertheless there is no good evidence that money has ever actually been the means of spreading contagious disease. If money is frequently a carrier of infection, persons who handle a great deal of money ought to be particularly subject to infectious disease. This does not seem

[1] Doty, Med. Rec., N. Y., 1900, LVIII, 681.

[2] Remlinger, Hyg. gén. et appliq., Par., 1907, II, 257.

to be the case, though there are unfortunately no good published statistics bearing on the subject. However, it is the business of the supporters rather than the opponents of the theory to produce the figures. I have been on the lookout for contagious disease among bank clerks, but the very few cases that have come to my knowledge during the past twenty-five years have evidently been contracted in other ways. According to Hilditch,[1] the "United States treasurer, who has given the subject long and careful consideration, is emphatic in his statement that 'there is not the slightest evidence to show that the employees in his department contract infectious diseases any oftener than others who are not in this line of work.'" It may be argued, and there is some truth in this, that tellers are accustomed to take considerable precaution, such as keeping the fingers away from the lips and washing the hands before eating. Tram-car conductors are, however, I know from observation, particularly prone to hold bills and coins between the lips, and are in other ways extremely careless, yet they certainly show no excess of scarlet fever, diphtheria or smallpox. A bacteriological study of paper money has been made by Hilditch above referred to. He examined twenty-four bills and found the number of bacteria varied from 14,000 to 586,000 per bill. Pus bacteria were found, as was to have been expected, but no other pathogenic forms. Hilditch could find accounts of only four other similar investigations, none of which, however, were as thorough as his. Bacteria are not found in any large numbers on coins, chiefly because of the germicidal action of the metal, as shown by the researches of Park,[2] Vincent [3] and Bolton.

Much Evidence Unsatisfactory. — It would be easy to find hundreds of alleged instances of fomites infection, in some of which the infection was supposed to have persisted for

[1] Hilditch, Pop. Sc. Month, N. Y., 1908, LXXIII, 157.
[2] Cited by Hilditch.
[3] Vincent, Abst. Med. News, N. Y., 1892, LXXX, 275

years. Those mentioned in the preceding pages are only a few which I happened to have at hand. In most of them there is no real evidence that the disease was produced in the manner claimed. The error made in claiming so much for fomites infection in yellow fever shows how great is the liability of error for other diseases.

Persons, not Things, are Dangerous. — It must also be borne in mind that in very many of the reported cases the supposed infected articles were carried by some person. That the person may be the "carrier" of living germs on his own mucous surfaces, though showing no symptoms, we now know full well. Until recently this was not known, hence it was universal to consider things, not persons, as the bearers of infection. We can now see that persons in whom the germs are growing are much more likely to be the agents of infection than are things on which the germs are dying. Some of the instances of alleged fomites infection, such as the room infection in scarlet fever referred to, are doubtless really instances of carrier infection.

Fomites and Tetanus. — It is not for a moment to be assumed that there are no instances of fomites infection. It is not impossible, or at all improbable, that occasionally typhoid fever, smallpox, diphtheria and other diseases are caused by material things holding the living bacteria for some weeks or even for months. In some instances the clinical evidence of fomites infection is very strong, though perhaps it can rarely if ever be in any individual instance entirely conclusive. If it can be substantiated by bacteriological evidence, it becomes so much the stronger. The strongest evidence we have of fomites infection is concerning anthrax and tetanus. This is not surprising when it is recalled that the bacilli of both of these diseases are spore-forming and capable in that state of resisting unfavorable conditions of life for years. Thus Smith[1] finds that tetanus bacilli will survive boiling for sixty minutes at a time, or twenty minutes on

[1] Smith, Theobold, J. Am. M. Ass., Chicago, 1908, L, 929.

each of three successive days. This explains why they have been found alive and virulent in commercial gelatine and in that situation have been known to give rise to the disease in human beings.[1] Of six samples of cotton lamp wick purchased in various shops in Havana, five were shown by the inoculation of white mice to be infected with tetanus. This material was used by midwives for tying the umbilical cord, and after sterile material was furnished them by the department of health it is said that almost no deaths from infantile tetanus occurred in Havana.[2] The number of deaths from tetanus in children under one year of age in Havana decreased from 128 in 1901 to 18 in 1908. Some of the Fourth of July tetanus is believed to be due to the presence of the spores in the wads of blank cartridges, and they were demonstrated in them by Dolley,[3] and are said to have been found in cartridges in Germany by Musehold of Strassburg and others, but several other American observers failed to find tetanus germs in a total of 759 cartridges examined.

Fomites and Anthrax. — The spores of anthrax are so resistant that they have been kept for ten or twelve years, but the bacilli themselves do not survive any longer than typhoid bacilli. Anthrax, though rather rare in the United States and England, is very common in some parts of the world, particularly in Asia, and the spores are frequently imported in dry animal products from Asiatic countries. Legge[4] cites from several observers who recovered the spores from hair and hides imported from China and Siberia. More recently Eurich[5] has examined nearly 750 specimens of wool, hair and dust from these materials. In over 600 specimens

[1] Tuck, Jour. Path. & Bacteriol., Edinb. & Lond., 1904, IX, 38.

[2] Junta Sup. de San. de la Isla de Cuba, Supplemento y Note Adicional, 1902–03, 4.

[3] Dolley, J. Am. M. Ass., Chicago, 1905, XLIV, 466.

[4] Legge, Lancet, Lond., 1905, I, 694, and Rep. Insp. of Fact., Lancet, Lond., 1904, I, 1206.

[5] Rep. Anthrax Investigation Bd., Bradford, Eng., No. 3, 1908, 8.

free from blood he found no anthrax germs, but he did find them in 20, or 14.4, per cent, of 139 bloodstained specimens. These findings are substantiated in his last report (1909), and he speaks of a case of anthrax in a man who handled wool in which anthrax spores were actually found. In 64 samples of dust, anthrax germs were demonstrated only once.[1] Page[2] also gives references to other similar findings. But such observations are not necessary to show that the disease is transported in this way, for there is ample clinical evidence that such goods are the direct cause of anthrax in men and animals. In fact, most industrial anthrax in Western Europe and North America is caused by handling wool, hair and hides imported from anthrax-infested countries.

Fomites and Typhoid Fever. — One of the most remarkable of the authenticated instances of fomites infection is the transmission of typhoid fever by means of army blankets from South Africa.[3] These blankets came from Africa in October, 1902, and were then sold. They went to 290 different parties. One lot used on the transport *Cornwall* apparently gave rise to the disease in May, 1903; the use of another lot in England was also followed by typhoid fever. Some of the blankets were considerably soiled, and living bacilli were found on several that were examined in London.

Fomites and Diphtheria. — A young man working in a laboratory in an American city spilled some bouillon culture of diphtheria bacilli on his coat. This coat, without disinfection, he wore when calling on the young woman to whom he was engaged, and she developed diphtheria two days later. The culture which was spilled contained only the branching forms of the diphtheria bacillus, and the culture from the patient's throat showed the same forms.

But very few instances other than the above are on record

[1] Rep. of Chief Inspector of Factories and Workshops, 1907, 57.

[2] Page, J. Hyg., Cambridge, 1909, IX, 357.

[3] Parkes, Practitioner, Lond., 1903, LXXI, 297.

where pathogenic bacteria have actually been found on materials which presumably have carried infection. According to Simpson,[1] plague bacilli were found by Kitasato on cotton goods imported into Japan, and this was thought by Kitasato to be the way in which the disease was introduced into that country, but from what is now known about the mode of extension of the disease this seems highly improbable.

Few Instances of Fomites Infection. — But while we may admit that occasionally the virus of even many of the commoner diseases may be retained on fomites for a considerable length of time, and ultimately give rise to new cases, there is no clinical evidence to show that such instances are at all common. Even when carefully sought for, fomites infection is not very often found. In my early work as health officer I firmly believed in the importance of this factor, and diligently sought for evidence. The fact that I found very little was one thing which led to a more careful consideration of the subject. Of 13,970 cases of scarlet fever reported in Michigan,[2] only 335 were attributed to fomites infection. To an even less degree are diphtheria and measles attributed in this report to fomites infection. Of 221 cases of bubonic plague in Natal,[3] only 8 were by Hill attributed to fomites infection, and Mitchell in Port Elizabeth attributed only 6 of 337 cases to the same source. When we consider that most of the evidence is extremely flimsy, and that much of the alleged fomites infection is probably carrier infection, and remembering also how the history of yellow fever has taught us to be wary of such proofs, we are forced to the conclusion that there is little in the history of the more prevalent infectious diseases to indicate that fomites infection is at all common.

Reasons for Belief in Fomites. — One reason why fomites infection looms so large in the minds of health officers, as

[1] Simpson, Treatise on Plague, Cambridge, 1905, 204.
[2] Rep. St. Bd. Health, Mich., 1906, 134.
[3] J. Hyg., Cambridge, 1907, VII, 712.

well as of the laity, is that the striking character and air of mystery about the alleged incidents are so impressive. "Death in a Toy," or "A Child Succumbs to the Dread Disease from Infection Lurking in its Mother's Shawl," appeal to the imagination. That the invisible emanations of disease should cling to a garment for years is too near akin to the stories of the Arabian Nights not to impress the average mind. Hence it is that the comparatively few instances of real fomites infection have far more than their due weight in our estimation of the relative importance of different modes of infection.

Even if all the alleged instances of fomites infection were true, the amount of disease apparently caused in this way is relatively very small. The frequency with which contagious disease can be traced to fomites is not the reason for the general belief in the importance of this mode of infection. The real reason, I have no doubt, is, that until very recently there seemed to be no other way of explaining isolated cases of disease. As a rule it is impossible, even with modern aids to the diagnosis of obscure cases, to trace the source of infection of most cases of contagious disease, particularly in cities. The theory of long persistent fomites infection seemed to offer a reasonable solution, and hence met with universal acceptance. The theory was almost a necessity to explain the facts as they were formerly understood. Now we have no need for such a theory, and a much more satisfactory explanation is at hand.

Evidence against Theory. — It is only within a very few years that the frequency with which mild atypical cases of disease occur has been recognized, and the existence of numerous entirely healthy carriers is a modern discovery, which is even now denied by some. The more carefully individual cases and outbreaks of disease are studied, the more often are they traced to missed cases and carriers. It is not probable that we shall ever be able to discover the origin of all our contagious disease. We can only infer its source from the data we have. As was shown in the first chapter, there is every reason for thinking that disease germs rarely grow outside of a living body. Two other theories are open to us. Disease may be due to the persistence of infection on things, or it may be due to exposure to mild cases or carriers. There should be no hesitancy in choosing between the danger from rapidly dying germs on books, money, furniture or clothes, and rapidly growing germs in the mouth, nose and intestines of persons. Moreover things must be carried, people move freely at will.

If the danger from fomites infection were as great as is generally believed, the contagious diseases would be much more common than they are. The advocates of this theory are constantly telling us how easily everything near the sick becomes infected and how long the infection lasts. Every one knows that at the best disinfection is imperfect, and that much that passes for disinfection is no disinfection at all. Then the missed cases, which all admit occur in considerable numbers, to say nothing of the carriers, are constantly infecting large numbers of things which are not subjected to any disinfection. Yet our scarlet fever and diphtheria are not increasing, which means that one case of the disease gives rise to no more than another case. If fomites infection occurred as easily as is alleged, each case would ramify through fomites into a dozen more cases. One reason for doubt about the prevailing ideas of fomites infection is this: if fomites infection were as common and as easy as is alleged, few could escape it, and the infectious diseases would be much more prevalent than they are. As was shown in Chapter IV, the chances for the transfer of fresh infective material are so extremely numerous that there is no necessity for assuming the far more difficult and uncertain modes of aerial convection and transmission by fomites, and indeed there seems to be little opportunity for their action.

Bacteriological Evidence. — Having considered some of the clinical evidence of the part played by fomites in the transmission of infection, it is desirable to inquire what light the laboratory study of disease has thrown on the problem. One of the first labors of the discoverer of a pathogenic organism is to determine its resistance to various hostile influences, such as heat, cold, drying, light and disinfectants.

The Effect of Drying upon Bacteria. — Drying, exposure to light and lack of nourishment are the principal factors which determine the life of micro-organisms on fomites. Besides the study of the germs of special disease by those particularly interested, Germano, whose work is mentioned in the chapter on aerial infection, Ficker,[1] Zonchello,[2] Heim,[3] and Buckley,[4] among others, have given careful and systematic attention to the effect of drying on the vitality of bacteria. Exceedingly divergent results have been reported by these different observers. This, however, is not surprising if the number of factors involved is taken into consideration. Among the most important of these factors is the amount of light. Germs that are killed in a few minutes in direct sunlight may live for weeks in a dark place or even in diffused light. The thicker the layer of infectious material, the longer is its virulence likely to be maintained. This thickness depends largely upon the nature of the medium. In a dried watery medium, bacteria may die quickly, while they may survive long in sputum or feces. The more complete the drying, the shorter the life, and alternate drying and dampening is unfavorable. The higher the temperature, the sooner the germs perish. Their vitality also varies with the rapidity of the drying process and the material on which they happen to be. Old cultures die sooner than fresh ones, and different strains have different powers of resistance. The chemical composition of the medium and

[1] Ficker, Ztschr. f. Hyg. u. Infectionskrankh., Leipz., 1908, LIX, 367.

[2] Zonchello, Giornale della Real Soc. Ital. d' Igiene, 1905, XXVII, 489, 537.

[3] Heim, Ztschr. f. Hyg. u. Infectionskrankh., Leipz., 1905, L, 122.

[4] Buckley, Pub. Health, Lond., 1906–07, XIX, 290.

the presence or absence of other organisms may have an influence.

The spores of bacteria are so resistant that we should naturally expect the diseases caused by the spore-forming kinds to be readily carried on fomites. As has been shown, this is true of anthrax and tetanus, diseases which belong to this class.

Typhoid Bacilli. — Among the more hardy non-spore-forming bacteria is the bacillus of typhoid fever. In the first chapter it was shown that in the presence of moisture, as in privy vaults, the soil, milk, water, etc., this bacillus sometimes lives for some months, though it often dies out in a much shorter time. It remains to consider the duration of its life when in a more or less dry condition.

Firth and Horrocks[1] found that typhoid bacilli would live on khaki for 78 days, in feces dried on serge for 9 to 17 days, on serge for 10 days after it had been exposed to direct sunlight for 50 hours. Pfuhl[2] says that dried on linen they lived 97 days. Germano[3] cites Gaffky as reporting that the typhoid bacillus would live for 3 months when in a dry condition, and that Uffelmann recovered it from various dry materials after a period of from 21 to 80 days. But Germano suspects that the substances were not perfectly dry. Germano himself was able to preserve typhoid bacilli dried on wood or linen for 90 days, but when he inoculated sterile dust with a bouillon culture, the bacilli did not survive over 4 days and sometimes perished in 1 day. Most of them died off very rapidly. Buckley[4] found they would live for from 5 days when dried on paper in a room to 119 days when kept on wood in a moist chamber. The consensus of opinion seems to be that while under unfavorable conditions,

[1] Firth and Horrocks, Brit. M. J., Lond., 1902, II, 936, 1094.

[2] Pfuhl, Ztschr. f. Hyg. u. Infectionskrankh., Leipz., 1902, XL, 555.

[3] Germano, Ztschr. f. Hyg. u. Infectionskrankh., Leipz., 1897, XXIV, 403.

[4] Buckley, Pub. Health, Lond., 1906–07, XIX, 290.

as when quite dry and exposed to light, the typhoid bacillus may die in a few days, yet under conditions which must frequently prevail it may remain alive on such things as clothing and bedding for some months.

Mediterranean Fever. — The micrococcus of Mediterranean fever has about the same resistance as that of typhoid fever. Like the typhoid bacillus, it is killed in an hour or two in direct sunlight. Dried on glass it survives 16 days, in moist soil 72 days and on a blanket 80 days.[1]

Diphtheria. — Loeffler kept dry diphtheria bacilli alive for from 9 to 16 weeks, Roux and Yersin for 5 months, D'Espine and Morignac for between 3 and 4 months, and Park for 4 months.[2] Germano[3] found that they would retain their virulence after remaining in dry earth or dust for 20 to 40 days, and Reyes[4] found them virulent in sand and on cloth after 14 days. Buckley[5] recovered living bacilli, when dried in the air on paper, after 6 days, on wood after 8 days, on cotton and on glass after 24 days, and on plaster after 37 days. Hill[6] exposed to ordinary room conditions, glass rods which had been rubbed on a culture of diphtheria bacilli. Of these 28 per cent survived 14 days and 9 per cent 20 days. Houston[7] found that they died very quickly in earth. Leighton[8] recovered them from warm moist modeling clay up to 18 days. Williams[9] could not recover the germs after 24 hours from pencils moistened by the lips of patients who had the bacilli in the throat.

[1] Horrocks, Rep. Commission Roy. Soc., Pt. I, 1901.

[2] Cited by Germano.

[3] Germano, Ztschr. f. Hyg. u. Infectionskrankh., Leipz., 1897, XXV, 439.

[4] Reyes, Jahrb. u. d. Fortschr. . . . d. path. mik., Baumgarten, 1895, XI, 203.

[5] Buckley, Pub. Health, Lond., 1906–07, 290.

[6] Hill, Am. Pub. Health Ass. Rep., 1902, XXVIII, 209.

[7] Houston, Rep. Med. Off. Loc. Gov. Bd., Lond., 1898-99, XXXIII, 413.

[8] Leighton, Pediatrics, 1901, XII, 360.

[9] Williams, N. Y. Health Dept., Sci. Bull. 2, 1895, 16.

Dysentery Bacilli. — According to Pfuhl[1] the bacillus of dysentery may remain alive for 17 days when dried on cloth, or 10 days when in dry sand. In direct sunlight it dies in 30 minutes.[2] Kruse[3] claims that when dry it will retain its vitality for months.

Tubercle Bacilli. — More attention has been paid to the vitality of the tubercle bacillus than to that of other bacteria. It is generally believed to be one of the most resistant, but Hill[4] has shown that under the same natural conditions of dryness, light, etc., the diphtheria bacillus will outlive it. Many of the earlier writers claimed a very considerable longevity for the tubercle bacilli in dried sputum. Villemin, Schill, Fischer, Koch, De Thoma, Sormani, Maffuci and Cadéac and Malet claimed a life of from 1 to 9 months.[5] Ransome and Delépine[6] found that the bacilli if exposed to air and light would not survive 45 days, but if kept in dim light they did survive. Twichell[7] placed sputum in a folded handkerchief, in a folded carpet, and spread on wood, and exposed it to the air at ordinary temperatures and in diffused light. The bacilli survived for 39 to 70 days. In sunlight they died in a few hours. Migneco[8] found that when dried on cloth in the sun they lived from 20 to 30 hours.

Not so Resistant as Believed. — Many recent observers do not find this bacillus so resistant as has been supposed. That it perishes in direct sunlight in less than an hour seems certain. Weinzirl,[9] using improved methods, finds that it will not survive 10 minutes, and frequently dies in 2 minutes.

[1] Pfuhl, Ztschr. f. Hyg. u. Infectionskrankh., Leipz., 1902, XL, 555.
[2] Shiga, Deutsche med. Wchnschr., 1901, XXVII, 765, 783.
[3] Kruse, Deutsche med. Wchnschr., 1901, XXVII, 370, 386.
[4] Hill, Am. Pub. Health Ass. Rep., 1902, XXVII, 209.
[5] Kolle and Wasserman's Handbuch [etc.], Jena, 1903, II, 108.
[6] Ransome and Delépine, Proceedings Royal Society, No. 336.
[7] Twichell, Med. News, N. Y., 1905, LXXXVII, 642.
[8] Migneco, Arch. of Hyg., München u. Leipz., 1895, XXV, 361.
[9] Weinzirl, J. Infect. Dis., Chicago, 1907 [Suppl. No. 3], 128.

Cadéac [1] spread sputum on marble and could find no living germs after the fourteenth day. On a porous plaster plate they died within 2 days. Hill [2] dried sputum on glass rods in the air under ordinary room conditions, and found no living bacilli at the time of his first test, which was made after 16 days. Rickards, Slack and Arms [3] have made very careful tests by exposing sputum on wood and cloth in the rooms of ordinary tenements. They find that when dry and kept in diffused light the bacilli will live about 1 month, in dark and dry rooms up to 85 days; another strain survived only 45 days under the latter conditions. Rosenau [4] says that further work upon the viability of the dried tubercle bacillus may change our views as to its hardiness, and failure to recognize lesions produced by the dead bacillus is responsible for some of the false conclusions reached by certain experimenters.

Plague Bacilli. — Simpson [5] states that the German Plague Commission found that in a large number of experiments with sputum, blood, etc., dried on all sorts of materials, under natural conditions, the bacilli of bubonic plague do not survive over 8 days. Of many specimens of the organism dried on cover glasses and sent to England, none survived the journey. Kitasato [6] found that plague pus dried on cover glasses lost its virulence, when exposed to the sun, in from 3 to 4 hours, and this has been substantiated by others. As was referred to in the first chapter, the work of the last English Plague Commission shows that virulent plague bacilli cannot be found in the dirt floors of native houses after 48 hours. According to the careful experiments of Buckley,[7]

[1] Cadéac, Lyon méd., 1905, CV, 865, Abst. Brit. M. J., Lond., 1906, I.

[2] Hill, Am. Pub. Health Ass. Rep., 1902, XXVIII, 209.

[3] Rickards, Slack and Arms, Am. J. Pub. Hyg., Bost., 1909, V, 586.

[4] Rosenau, U. S. Pub. Health and Mar. Hosp. Serv. Hyg. Lab. Bull. No. 57, 1909.

[5] Simpson, Treatise on Plague, Cambridge, 1905, 96.

[6] Kitasato, Lancet, Lond., 1894, II, 428.

[7] Buckley, Pub. Health, Lond., 1906–07, XIX, 290.

plague bacilli remain alive after drying in the air, for 11 hours when dried on cotton, 2 hours on wood, 5 hours on plaster, 2 hours on glass, and 3 hours on paper. When kept in a desiccator they survived on cotton for 22 hours, and in a moist chamber for only 36 hours. Gotschlich,[1] by folding material containing the germs in cloth, could preserve them alive for from 3 to 4 weeks. Simpson[2] reports that infected cloth may retain its virulence for 80 days. According to Verjbitski,[3] the crushed viscera of experimental animals and the crushed bodies of fleas when smeared on cloth and dried will preserve the bacilli alive for 130 days at a temperature of 4–5° C., and for 35 days at room temperature. Bandi and Stagnitta-Balistreri state that these bacilli may survive in the bodies of dead rats for 2 months. The vitality of the plague bacillus has been carefully investigated by Rosenau,[4] who does not consider it a frail organism. Temperature is the most important factor in its life. It may lose its virulence before it loses its vegetability. It dies in a few days on the dry surface of hard objects and on paper. Rosenau says that bedding may harbor the infection for a long time. Tidswell,[5] experimenting with a large number of materials, found that plague bacilli dried under natural conditions lived only from 3 to 4 days, but when dried slowly on muslin they might live for 21 days. The colder the climate the greater is the chance of the persistence of infection. In this all are agreed.

Pus-forming Bacteria.—The pus-forming bacteria are quite resistant to drying. According to Germano,[6] streptococcus

[1] Gotschlich, cited by Kolle and Wasserman's Handbuch [etc.], Jena, 1903, II, 496.

[2] Simpson, Treatise on Plague, Cambridge, 1905, 93.

[3] Verjbitski, J. Hyg., Cambridge, 1908, 203.

[4] Rosenau, U. S. Pub. Health and Mar. Hosp. Serv. Hyg. Lab. Bull. No. 4, 1901.

[5] Tidswell, Report on Plague in Sydney, J. A. Thompson, 1902, 67.

[6] Germano, Ztschr. f. Hyg. u. Infectionskrankh., Leipz., 1897, XXVI, 66.

withstands drying for a month, but different strains have varying degrees of resistance. See also Heim[1] and Neisser,[2] who found that these organisms would withstand drying for a long time. Buckley[3] could keep staphylococcus alive for only 7 days when on paper in the air, and on other substances and under different conditions for varying times, up to 130 days on cotton kept in a desiccator.

Cholera Spirilla. — Germano[4] in a number of experiments found that the cholera spirillum in dried feces lived only 3 days and in other experiments only 1 day. He also cites Zonchello as reporting that it is among the least resistant bacteria. Kitasato[5] states that it may retain its virulence up to 8 days, but that it may die sooner, especially when dried on glass. Usually it lives from a few hours up to 4 days. Koch and Gaffky[6] state that when dried on glass it survives only a few hours, but when dried on fabrics it may retain its virulence up to 4 days. Buckley[3] found that cholera germs would survive when dried in the air, 9 hours on cotton, 8 hours on wood, $1\frac{3}{4}$ hours on glass, and 5 hours on paper. They did not survive nearly so long when dried in a desiccator. This is contrary to the experience of others, for as a rule bacteria live much longer when dried in a desiccator than when dried in the open air under natural conditions. Gotschlich[7] says that cholera germs will live in dejecta dried in the air on clothing for 36 days, and when damp, according to Karlniski's observations, for 7 months. He considers that such a long life is exceptional, and that generally the spirillum dies in a few days. A duration of only a few days, or even hours,

[1] Heim, Ztsch. f. Hyg. u. Infectionskrankh., Leipz., 1905, L, 122.

[2] Neisser, Ueber Luftstaub-Infection, Inaug. Dis., Breslau, 1898.

[3] Buckley, Pub. Health, Lond., 1896–97, XIX, 290.

[4] Germano, Ztschr. f. Hyg. u. Infectionskrankh., Leipz., 1897, XXIV, 403.

[5] Kitasato, Ztschr. f. Hyg. u. Infectionskrankh., Leipz., 1885, V, 134.

[6] Koch, Arb. a. d. k. Gesundsamte, Berl., 1886, I, 199.

[7] Gotschlich, Kolle and Wasserman's Handbuch [etc.], Jena, 1902, I, 211.

was also found by Gamaleia,[1] Hesse[2] and Koch and Gaffky.

Pneumococci. — The pneumococcus is widely distributed in healthy human mouths, and the opportunities for the direct transference of fresh secretion are so numerous that it probably is of no importance whether this organism lives long or not. Wood[3] found that while pulverized sputum lost its virulence in a few hours when dried in mass, it might, under favorable conditions, retain it 35 days. Buerger[4] recovered the pneumococci from a handkerchief 7 days after it had been in use. Germano[5] and some others claim a considerably greater resistance. Germano kept it alive in dust for 140 days, but the tendency of later observers is to consider it a much feebler organism.

Influenza Bacilli. — According to Pfeiffer,[6] the influenza bacillus retains its vitality when dried in sputum for 36 to 40 hours. When dried on a cover glass and kept at 37° C., it survives for only 2 hours, and when kept at room temperature for from 8 to 20 hours.

Meningococci. — The evidence in regard to the germ of cerebro-spinal meningitis appears to be somewhat conflicting. Germano and Neisser claim considerable resistance for it, as also does Jaeger.[7] Germano said it would live for 80 to 90 days, but it is said that he did not work with the true meningococcus.[8] More careful and recent observers do not find it so resistant. Councilman[9] found that it would live when dry

[1] Gamaleia, Deutsche med. Wchnschr., 1893, XIX, 1350.

[2] Hesse, Ztschr. f. Hyg. u. Infectionskrankh., Leipz., 1893, XIV, 30.

[3] Wood, J. Exper. M., N. Y., 1905, VII, 592.

[4] Buerger, J. Exper. M., N. Y., 1905, VII, 518.

[5] Germano, Ztschr. f. Hyg. u. Infectionskrankh., Leipz., 1897, XXVI, 66.

[6] Pfeiffer, Nothnagel's Encycl. Pract. Med., Phila. and Lond., Influenza, 1895, 584.

[7] Jaeger, Med. Klin., Berl., 1905, I, 990, 1011.

[8] Arkwright, J. Hyg., Cambridge, 1907, VII, 193.

[9] Special Report on Cerebro-spinal Meningitis, Mass. St. Bd. Health, 1898, 78.

in a dark room less than 72 hours. Albrecht and Ghon [1] could keep it only 24 hours in the dark, and Bettencourt and Franca [2] less than 9 hours. Kache,[3] Kutscher [4] and Flügge [5] had similar results, and Arkwright [6] succeeded in keeping the organism alive only from 20 to 48 hours. Lingelsheim [7] says that in culture media it dies in a few hours, but in sputum it may be kept alive for 5 days.

Gonococci. — According to Schaffer and Steinschneider,[8] and Ullmann [9] the gonococcus lives only a few hours on textiles, at most 36 hours, and often dies as soon as thoroughly dry.

Hertmanni [10] from his own observations and those of others, whom he cites, concludes that the *Tryponema pallida* of syphilis may retain its motility for some months if left moist and in the dark. Drying quickly kills it.

Bacteria on Fomites. — Pathogenic bacteria have frequently been sought for on various articles believed to be likely to be the means of transporting disease, but with the exception of the spores of anthrax and tetanus they have rarely been found. The finding of anthrax and tetanus spores has already been referred to. Besides the places mentioned, tetanus germs have been found in the soil in various places, in the dirt filling between the floors of houses [11] and in one

1 Albrecht and Ghon, Wien. klin. Wchnschr., 1901, XIV, 984.

2 Bettencourt and Franca, Ztschr. f. Hyg. u. Infectionskrankh., Leipz., 1904, XLVI, 463.

3 Cited by Flügge.

4 Kutscher, Deutsche med. Wchnschr., 1906, XXXII, 1071.

5 Flügge, Klin. Jahrb., Jena, 1905, XV, 373.

6 Arkwright, J. Hyg., Cambridge, 1907, VII, 193.

7 Lingelsheim, Klin. Jahrb., Jena, 1905, XV, 373; Ztschr. f. Hyg. u. Infectionskrankh., Leipz., 1908, LIX, 457.

8 Verhandl. d. IV Kong. d. deutsch. dermatol. Gesellsch., Breslau, 1904.

9 Ullmann, Wien. med. Blätter, 1897, XX, 703 et seq.

10 Hertmanni Dermat. Ztschr., Berl., 1909, XVI, 633.

11 Heinzelmann, München med. Wchnschr., 1891, XXXVIII, 185, 200.

instance in a house where there had been a death from tetanus.[1]

Distribution of Germs of Suppuration. — The pus organisms are quite resistant to drying, and if they were not, they are so widely distributed, being found constantly on the skin and mucous surfaces of human beings, that their presence might be expected wherever human beings are found. They have as a matter of fact been found almost wherever sought, as on clothing, books, money, instruments, floors and woodwork, and indeed on anything that is touched by the hand of man.

Diphtheria Bacilli on Fomites. — Diphtheria bacilli have been frequently searched for on all kinds of objects and frequently found. Abel[2] and Wesbrook[3] found them on toys, and in Abel's case it was 86 days after infection. Trevelyan[4] recovered them from a handkerchief 11 weeks after it had been used by a diphtheria patient. Park[5] took cultures which proved positive in almost every instance, from dried stains on bedclothing soiled by children sick with diphtheria. He also found the bacilli alive in a piece of membrane after 4 months. Wright and Emerson[6] made 20 cultures from various articles in the Boston City Hospital, and found 5 positive. Of these 3 were from the shoes, 1 from the hair of an attendant, and 1 from a floor brush. Schumburg[7] in 40 cultures from a room occupied by a diphtheria patient recovered virulent bacilli from a drinking glass and the handle of a mirror. In 2 of the 5 cultures the virulence of the organism was low.

[1] Gotschlich, Kolle u. Wasserman's Handbuch [etc.], Jena, 1902, I, 210.

[2] Abel, Centralbl. f. Bakteriol. [etc.], I Abt. Orig., Jena, 1892, XIV, 756.

[3] Wesbrook, Wilson and McDaniel, Am. Pub. Health Ass. Rep., 1899, XXV, 546.

[4] Trevelyan, Lancet, Lond., 1900, I, 1443.

[5] Park, Med. Rec., N. Y., 1892, XLII, 116.

[6] Wright and Emerson, Centralbl. f. Bakteriol. [etc.], I Abt. Orig., Jena, 1894, XVI, 412.

[7] Schumburg, Ztschr. f. ärztl. Fortbild., Jena, 1905, II, 567.

Weichardt[1] took 300 swabbings from various things in a sick-room and 250 from other parts of the house, and found diphtheria germs 3 times on objects which had been in contact with the patient's mouth. Hill[2] took 532 swabbings from a room occupied by a diphtheria patient, and obtained 4 positive results, all of which were from objects handled by the patient. In Providence about 200 swabbings taken under similar circumstances showed no diphtheria bacilli. These last three observations indicate that diphtheria bacilli are not very numerous, even on objects brought into close contact with the patient. Kober[3] could find no bacilli on the floor, bed linen, etc., of 10 houses in which there had been diphtheria, and he states that Heymann did not find them in the Hygienic Institute at Breslau. Klein could not find them on telephones in London,[4] and Hill in Boston[5] could not find them on 24 mouthpieces of lung-testing machines.

Tubercle Bacilli on Fomites. — While the tubercle bacillus is not so resistant to drying as was formerly thought, it is discharged in such numbers in the sputum that it has been found outside of the body more often than have any other organisms except the pus-forming bacteria. Reference to finding it in dust will be given in the next chapter. When in considerable masses of sputum, and kept damp, the bacillus will survive longer than when mixed with dust. Besides on the floors and various articles in rooms, the bacillus has been found in books which were in use for some years in a circulating library.[6] Petersson[7] examined the history charts kept by the bedside of tuberculous patients and put away for

[1] Weichardt, Jahresb. u. d. Fortschr. . . . d. path. Mik., Baumgarten, 1900, XVI, 197.

[2] Hill, Am Pub. Health Ass. Rep., 1902, XXVIII, 209.

[3] Kober, Ztschr. f. Hyg. u. Infectionskrankh., Leipz., 1899, XXXI, 449.

[4] Klein, Abst. J. Am. M. Ass., Chicago, 1905, XLIV, 1866.

[5] Hill, Rep. Bd. Health, Boston, 1906, 91.

[6] Mitulescu, Ztschr. f. Hyg. u. Infectionskrankh., Leipz., 1903, XLIV, 397.

[7] Petersson, Ztschr. f. klin. Med., Berl., 1907, LXIII, 346.

periods varying from months to years. He found by microscopic examination tubercle bacilli on two books that were kept for six years. Bissell [1] washed the pockets of some uniforms that had been used by soldiers sick with consumption, and obtained two positive results by guinea-pig inoculation. Friberger [2] used a vacuum cleaner to remove the dirt from clothing fresh from use by tuberculous patients, and found virulent bacilli in 3 of 12 tests.

Cholera Spirilla. — Although the life of the cholera spirillum outside of the body appears to be short, usually only a few days and often less, some early observers, as Babes,[3] claim to have found it on the personal effects of cholera patients.

Resistance of Protozoa. — There is no theoretical reason why the protozoan blood parasites might not, in a spore-like, resistant stage, withstand drying and remain alive for some time outside of the body. But there is no experimental evidence to show that in any of the well-known protozoan diseases such spores are formed. There is certainly no clinical evidence to show that such diseases are ever carried on fomites, and for malaria, yellow fever, sleeping sickness and Texas cattle fever there is convincing evidence that they are not so carried.

Resistance of Vaccine Virus. — With two exceptions, practically no experimental work has been done with the virus of any of the infectious diseases, a specific organism for which has not been determined. Vaccine virus has an extensive use, and it is desirable to store it and transport it long distances, so that its keeping qualities have received considerable attention. When the infectious material dries naturally in the crust which forms from the vesicle, it retains its virulence for a considerable time. These crusts were largely used in

[1] Bissell, Med. News, N. Y., 1899, LXXIV, 156.

[2] Friberger, Ztschr. f. Tuberk. u. Heilstältenw., Leipz., 1908–09, XIII, 37.

[3] Shakespeare, Report on Cholera in Europe and India, U. S. Gov. Print. Off., 1890, 606.

Providence for maintaining the Jennerian strain of vaccine, which was used in the health department for nearly fifty years. The crusts, when taken from the arm and kept wrapped in paper in a dark place, could be relied upon to retain their virulence for a month, and often did retain it longer. When kept in a tightly corked bottle in a refrigerator, they will generally remain virulent over 6 months. If exposed to light and air and varying temperature, the virulence may be lost in less than a month. A thin layer of the same lymph on a quill does not remain active when exposed to the air for more than a week or ten days. The ivory points covered with vaccine matter, which were so much used a few years ago, were usually guaranteed to keep 3 weeks, and often did remain virulent a month or more. But there was usually more than one layer, and the thickness of the material was further increased by the presence of blood and leucocytes. According to Seaton,[1] dried vaccine matter on points may keep for from 6 or 9 months or more, and he quotes Husband as securing successful vaccinations from 7 of 93 dried points kept for periods varying from 6 to 30 months. Vaccine matter in powder also has been kept by Warlomont and others for several months.[2] Recently Green[3] has kept dried pulverized vaccine matter in sealed tubes for periods varying from 20 days at 37° C. to 252 days at 10–15° C. and 301 days at 4° C. Although under exceptional circumstances dried vaccine matter may be kept a considerable time, it requires great care and often results in failure. Hence early in the nineteenth century, in order to introduce vaccination into her American possessions, the Spanish Government[4] sent out a ship with a number of children on board, so that by successive arm-to-arm vaccinations fresh lymph might be carried across the seas. At the end of the nineteenth century, when Porto

[1] Seaton, Handbook of Vaccination, 1868, 172.
[2] Warlomont, Manual of Animal Vaccination, Phila., 1886, 139.
[3] Green, J. Hyg., Cambridge, 1908, VIII, 528.
[4] Life of Jenner, Baron, I, 606; II, 78.

Rico came under the control of the United States, the difficulty of transporting vaccine virus to the island became so great, so little active virus surviving even this short voyage, that it was necessary to establish a vaccine farm on the island. In the Philippine Islands it was found to be necessary to transport the virus packed in ice to inland villages.[1]

Resistance of Smallpox Virus.—It is a common belief that the crusts in variola are infectious, and they are supposed to have been used at times in the practice of inoculation. I do not remember to have seen any evidence of this till I came across the work of Brinckerhoff.[2] He refers to a rather limited literature, and details his own experiments, which determined a persistence of virulence in the crusts for periods of from 22 to 52 days, and in one instance to 88 days.

Comparative Resistance. — Experiment shows that some pathogenic organisms, like those of gonorrhea and cerebrospinal meningitis, are of such feeble resistance that infection by fomites, as ordinarily understood, is in these diseases highly improbable. It is also shown that certain other bacteria, as those of diphtheria, typhoid fever and tuberculosis, are resistant enough to make infection by fomites very possible. But it appears that all known pathogens, except those having spores, tend to die off quite rapidly outside of the body, and that under natural conditions it is rather the exception for them to persist for any great length of time. It is worth noting that the typhoid bacillus is more resistant than any other pathogenic organism referred to. Yet we hear almost nothing about fomites infection in that disease. Is it not because attention has been directed to other sources which have been believed to be sufficient, so that there has been little temptation to assume infection by fomites ? Infection by fomites has, on the other hand, been considered of much importance in cholera, the spirillum of which is far less resistant than is the bacillus of typhoid fever, probably because

[1] Rep. Bd. Health, Philippine Isl., 1904–05, 23.
[2] Brinckerhoff, J. Med. Research, Bost., 1904, XI, 284.

in the absence of the knowledge of carriers which we now possess the world-wide diffusion of this disease seemed inexplicable except by means of fomites.

Experiments with Yellow Fever. — With a few notable exceptions, little experimental work has been done to determine the part played by fomites in the spread of disease. When Reed, Carroll Lazear and Agramonte proved that yellow fever is transmitted by the mosquito, it still remained uncertain whether it might not also be carried in other ways, and sanitary officials were generally so convinced of the overwhelming evidence of the great part played by fomites, that definite proof or disproof of the fact was earnestly desired. The complete failure of the commission to produce the disease in human beings by fomites is well known, and their experimental work has now been corroborated by abundant clinical evidence from all the great endemic foci of this disease. In these experiments, non-immunes were confined in a small room for a number of days in close contact with bedding and clothing fresh from yellow-fever cases, most of which was soiled with excreta and vomitus.[1] The experiments were repeated a number of times, but in no instance did the disease develop. When not long after I stood in one of those dirty little rooms in company with Dr. Finlay and Dr. Gorgas, and saw some of the old bedding lying in the corner, I realized as never before how very much greater are the difficulties in observation than in experiment, and it seemed that the time had come when the prevailing views as to the importance of fomites infection in other diseases than yellow fever should be seriously reviewed.

Observations on Plague. — In another disease, bubonic plague, exceptionally brilliant work, from the purely epidemiological standpoint, has been done by Thompson in Australia. It is true enough that conditions are much more favorable for observation when a disease first invades a country than when it has become as widespread as plague is in India, but in no

[1] Phila. M. J., 1900, VI, 790.

place have they been taken advantage of as they were in Sydney. Thompson [1] showed conclusively that rat plague preceded human plague, that the flea was the intermediary between rat and man, and that in New South Wales, at least, fomites had no part in the diffusion of the disease. These observations have been confirmed in other parts of Australia.[2]

Experiments with Plague. — The present English Plague Commission have, by their ingenious and painstaking experiments and observations in India, confirmed Thompson's work. Reference will be made in another chapter to the experiments on the transmission of the disease by the air, in which they definitely proved that aerial infection does not take place. They also studied experimentally the conditions of house infection, and their work is among the best planned and executed and the most convincing of any that has ever been attempted for any disease. Besides much other work, they placed guinea pigs in the houses of an Indian village just vacated by the inhabitants because of plague, thus substituting an experimental population under control for the normal human population.[3] The results were in every way in accord with the view that plague is primarily a rat disease, and is transmitted from rats to man, or to other animals, by means of fleas. In these and in similar less extensive experiments [4] there was evidence to show that the animals could not contract the disease from the dwellings themselves. To test more definitely the possibility of transmission by fomites other experiments were made. The floors of houses were soaked with cultures of the bacilli, and guinea pigs placed upon them. Of 24 exposed during the first hour after infection 4 died; of 12 exposed up to six hours 4 died; but during all this interval pools of the culture were upon the floor. Of 24 animals exposed after twelve hours only 1

[1] Thompson, J. Hyg., Cambridge, 1906, VI, 537.
[2] Ham, Rep. on Plague in Queensland, 1900–07, Brisbane, 1907.
[3] J. Hyg., Cambridge, 1907, VII, 799–875.
[4] J. Hyg., Cambridge, 1906, VI, 450–482.

succumbed. Guinea pigs were also allowed to run freely about hospital wards in which cases of bubonic plague were being treated, and 15 were confined in a room with freshly soiled bedding, which was renewed every day for six weeks. In none of the animals did the disease develop. Again (p. 887), clothing from infected houses, removed without precautions to prevent the transport of fleas, was placed in cages containing 26 guinea pigs, 1 of which died of the plague. A few fleas which had been brought in the clothing were found in the cages. It seems to be quite clear from these experiments that while infection by fomites is possible, it is probable only when the infection is exceedingly gross and the contact is intimate, as in the case of the infected floors referred to above; or it may also be possible when infected fleas are transported in the goods. How common this is has not yet been determined.

Tuberculosis. — I know of no other diseases in which serious experimental work has been done to determine the part played by fomites in their diffusion. It is particularly remarkable that tuberculosis has not been thus critically studied. Every one has been calling for room disinfection as a powerful means of combating this disease, yet it does not seem to have occurred to anyone to place susceptible animals in a series of supposedly infected rooms (as was done in the case of plague in India) to determine if possible how great the danger from room infection really is.

Disinfection Unnecessary after Diphtheria. — By a study of the facts presented in this chapter the writer was convinced some time since that the danger from fomites infection is for most diseases very much less than is generally believed. In diphtheria particularly it appeared that little if any sickness could be due to infection remaining about the house or its contents after the termination of isolation. As isolation is almost invariably terminated without any reference to the presence of carriers in the family, it appeared to be absurd to disinfect the material things in the house when in all probability some carrier was still growing the bacilli. Hence in March, 1905, terminal disinfection was abandoned in Providence, except in those very few instances in which the family was willing to wait for two successive negative throat and nose cultures from each of its members. The attempt was thus made to test the importance of fomites infection by abandoning disinfection and noting any change that might occur in the prevalence or distribution of the disease. One obvious way of testing the influence of disinfection is to compare the recurrence of the disease after disinfection with the amount which occurred after the warning placard was removed without disinfection. The following shows the number of recurrences within 60 days after disinfection, the number of infected families and the ratio between the two, during the years 1902 and 1905.

Year.	Infected Families.	Recurrences.	Ratio.
1902..........	358	6	1.67
1903..........	453	7	1.54
1904..........	559	10	1.78
1905..........	87	2	2.30
Total.......	1457	25	1.71

The following shows the same facts where there was no disinfection.

Year.	Infected. Families.	Reçurrences.	Ratio.
1905..........	258	4	1.55
1906..........	259	4	1.55
1907..........	343	7	2.04
1908..........	687	17	2.34
1909..........	472	10	2.12
1910..........	431	4	.93
1911..........	550	8	1.49
Total.......	3000	54	1.80

The period from 1902 only is taken, because previous to that time the duration of isolation was somewhat longer, but there has been no change since. Very few health officers keep any record of the recurrences in diphtheria and other infectious diseases, but such records are kept in Baltimore, where terminal disinfection is practiced in an unusually thorough manner, and is in a large majority of cases tested for its efficiency. In order to make the Providence figures comparable to those of Baltimore, it was necessary to include recurrences in other families in the house as well as in the family first invaded, and to calculate the percentage on total cases, rather than on invaded households. The following are the figures and there is nothing in them to indicate that terminal disinfection is of any value in preventing recurrences.

BALTIMORE. DISINFECTION.

Years.	Cases.	Recurrences.	Ratio.
1903–1909.....	6931	122	1.76

PROVIDENCE. NO DISINFECTION.

Years.	Cases.	Recurrences.	Ratio.
1905–1911.....	4189	69	1.64

Again, it may be objected that recurrence in the family is no criterion of the infection of the house, for it may be that the family is largely immune. This would certainly be much less true of those members of the family who went away during the sickness. Of 634 minors who thus returned to the non-disinfected house only 2 were taken sick. So, too, if terminal disinfection is such an important matter, its neglect should be followed by an increase in the disease. As a matter of fact, after disinfection was abolished diphtheria diminished, until at one time in the following August there was not a single reported case in the city. Again in August, 1908, the disease was reduced to a single recognized case. There has been a marked increase since, common to many parts of New England, and the excess in Boston, where disinfection is practiced, has been greater than in Providence. Still another test of the danger from the omission of disinfection is the extension of the disease to other families in the same house. Of 2592 such families with susceptible children only 19 or 0.73 per cent were invaded by the disease within two months after the termination of isolation in the non-disinfected apartment. It may be suggested that, though no official disinfection was practiced, the houses were perhaps thoroughly cleansed by the occupants. I must confess that I hoped that the abandonment of official disinfection would cause people to do more cleansing for themselves, but there has thus far been little improvement, and as a large part of our diphtheria occurs among poor and ignorant people, many of whom are recent immigrants, house cleaning by the family can scarcely be expected to be very efficient at present. It appears, then, that this experiment shows that house infection in diphtheria is in Providence a negligible factor in the dissemination of the disease.

Disinfection Unnecessary after Scarlet Fever. — So similar, from an epidemiological standpoint, are scarlet fever and diphtheria that I have been gradually abandoning disinfection after the former disease also. The following shows the recurrences where there was and where there was not official disinfection.

The first table shows the number of recurrences within 60 days after disinfection for scarlet fever, the number of infected families, and the rate of recurrence during the years 1904–09.

Year.	Infected Families.	Recurrences.	Ratio.
1904..........	868	12	1.38
1905..........	298	2	.67
1906..........	398	9	2.26
1907..........	540	8	1.48
1908..........	273	3	1.09
1909..........	52	3	5.77
Total.......	2429	37	1.52

During the last four years the recurrences where there was no disinfection were as follows:

Year.	Infected Families.	Recurrences.	Ratio.
1908..........	40	1	2.50
1909..........	377	10	2.65
1910..........	389	5	1.29
1911..........	434	4	.92
Totals......	1240	20	1.61

As in diphtheria so in scarlet fever the infection of well persons who return to the house after the termination of isolation may perhaps be a measure of the value of terminal disinfection. In Providence, during the years 1887–89, of 1816 persons, mostly under 14 years of age, who had never had scarlet fever, and who returned home after disinfection, 33, or 1.8 per cent, developed the disease. Of 207 persons who, since 1908, have returned to non-disinfected houses, 3, or 1.4 per cent have contracted scarlet fever. During the years 1908–10, of 138 persons so returning none were attacked. The only apparent recurrences were in 1911.

Again one may examine the recurrences in other families in the same house. Of 1329 such additional families in 1904–08 there was recurrence within two months after disinfection in 21, or 1.6 per cent. Of 1005 families in 1909–11, living in houses where there had been no disinfection, there were recurrences in 15, or 1.5 per cent.

A further comparison showing the results with and without disinfection can be made with the data from Baltimore. To make these comparable to the Providence figures there have been included, in the latter, recurrences in other families in the same dwelling. The ratio is calculated on the number of cases instead of on the number of families as in the table next preceding.

BALTIMORE. DISINFECTION.

YEARS.	Cases.	Recurrences.	Ratio.
1903–09.......	5792	84	1.44

PROVIDENCE. NO DISINFECTION.

YEARS.	Cases.	Recurrences.	Ratio.
1908–11.......	1801	31	1.72

The health commissioner of Buffalo [1] reports, as illustrating the efficacy of disinfection, that after 3029 cases of scarlet fever where terminal disinfection was practiced and tested, there were 117 recurrences, or 3.8 per cent.

Disinfection Unnecessary in Other Diseases. — In any disease which is widely distributed, and in which there is ample opportunity for extension from mild cases, from carriers, from cases in the early stages, and from convalescents, the absolute disinfection of all possible fomites at the assumed termination of the sickness will probably have no influence in checking the disease. Thus I can see no use in disinfecting after measles, whooping cough, influenza, pneumonia or cerebro-spinal meningitis, and I think that this

[1] Rep. Dept. of Health, 1909, 20, 44.

view is held by the majority of our health officers and epidemiologists. In fact it is the expressed opinion of most health officers that disinfection after measles is unnecessary, as there is no evidence that fomites are a factor in the spread of the disease. Disinfection after measles, which was practiced in Aberdeen for twenty years, had no influence on the prevalence of the disease. When official disinfection after measles was temporarily suspended in New York from January 10, 1908, to March 1, neither the suspension nor the resumption of the practice appeared to have any effect on the epidemic curve. Disinfection after cerebro-spinal meningitis is also absurd, as the meningococcus lives only a few hours, and carriers are almost the sole means by which this disease is spread. This is coming to be the accepted view and in a recent publication of the U. S. Public Health Service [1] Frost makes no mention of terminal disinfection among prophylactic measures. Much disinfection after tuberculosis is also without reason. If a patient has been living with his family and taking no precautions, certainly no amount of terminal disinfection will atone for long-continued sanitary sin. If precautions are taken, the phthisiologists tell us that there is no danger in living with the patient, and if so, certainly there can be no possible danger in living in his house after he is dead. The only occasion for disinfection after consumption, then, is when the apartments of a careless patient are to be occupied by another family, and, after all, we have no evidence to show how much danger there is even then. Yet many health officers make disinfection after every death from consumption the first and often the only measure taken to restrict tuberculosis.

Dr. William C. Woodward of Washington in the discussion of a paper read before the American Public Health Association presented some figures which he believes indi-

[1] U. S. Pub. Health and Mar. Hosp. Serv., Pub. Health Rep., 1912, XXVII, 97.

cate that terminal disinfection after tuberculosis is a valuable prophylactic measure. He says that during a period of about two years ending in May, 1910, 1650 houses in Washington were disinfected because of tuberculosis. Subsequent to the disinfection there were reported from the disinfected houses cases of tuberculosis sufficient to give an annual attack rate of 223 while the attack rate throughout the remainder of the population was 414.

Even in smallpox there are bits of evidence to show that fomites play an unimportant part. Jordan [1] refers to two unvaccinated men who fumigated and handled infected smallpox clothing for two months without contracting the disease but who succumbed to it as soon as they came in contact with patients.

School Disinfection. — When a number of cases of scarlet fever or diphtheria develop in a school, the public is inclined to consider room infection the source and to demand "disinfection." This subject has lately, perhaps owing in part to the efforts of sellers of disinfectants, been much discussed in England, but fortunately the leading officials refuse to be influenced by public clamor. Among others, Kerr [2] has clearly set forth the reasons why the room can rarely be at fault in school outbreaks of the contagious diseases. In another place Kerr [3] reports 26 instances in which scarlet fever patients in the desquamating stage were found in school. In 2 instances the room was disinfected after their removal and in 1 of these a secondary case developed 9 days later. In the other 24 instances there were 2 secondary cases. Hope[4] says, "All evidence points strongly to the fact that when children contract infectious disease in school the channel of infection is not by means of school desk or floor but by the personal infection of another child."

[1] Jordan, Am. J. Pub. Hyg., 1910, VI, 755.
[2] Kerr, Pub. Health, Lond., 1909, XXIII, 49.
[3] Kerr, Rep. Med. Off. Education, Lond., 1909, 59.
[4] Hope, Rep. to Education Authority, Liverpool, 1909, 9.

French Views on Disinfection. — Recently,[1] at a discussion in Paris, Comby, Courmont and Lemoine took the ground that the active disinfection which has been insisted on in that city in recent years has not reduced the mortality from scarlet fever, diphtheria or measles, for which diseases it is required. Comby [2] is emphatic in his contention that it is persons, not things, that are the bearers of contagion. The same position was taken by *Semaine médicale* for February 14, 1906. Lemoine [3] has found disinfection not so essential as has been claimed. At the hospital at Val de Grâce certain rooms were used for isolating single cases of contagious disease. There was often such demand for their use that cases of different diseases quickly succeeded one another, sometimes without any disinfection and often with slight disinfection by washing the walls as high as could be reached. Sixty-five cases of scarlet fever, 41 of measles, 25 of mumps, 31 of diphtheria, 4 of smallpox, 1 of chicken pox and 136 of other diseases are reported as rapidly succeeding one another in these rooms. One case of measles and 4 of scarlet fever developed in the rooms. Often it was necessary to shift entire wards of twenty to thirty beds, with only a slight attempt at disinfection. This was done a good many times during nine years without bad results. We have had a similar experience at the Providence City Hospital where no attempt is made to disinfect the walls and ceilings of the cubicles in which different diseases rapidly succeed one another, and there has never been an instance in which infection could possibly be attributed to neglect of this rite.

English Views. — There is a growing tendency on the part of many English health officials to attach less importance to the part played by fomites in the spread of disease and consequently less value to terminal disinfection as

[1] Bull. et mém. Soc. méd. d. hôp. de Par., 1909, n. s., XXVII, 585.
[2] Comby, Presse méd., Paris, 1909, XXVII, 249.
[3] Lemoine, Rev. d'hyg., 1907, XXIX, 1057.

ordinarily practiced. Richards[1] does not consider disinfection of the room necessary, provided the floors are washed and things which came in contact with the patient are cleansed and disinfected. Butler, Barlow, Hogarth and others have expressed a growing belief that fomites play a comparatively unimportant part in the spread of disease. The views of Hope and Kerr are referred to above. The writer has received a number of letters from English and Colonial medical officers of health indicating agreement with the main proposition of this chapter.

American Views. — It is not, of course, to be expected that the majority of health officers would be willing to abandon terminal disinfection as now practiced. There are, however, very many of the most thoughtful, and at the same time most conservative, who agree that the present methods of disinfection should either be made really efficient or else given up. They are ready to admit that fomites are a far less important factor in the spread of disease than was formerly thought, but they think that even minor factors should if possible be efficiently controlled. A few health officers are willing to test the matter for themselves and have given up or are gradually omitting gaseous disinfection after scarlet fever and especially after diphtheria. The health officer of one important American city was trying gradually to abandon terminal disinfection until his progressive attitude was frowned upon by the state health officials. In Newton disinfection is not compulsory.

When Terminal Disinfection is Desirable. — When a new or rare disease invades a locality, it may at times be desirable to take extraordinary precautions to prevent its extension, which would be entirely useless if the disease were established. This, it is true, is not the popular or legal way of regarding preventive measures, but it is the scientific one. If a case of smallpox should occur in Providence,

[1] Richards, Pub. Health, Lond., 1909, XXIII, 42.

which has been free from it for several years, it would be worth while, perhaps, to expend considerable time and money in disinfection, even though the chance of infection from the room or goods might not be one in a thousand. But if there were hundreds of cases of measles in the city, it would be folly to go to the same trouble and expense for each case, even if the chance of infection were ten times as great. A spark in the dry grass should be stamped out at any cost, but it is useless to waste time in extinguishing the smoldering flames left here and there as the line of fire is sweeping across the prairie.

Objections to Disinfection. — There are several objections to the present practice of terminal disinfection. One is that it only partially disinfects. If disinfection is to be honestly and efficiently applied, methods must be changed. But even as now practiced, disinfection is expensive. Many cities employ disinfectors, with horses and apparatus, while their laboratory languishes, their medical inspection is poor and their diphtheria patients must secure antitoxin as best they can. Another serious objection to routine terminal disinfection is that it misleads the public. They are given a false sense of security, and they are encouraged in the old belief that it is things, not persons, which are dangerous. We can never successfully preach the truth about carriers, or teach the necessity for stricter personal cleanliness, so long as we continue to make so much of a fetish of the practice of disinfection.

Cleanliness versus Disinfection. — I am here referring to terminal disinfection, which is often only a fumigation, or smell-producing process. The continued practice of cleanliness all through the sickness, and indeed at all times, by which the transference of fresh infective material may be prevented, is another matter, the value of which was considered in the preceding chapter.

Conclusions. — It seems to me, in view of the considerations here presented, that we are justified in concluding that,

1. There is no good epidemiological evidence that any diseases except those due to spore-forming bacteria are to any great extent transmitted by fomites.

2. Judging from our experience with yellow fever most of the alleged evidence of infection by fomites is not to be relied upon.

3. Even if all the alleged fomites infection is real, only a very small part of contagious disease is traceable to this source.

4. The theory of fomites infection was an *a priori* not an *a posteriori* theory, and is no longer demanded.

5. Other modes of transmission so much more satisfactorily account for the spread of disease, that there seems to be really little opportunity for infection by fomites.

6. Laboratory investigation shows that fomites infection with spore-forming bacteria is common; that such infection in typhoid fever, tuberculosis, diphtheria and with other resistant organisms doubtless sometimes takes place; that it is possible in cholera and plague, while such infection in gonorrhea, influenza, cerebro-spinal meningitis and pneumonia must be practically impossible.

7. Experiment and epidemiological observation have demonstrated that fomites infection is practically unknown in yellow fever and is probably so in the other diseases carried by flying insects.

8. Experiment and observation show that fomites are of little moment in the diffusion of bubonic plague, and of no moment in the extension of Mediterranean fever, both formerly believed to be spread in this way.

9. Observations made in Providence indicate that fomites infection is of no practical importance in the diffusion of diphtheria.

10. Observations in Providence indicate that fomites are of no practical importance in the diffusion of scarlet fever.

Finally, it may be affirmed that the evidence has been rapidly accumulating that fomites infection is of very much less importance than was formerly believed.

CHAPTER VI.

INFECTION BY AIR.

Reasons for Former Belief. — From time immemorial the air has been considered the chief vehicle of infection. This was but natural, for until recently the virus of the infectious diseases was believed to be gaseous, or at least readily diffusible, and readily borne by air currents. The infective material was supposed to be given off in the expired breath, and to emanate from the surface of the body and from moist soil and decomposing matter of all kinds. Contagious diseases were known to arise without any apparent connection with other cases, and what could be more natural than to assume that the invisible, imponderable *materies morbi* is mixed with and carried by the air? Moreover one of the most widespread and best known diseases, malaria, was shown by a great mass of clinical evidence to be an air-borne disease, and yellow fever, another infectious disease of great importance, was also on good grounds believed to be transmitted in the same manner. What seemed to be well established for these two diseases was assumed on much more slender evidence to be true of most, if not all, the infectious diseases. It is true in a certain sense that the two diseases just mentioned are air-borne, that is, they are transmitted by small insects, which "diffuse," as it were, from their breeding places and are readily wafted by air currents. It is not in this sense that the term air-borne is used in this chapter, but the inquiry here made is whether the virus of the infectious diseases is borne by the air, either free or attached to small particles of inanimate matter.

Then, again, the first symptoms of measles, and often of influenza, are connected with the nose, diphtheria appears to be a throat disease, while consumption and pneumonia infect the lungs. What is more natural than to assume that the air which bathes these parts is the vehicle of infection? But since it has been shown that the pneumococcus is constantly found in the blood in pneumonia, and has been demonstrated before the initial chill, and since tubercle bacilli readily reach the lungs through the circulation, the force of this argument is lost.

Omitting the insect-borne diseases, let us see first what epidemiological evidence there is that the contagious diseases are air-borne.

Smallpox Air-borne from Hospitals. — Smallpox is believed to be more widely air-borne than is any other disease. The modern doctrine of the aerial transmission of smallpox received its greatest support from the investigations of Power[1] in 1881 concerning the conditions about the Fulham Hospital in London. That smallpox could be carried by the air long distances had been claimed by many before that time, for Dr. Waterhouse of Cambridge, more than one hundred years ago, believed the disease had been wafted across from Boston to Charlestown, though later he was inclined to deny this mode of transmission. Power showed that smallpox had not prevailed to any extent in the vicinity of the Fulham Hospital before the hospital was opened, and that on a number of occasions soon after it was occupied by a considerable number of patients the disease began to develop in the neighborhood. Furthermore he showed that there was a progressive decrease in the amount of smallpox as the distance from the hospital increased, the alleged influence of the hospital extending to at least one mile. It was furthermore shown by the doctor that this distribution of the disease was uniform in every direction from the hospital, that is, in every quadrant of the circle surrounding it. Later investigations at this hospital yielded similar data.[2] Smallpox almost always developed in the vicinity whenever the hospital was occupied by from

[1] Rep. Med. Off. Loc. Gov. Bd., Lond., 1880–81, X, Supl. 302.

[2] Rep. Med. Off. Loc. Gov. Bd., Lond., 1884–85, XIV, 55, 1885–86, XV, 111.

eighty to one hundred acute cases. But on one occasion, at least, there was no outbreak even when the hospital was fully occupied. The conclusion was that when a considerable number, eighty to one hundred, acute cases of smallpox are gathered in a hospital, there is great danger that the virus of the disease will be carried by the air a mile or more from the hospital in quantity sufficient to infect persons at that distance. Power considered that the hospital was thus the focus of infection on one occasion when there were only twenty patients, and at another time when there were only nine, of which five were acute. It was thought, from a study of the conditions at the time of the outbreak, that the dissemination was favored by still, damp weather. A somewhat similar though not generally so well defined or nicely graded distribution of smallpox around hospitals was believed by many to have been demonstrated in the cases of the Homerton, Deptford, and Hempstead hospitals. It was natural that twenty-five years ago, when knowledge of modes of infection was far more vague than at the present time, and with such evidence at hand, the officers of the Local Government Board should have been firmly convinced of the importance of aerial transmission in the spread of smallpox, and that this opinion should have been shared by many medical officers of health. Subsequent to the investigations referred to above, outbreaks due to the spread of this disease from hospitals are said to have occurred, among other places, at West Ham, 1884–85,[1] Nottingham, 1887–88,[2] Oldham, 1888 and 1892,[3] Warrington, 1892–93,[4] Bradford, 1893,[5] Liverpool, 1902–03,[6] and in Gates-

[1] Rep. Med. Off. Loc. Gov. Bd., Lond., 1886–87, XVI, 97.

[2] Whitelegge, Practitioner, Lond., 1888, XLI, 65.

[3] Report on the Health of Oldham, 1892, by Niven; also Niven, Pub. Health, 1892–93, V, 324, 366.

[4] Gornall, Rep. on the Epidemic of Smallpox in the years 1892–93 in Warrington, 1885, 111.

[5] Evans, Brit. M. J., Lond., 1894, II, 356.

[6] Reece, Special Rep. Loc. Gov. Bd., Lond., No. 208, 1905, Smallpox in Liverpool.

head and Felling, 1903–04.[1] In Glasgow[2] Chalmers states that smallpox seemed to develop around the hospital when it contained many patients, but that this did not invariably occur. When the hospital was removed to another location, it again appeared to be a focus of disease. Much has been made of the alleged aerial transmission of smallpox from the ships lying in the Thames below London and used for the reception of cases of that disease from the metropolis. Buchanan[3] and Thresh[4] attempt to show that after the ships were brought into use the disease was carried by the air to the Essex shore at Purfleet and West Thurrocks in the Orsett Union. It is true enough that the incidence of the disease was very great in these districts, but it is difficult to understand why it is not as well explained by contact infection, as were hundreds of similar outbreaks in England and the United States. The chief evidence on which the theory of aerial infection is based is the existence around the hospital, in every quadrant, of a graduated incidence of the disease. No such evidence is presented in this instance, and the area of infection attributed to the ships lies only in one direction from them. Smallpox appeared on the shore nearest the ships, and then gradually extended to a distance of two or three miles. This sort of extension is just what would be expected in contact outbreaks. If air-borne, the near and distant communities should have been affected at the same time. It was claimed by Dr. Thresh that the influence of the ships could be noted at a distance of four or five miles. It was also claimed that several vessels anchored near the hospital ships developed smallpox twelve days later. That ships leaving London during the period of the extensive out-

[1] Buchanan, Special Rep. Loc. Gov. Bd., Lond., Smallpox in Gateshead and Felling, 1904.

[2] J. Royal San. Inst., 1905, XXVI, 212, and Tr. Epidemiol. Soc., Lond., 1904–05, n. s., XXIV, 151, 244.

[3] Rep. Med. Off. Loc. Gov. Bd., Lond., 1902–03, XXXII, 81.

[4] Thresh, Tr. Epidemiol. Soc., Lond., 1902, n. s., XXI, 101.

break in that city should occasionally carry smallpox with them is not remarkable. Finally it was admitted that surreptitious communication with the ships occasionally occurred.

Aerial Convection Denied by Some. — Many sanitary officials did not, and do not, accept these conclusions, and numerous instances are given where the disease has not extended from hospitals. Thus Renney[1] says that in 1883–84 he saw 300 cases of smallpox treated in wards which were situated between twenty and two hundred and twenty-four feet of other hospital wards, schools and houses, without any extension, though only the school was protected by vaccination. At another time he saw a considerable number of cases cared for without harm in a ward from forty to one hundred and thirty-eight feet from other occupied buildings. So Wilson at Rugby[2] had a hospital within a few yards of a much frequented road with no untoward results. At many other times he has seen smallpox hospitals maintained in close proximity to other occupied buildings without aerial transmission resulting. Boobbyer[3] treated 20 cases near a highway where a thousand workmen passed daily, and not a case was contracted from them. Ker[4] at Edinburgh had a smallpox hospital in connection with a general hospital, and close to other institutions, and with a population of 3000 persons living within a mile circle. There were only 4 cases within this circle, of which 2 were known to be contracted elsewhere. Dr. Thorne Thorne[5] stated that in two instances only had he seen evidence of the aerial extension of smallpox from a hospital, namely, at Maidstone and at Stockton, while he had seen numerous instances where there was no extension, notably at Leeds and Nottingham.

[1] Renney, Jour. Roy. San. Inst., 1905, XXVI, 210.
[2] Wilson, Brit. M. J., Lond., 1905, II, 630.
[3] Boobbyer, Tr. Epidemiol. Soc., Lond., 1905, n. s., XXIV, 219.
[4] Ker, Tr. Epidemiol. Soc., Lond., 1905, n. s., XXIV, 174.
[5] Thorne Thorne, Rep Med. Off. Loc. Gov. Bd., Lond., 1880–81, X, Supl. 40.

At Manchester Niven[1] reported only 13 smallpox cases out of a population of over 40,000 living within a half mile to a mile area around the hospital and none among the 606 persons living within the half-mile circle. Other instances can be given where smallpox hospitals have not infected their neighborhood, and these facts should have some weight, though according to the advocates of the theory aerial transmission is to be expected only under certain conditions of the atmosphere. There is not much evidence bearing upon this subject to be obtained in the United States, partly because smallpox hospitals have been much more rarely situated in thickly populated districts and partly because less attention has been given to the subject here than in England.

American Evidence against Theory. — In Philadelphia it is claimed[2] that the hospital has been the source of smallpox in its neighborhood. Thus in one outbreak in the municipal ward in which the hospital was situated the case rate was 61 per 10,000, nearly twice that of any other ward, and it decreased as the distances from the hospital increased. The same conditions were noted in another outbreak.

In Boston in 1902–03 there was some discussion as to whether the disease spread from the hospital, which was on a busy street and near many occupied buildings. The evidence was that there was not much smallpox in the neighborhood, and also that contact infection from the hospital could not be excluded.

In New Orleans[3] a large number of cases of smallpox were in 1900 treated in a hospital in close proximity to a dense population, but without evidence of extension. Dr. Théard writes me that his observations, extending over nine years since that time, have only strengthened his views then expressed, namely, that smallpox virus is not carried from hos-

[1] Niven, Tr. Epidemiol. Soc., Lond., 1905, n. s., XXIV, 157.
[2] Rep. Bu. of Health, Phila., 1903, 29.
[3] Rep. Bd. Health of the City of New Orleans, 1900–01, 33.

pitals by the air. In Brooklyn smallpox is cared for at the contagious-disease hospital, in pavilions about twenty feet from those occupied by measles and scarlet-fever patients. There has been no extension of the disease, though this may be largely due to the effort to keep the other patients well protected by vaccination. But there is also a considerable population within a mile of the hospital which has never been injuriously affected by it. In Providence the smallpox hospital is distant only four hundred or five hundred feet from a number of cottages and an excursion ground frequented by hundreds of persons daily. It is true that only about a dozen patients have ever been there at one time, but it is hard to understand why ten patients should not be more dangerous at five hundred feet than one hundred patients a mile distant. In Detroit, Dr. Kiefer writes me, there has been no extension from the hospital, and in Chicago [1] there was less smallpox around the hospital than in other parts of the city.

Theoretical Objections. — I have been led to question this theory of the aerial transmission of smallpox for various reasons. From what is known of the nature of the virus of so many other diseases it seems highly improbable that they are carried any great distance by the air, and in fact it is only for smallpox that this mode of transmission is claimed. But smallpox virus is certainly solid matter, and it certainly after a time loses its vitality, and in all respects other than the one under consideration it behaves not unlike the *materies morbi* that we are better acquainted with. Again, it would be most remarkable, if the disease extends from, say, one hundred cases to the distance of a mile with sufficient intensity to infect many persons, that it should not extend one hundred feet from ten cases or even from one case. Why should we not expect aerial infection frequently to operate at short distances from single cases? Yet such transmission does not occur unless it be with great rarity. How rare it is for any claim to be made that this disease has been carried

[1] Rep. Health Dept., Chicago, 1907–10, 60.

across the street from house to house, and how unique a rigid demonstration of such an occurrence would be! How often a single case in a crowded lodging house, ship's steerage, or hospital ward, fails to infect others! Yet we are asked to believe that one hundred cases can give rise to a whole circle of cases a half mile away. Either the amount of virus must depend upon the number of patients, or it must under hospital conditions develop in some marvelous way outside of the body.

Contradictions in Claims. — If the evidence adduced in favor of this theory is examined, several suspicious circumstances are noticed. It is very curious that a material substance should be borne by the air without reference to air currents; yet in the earlier reports by Powers all evidence of such currents was lacking. It is true that in later reports the wind has been claimed as a factor, as at Gateshead and Felling, but the evidence in this case has been made valueless by more detailed search for the origin of the cases. At Liverpool the disease was distributed in different directions around the three hospitals, so that if air-borne it must have been independent of air currents. Savill at Warrington even claimed that the virus diffused against the wind. The reports of the Fulham Hospital give one the impression that the virus of smallpox must diffuse like a gas, which certainly is not thinkable. If air-borne at all, it must be carried as is dust or as are liquid particles. If the virus does diffuse in all directions like a gas, the intensity of the infection should diminish according to the square of the distance, which it did not do at Fulham and Liverpool. Whether it diffuses or is carried like solid particles, the houses nearest the hospital should be by far the most intensely infected. Solid particles are speedily, under ordinary conditions, precipitated to the ground, as one may easily note by observing a cloud of dust of any kind. The particles of smallpox virus ought, then, to work their chief havoc close to the hospital. Yet this incidence was not always the case, even at Fulham, and similar absence of near-by infection was noted at Stockwell[1] and Liverpool.[2] Again, quite a number of instances are given where large institutions, like schools, workhouses and general hospitals, have been located within the area alleged to have been severely infected from the hospital, and yet have nearly or entirely escaped. It is curious, too, that in the only instance I have noticed in which the sex of the patients in the infected area was given, namely Fulham,[3] twenty-four were male and seventeen female. As so many more men are away from their homes at work, a much larger female population must be exposed to the hospital influence, and the female patients ought to be more numerous than the male. In most outbreaks of smallpox the male patients are more numerous, because the men move about more, and are thus more likely to be exposed to cases of disease. Again, it is remarkable that extension should be more likely to take place from acute than from chronic cases. In the former it is probable that the moist mucous membrane is the only source of infection, while in the latter the dried crusts are known to be infectious.

Distribution of Cases Opposed to Theory. — It is thus seen that there are a number of facts and a number of theoretical considerations opposed to the theory of aerial transmission. That smallpox is distributed with decreasing intensity around smallpox hospitals is not a demonstration that the hospital is the cause, for as even the advocates of the theory admit, such circles of infection can be drawn around other points in a city during epidemic times, as was indeed shown by Hope in Liverpool in 1902–03 and Clayton at Gateshead in 1903–04. In fact most outbreaks, not only of smallpox but also of scarlet fever and diphtheria, are in a general way arranged around a center, with more cases toward the center

[1] Rep. Roy. Com., Smallpox and Fever Hospitals, Lond., 1882, 92.
[2] Hope, Observations by the Med. Off. Health on the Report of Dr. Reece on Smallpox at Liverpool. C. Tinling & Co., 1905, 11.
[3] Rep. Med. Off. Loc. Gov. Bd., Lond., 1880–81, X, Supl.

and fewer toward the periphery. It is not remarkable that occasionally a smallpox hospital is found near the center of such a localization of disease. As favoring this chance, it must be remembered that the population near a smallpox hospital is likely to be of the poorer classes, upon whom the weight of this disease most often falls. That surrounding outbreaks occur chiefly after the hospital has been occupied, is only to be expected, as the hospital is occupied by a number of cases only in epidemic times. Much stronger evidence would be offered by the advocates of this theory if they could show that no other explanation of the origin of the cases could be found than hospital infection. This they are not able to do, and in the absence of such evidence, and in the face of the evidence against the theory, the theory must be considered not demonstrated.

Cases often traced to Other Sources. — A good deal of evidence in regard to the influence of hospitals in the spread of smallpox was collected in England at a time when there was no registration of the disease, when the frequency and importance of mild cases were not recognized as at present, and when its administrative control was not so complete. Thus it was stated that many cases of smallpox walked to the Homerton Hospital to apply for admission, ambulance drivers stopped at public houses, children of the neighborhood rode on the steps of the ambulance and the patient's friends inside. It would not be surprising if, under such conditions, smallpox spread by contact—and indeed it was admitted that this was a factor. It is interesting to note that even Power found personal exposure the cause of nine out of thirty-two cases near Fulham. In many outbreaks, where there is no question at all of hospital infection, to trace the source of such a proportion of cases is all that can be expected. Again, in the block of houses nearest the same Fulham Hospital Dudfield [1] showed that twenty of forty-one cases were due to

[1] Dudfield, Rep. Roy. Com., Smallpox and Fever Hospitals, Lond., 1882, 101.

contact infection. According to Clayton,[1] the medical officer of health of Gateshead, of the fifty-six cases of smallpox within one-half mile of the hospital, on which Buchanan bases his conclusion that the disease was carried by the air, fifty-two were traced to contact infection. Clayton in his report on this outbreak very clearly shows the fallacy of most of the arguments presented by Buchanan. In Liverpool it was shown by the advocates of aerial transmission that within one-quarter of a mile of the Parkhill Hospital the rate of incidence of smallpox was five hundred and twenty-six per ten thousand houses, while in the city outside of hospital areas it was only eighty-five. A detailed study shows that this apparent high rate depended on only nine patients in one hundred and seventy-one houses, and Hope shows that of these nine, four were known to be due to direct exposure to other cases. A careful study of the report by Reece[2] of this Liverpool outbreak is well worth while by all interested in this subject. A most ingenious use has been made of the facts, but an impartial critic must see that the conclusions arrived at are entirely unwarranted. If one is still in doubt, he should read the report of Hope,[3] the medical officer of health of Liverpool, which clearly and briefly refutes all the arguments of the government inspector.

Conclusions concerning Smallpox. — It appears that the evidence for the aerial transmission of smallpox from hospitals consists solely of the alleged distribution of the disease, at a gradually decreasing rate, around the hospital, the existence of the cases being assumed to be otherwise unexplained. It will be noted:

1. That there are comparatively few instances of such distribution recorded.

[1] Clayton, J. Roy. San. Ins., 1905, XXVI, 199.

[2] Reece, Rep. Local Gov. Bd., Lond., No. 208, Smallpox in Liverpool, 1905.

[3] Hope, Observations by the Med. Off. Health on the Report of Dr. Reece on Smallpox at Liverpool. C. Tinling & Co., Liverpool, 1905.

2. That many instances are noted where there was no such diffusion.

3. That in some of the alleged instances, as at Fulham, Gateshead and Liverpool, a large number of the surrounding cases have been shown to be due to contact infection.

4. That in the long run the amount of infection around the hospital should diminish according to the square of the distance. This it does not do, but it diminishes irregularly, just as it does in most outbreaks of this and other diseases due to contact infection.

5. There may sometimes be contact infection from the hospital. The surrounding population is often of the poorer sort, and is consequently particularly subject to the disease. Contact infection and chance may be sufficient to account for those instances where a smallpox hospital is the center of a local outbreak.

The evidence in favor of the aerial transmission of smallpox from hospitals is so slight that it should never influence a municipality in its selection of a hospital site.

Chicken Pox. — Caiger,[1] while able successfully to isolate scarlet fever, diphtheria and whooping cough in his hospital wards by the cubicle system, had several transfers of chicken pox, and concludes from his experience that this disease is frequently air-borne. Others in England and in the United States have had difficulties in isolating chicken pox. Goodall,[2] however, has isolated this disease in cubicles with only 1 cross infection which he does not think was air-borne.

Scarlet Fever believed to be Air-borne.—Scarlet fever also is generally believed to be an air-borne disease. One reason for this is doubtless because until recently the desquamating epidermis was considered to be the chief vehicle of infection. As the epidermis comes off to a large extent as very fine light particles, it was but natural to assume that these would be

[1] Rep. Metropol. Asylums Bd., 1907, 1908.

[2] Pub. Health, Lond., 1911–12, XXV, 17.

readily carried by the air. Recently much clinical evidence has accumulated which indicates that the epidermal scales are not infectious, and this has in turn developed doubts as to the disease being commonly air-borne. Whether or not the epidermis is infectious, there seems to be no really good evidence that the disease is caused by air-borne infection. On the contrary, there is considerable evidence that it is not air-borne.

Scarlet Fever in Hospitals. — The writer, like every health officer, has frequently noted that a case of this disease may remain in school or hospital ward for days, or sometimes for weeks, without another case developing, or at most only one or two cases. Such facts indicate that the disease is not easily air-borne. Visitors to fever hospitals do not contract scarlet fever. Thus, of three hundred to four hundred non-immune students who visited the scarlet-fever wards of the Philadelphia hospital, remaining in the ward from twenty minutes to an hour, not one contracted the disease.[1] Oftentimes scarlet fever does attack other patients in hospitals, but it is in a manner to indicate contact rather than air-borne infection. When contact infection is rigidly guarded against, as in the Pasteur Hospital in Paris and in many English hospitals, scarlet fever may be, and is, treated in the same ward with other diseases without cross infection. The failure of contagious disease to spread in hospitals when contact infection is guarded against was referred to in some detail in the chapter on contact infection, and is a striking demonstration of the small part played by aerial infection in the transmission of the common contagious diseases.

Scarlet Fever in Dwellings. — I have been much impressed by the fact that scarlet fever and likewise diphtheria do not extend from one family to another in the same house. Most people in Providence live in houses of two or three stories, rarely more, with one or two families on each floor. Of 4306

[1] Welch and Schamberg, Acute Infectious Diseases, Phila., 1905, 346.

"other families" living in the same house with scarlet-fever families, only 6.8 per cent were invaded. Investigation has shown that with very few exceptions the infection takes place through close intercourse before the disease is recognized or, more rarely, after the isolation has been terminated. Most of the disease in the "other families" develops within a few days after the report of the primary case, and is doubtless due to contact infection before the disease is recognized. Between the end of the second week and the termination of isolation, the disease extends to other families in the house in only 0.6 per cent of the cases, and in most of these it is known that isolation is not carried out, and that there is free intercourse between the families. If the disease were air-borne, it would certainly pass from one family to another in the house, which it does not do.

Scarlet Fever and Outdoor Air. — If scarlet fever is not air-borne from family to family in the house, one would not expect it to be borne from house to house by the air. Yet such a claim is sometimes made, and even that the virus of the disease may thus be transmitted a considerable distance. A number of the reports of the health department of Philadelphia contain shaded maps purporting to show an excess of this disease, as well as of smallpox, in those parts of the city near the hospital. I do not think that much value attaches to such maps, for there are too many factors involved, and very rarely is the intensity of the disease as great close to the hospital as the theory demands. Moreover, around very many hospitals no such distribution of the disease can be shown. Thus Tarnissier,[1] in Paris, found that the Enfants Malades and Trousseau hospitals could not be considered foci of infection. The same is true of the scarlet-fever wards in Providence, in Detroit and in Boston. In the latter city,[2] for the period studied, there were no cases of the disease within one-eighth of a mile of the hospital, while in the next

[1] Tarnissier, Semaine méd., 1903, 267.

[2] Med. and Surg. Rep., Bost. City Hosp., 1897.

eighth of a mile circle there were sixty-eight cases, in the next seventy-one, in the next seventy-five and in the next seventy-two.

Where various contagious diseases are treated in different wards of the same hospital there is sometimes cross infection. But this occurs so irregularly as to time and place, and is so limited in amount, that it can scarcely be attributed to anything but contact infection. As most of the physicians and nurses in our contagious hospitals have no appreciation of what true medical asepsis really means, it is surprising that we see as little cross infection as we do. If scarlet fever does not spread within the walls of the Pasteur Hospital, it would indeed be marvelous if it should extend to the neighboring houses. If it does not pass from family to family in the same house, it would be most surprising if it could be wafted by the air over large areas around the Philadelphia Hospital.

Diphtheria and Sewer Air. — Diphtheria was formerly believed to be a filth disease, and it was also believed that air, especially sewer air, was frequently the vehicle of infection. Graham-Smith refers to this,[1] and shows that there is no foundation for this belief, and that diphtheria bacilli have never been found in sewer air. He says that Shattock cultivated bacilli of low virulence in sewer air for two months, but could not thereby increase their virulence. As I was, years ago, prejudiced in favor of the filth origin of this disease, I gave the matter careful consideration in my investigation of cases, but was never able to find any evidence that sewer gas was an etiological factor. Indeed my observation of diphtheria and typhoid fever had as much to do with my discarding the filth and sewer-gas theories as had the slowly accumulating mass of bacteriological evidence.

Diphtheria in Hospitals and Dwellings. — From an epidemiological standpoint diphtheria and scarlet fever are much alike. As the latter disease has been supposed to be air-

[1] Nuttall and Graham-Smith, The Bacteriology of Diphtheria, Cambridge, 1908, 321.

borne from person to person, so has the former, and there is the same lack of positive evidence for both diseases; and the evidence against the theory is much the same for diphtheria as for scarlet fever. As is stated by Graham-Smith, bacteriological evidence is all against diphtheria being an air-borne disease except in rare instances, yet probably most medical men and most health officers consider that the disease is commonly spread in this way. But visiting students in hospital wards do not contract it, and it does not spread when cases of this disease are treated in pavilions together with other diseases. In Providence I am certain, from a careful study of about eleven thousand cases, that it practically never extends from one family to another in a house except by personal contact; and it does not extend from one hospital ward to another through the air. At North Brother Island in New York there is a diphtheria ward only a few feet from a tuberculosis ward, and Dr. S. A. Knopf tells me that there is no cross infection. Similar conditions are noted in many other hospitals. Yet Coutts[1] recently suggested, without any evidence, that certain cases of diphtheria were due to street dust, and Cornell[2] attempted to show that the development of the disease in a certain locality in Philadelphia was due to air-borne infection. At best there was in the instances reported by the latter only a possibility of aerial infection, with the probabilities very much against it, while the facts as stated did point very strongly to the existence of unrecognized cases probably spreading the disease by contact.

Typhoid Fever and Sewer Air. — During the heyday of the sewer-gas theory of disease, numerous outbreaks of typhoid fever were supposed to have been traced to infection by means of air from sewers and drains. A number of typical reports are given by Roechling,[3] and others may be found scattered through medical literature. In none of these is real

[1] Coutts, Pub. Health, Lond., 1906–07, XIX, 297.
[2] Cornell, N. York M. J. [etc.], 1905, LXXXII, 1318.
[3] Roechling, Sewer Gas and Health, Lond. & N.Y., 1898, 30.

proof given that the disease was thus caused; it was merely a plausible hypothesis. Now in the light of present-day knowledge of bacteria and sewer air it is no longer a plausible hypothesis. For years past we have been able to trace most of our outbreaks of this disease to water, milk, oysters or other food, or to contact infection. In most instances they could not be due to sewer air. Usually investigation shows that house or institution outbreaks cannot possibly be due to sewer air, and where such an hypothesis is permissible, it usually appears highly improbable. I see almost every year small house outbreaks of typhoid fever. There is rarely any evidence of the escape of drain air into the house, and in almost all instances such escape is impossible. Most of these house outbreaks indicate contact infection, and in none can contact infection be excluded. I have never seen the slightest evidence that typhoid fever is ever due to sewer air, though I began my public-health work with a fairly strong belief in the danger from this source and sought diligently for evidence of it.

Typhoid Fever and Dust. — It is also claimed that infected dust may be the cause of outbreaks of this disease. This mode of infection was considered to be of some moment in the Spanish-American and Boer[1] wars, and certainly bacteriological evidence points to its possibility. Many outbreaks supposed to be due to dust infection have been reported. Some of these are referred to by Germano[2] and Visbecq[3] and in the Report on Typhoid Fever in the war with Spain,[4] but if the original reports of these outbreaks are examined it will be seen that the evidence is very weak indeed. Because the houses

[1] Tooth, Brit. M. J., Lond., 1900, II, 1368; Tr. Clin. Soc., XXXIV, 1213.

[2] Germano, Ztschr. f. Hyg. u. Infectionskrankh., Leipz., 1897, XXIV, 403.

[3] Visbecq, Arch. de méd. et pharm. milit., Par., 1903, XLI, 536.

[4] Abst. of Rep. on the Origin and Spread of Typhoid Fever in U. S. Military Camps during the Spanish War of 1898, Wash., 1900, 215.

or apartments or barracks where an excess of typhoid fever appears are situated not far from a place where possibly infected feces are deposited, it is argued that the disease is caused by the wind blowing over the spot alleged to be infected. Quill[1] reports that typhoid fever was brought to a certain garrison in India by a company of five thousand Boer prisoners, many of whom were infected. The disease continued to spread among the prisoners for three months, until there were from six to eight hundred cases. Then it slowly appeared among the garrison, until there were twenty-four cases. It was supposed to be caused by dust blown from the latrines, though the possibility of fly-borne infection is mentioned; but an extraneous source, or unsuspected contact infection, is highly probable, though neither is excluded or even mentioned. Mewius[2] gives an excellent report of what he considers an air-borne outbreak, but it appears rather to have been due to contact infection, a typical outbreak of what Winslow calls prosedemic infection.

The fact that typhoid fever, dysentery and cholera[3] can be treated in a well-managed hospital without spreading to other patients is good evidence that these diseases are not air-borne under such circumstances.

Infantile Diarrhea and Dust. — Newsholme,[4] judging largely from the fact that the summer diarrhea of infants occurs with greater frequency during dry seasons, and in towns with poor scavenging, infers that it is due, to some extent at least, to the infection of milk and other foods by dust. This also is the view of Hope,[5] who states that in Liverpool in six Septembers with an average rainfall of 13.8 inches there were 373 deaths from diarrhea, while in four-

[1] Quill, Brit. M. J., Lond., 1902, I, 383.

[2] Mewius, Ztschr. f. Hyg. u. Infectionskrankh., Leipz., 1896, XXIII, 497.

[3] Woodruff, J. Am. M. Ass., Chicago, 1905, XLV, 1160.

[4] Newsholme, Pub. Health, Lond., 1899–1900, XII, 139.

[5] Hope, Pub. Health, Lond., 1898–99, XI, 435.

teen Septembers with 10.9 inches of rain the deaths numbered 573.

Influenza. — During the present pandemic of influenza, especially at its commencement, it was frequently stated that the disease was chiefly air-borne, and air-borne to great distances, even across the Atlantic. This view prevailed because the disease spread with such great rapidity, appearing on this side of the Atlantic at about the same time that it did in England, and developing almost simultaneously in a large number of localities. The subject has been thoroughly studied by Leichtenstern,[1] Parsons [2] and Schmid. The latter's observations were in Switzerland chiefly, where he had ample opportunity to study the outbreak in small isolated communities. His work is reviewed by Leichtenstern, who states that the disease never developed except after the advent of some stranger. Parsons studied the incidence of the disease on several thousand deep-sea fishermen and on four hundred offshore lighthouse keepers, and in no instance did the disease develop except as the result of contact with the sick or within two or three days after leaving shore. He says there is no evidence whatever that the disease is airborne. Leichtenstern studied the extension of the disease to distant countries, and found that all the evidence pointed to personal contact as the only factor in its spread. Thus careful epidemiological investigation is entirely in accord with the findings of bacteriology, for the weak resistance of the bacillus makes it difficult to understand how the disease can be carried by the air as readily as is often alleged. This feebleness of the germ renders it unlikely that influenza is a dust-borne disease. Of course it may spread by droplet infection, but the increased volume of the secretions, the persistence of the bacillus after recovery and the great number of carriers give such opportunities for contact infection that

[1] Leichtenstern, Nothnagel's Encycl. Pract. Med., Influenza, Phila. and Lond., 1905, 523.

[2] Parsons, Brit. M. J., Lond., 1891, II, 303.

it is hardly necessary to attribute much importance to aerial infection, as the term is generally used, or to fomites infection.

Poliomyelitis. — Hill,[1] from a careful study of this disease in Minnesota, was led to suggest the theory that this might be a dust-borne disease. He finds that usually outbreaks occur in hot, dry weather, and many cases had long exposure to dust infected with animal feces, especially those of the horse. Hill says that at Winona and some other places the disease ceased soon after the watering of the roads was begun. The fact that poliomyelitis occurs chiefly in the driest season of the year has led some others to accept Hill's proposition, and some have made similar observations as to the checking of outbreaks. Hillier[2] reports an outbreak at Stowmarket, Eng., brought to a sudden stop by the watering of streets. Experiments indicate that the virus has considerable resistance and may possibly be transported by dust. Landsteiner, Levaditi and Pastia[3] found that it was virulent after being dried thoroughly for 24 days. Neustadter and Thro[4] in at least one instance succeeded in causing the disease in a monkey by inoculating dust from a room occupied by a case of the disease. Fifty grams of dust were shaken up with 30 c.c. of water and 5 c.c. of the filtrate were used for the experiment.

Measles. — Measles is considered a typical air-borne disease, at least within doors, but the experience of the Parisian hospitals[5] shows that the danger of infection within wards decreases as the opportunity for contact infection is

[1] Hill, Northwestern Lancet, Sept. 1, 1909 [reprint].

[2] Hillier, Med. Off., 1912, VII, 78.

[3] Landsteiner, Levaditi and Pastia, Ann. de l'Inst. Pasteur, Par., 1911, XXV, 805.

[4] Neustadter and Thro, N. York M. J., 1911, XCIV, 614.

[5] Grancher, Cong. Internat. de méd., 1900, XIII, C.-r., Par., Sect. de méd. de l'enfance, 478. Moizard, Bull. et mém. Soc. méd. d. hôp. de Par., 1900, 3 s., XVII, 683. Martin, Rev. d'hyg., Par., 1903, XXV, 256; Bull. et mém Soc. méd. d. hôp. de Par., 1904, 3 s., XXI, 297.

lessened. Grancher was the first to avowedly disregard infection by air and to attempt to control the spread of disease by strict attention to medical asepsis. At l'hôpital des Enfants-Malades he did not at first use cubicles but merely wire screens or low partitions between the beds. During the 10 years when this experiment was going on measles was introduced 139 times and from these cases 115 cross infections resulted, less than one-third as many as occurred when attention was not focused on the prevention of contact infection. A suggestive instance is reported of a child with measles who remained for 24 hours in an open ward with many susceptibles, and it is stated that in the 3 cases which later developed there had been contact with the first patient, either direct, or by freshly infected fomites. At the Pasteur Hospital 126 cases of measles were cared for without a single cross infection. At the Providence City Hospital which was opened in March, 1910, many different diseases are cared for in rooms open most of the time into a common corridor as in the Pasteur Hospital, while other mixed cases are "barriered" in other wards, as described on pages 200 to 202. Up to September, 1911, 56 cases of measles had been admitted, with extension in only one instance to one child.[1] Since then there have been two small outbreaks which Richardson thinks were most likely not due to aerial infection but to some failure in technique. One of these outbreaks arose from a single case, though at other times several cases had been cared for at one time without extension. In this outbreak one of the cases was on a different floor from the infecting case. Rohmer[2] from his hospital experience at Cologne is satisfied that measles is not air-borne further than between adjoining beds.

English Hospital Experience. — Most English hospital superintendents who have tried cubicles and barriers do

[1] Richardson, Internat. Hosp. Rec., 1911, XV, 18.
[2] Rohmer, Jahrb. f. Kinderheilkunde, 1912, LXXV, 78.

not think that measles can be safely treated in this way because they consider it likely to be air-borne, or that is the explanation offered by some at least. Caiger,[1] Thomson,[2] Goodall,[3] Gordon[4] and Biernacki[5] may be mentioned as holding this view in regard to measles and chicken pox. All these and Crookshank[6] do not find that diphtheria is air-borne under the hospital conditions mentioned and uncomplicated scarlet fever usually is not. Caiger does not think that rubella and whooping cough are readily air-borne, while Thomson is inclined to think that they are. Biernacki agrees with Caiger as to rubella and also as regards whooping cough, if the beds are at least 12 feet apart so as to prevent droplet infection in coughing. Even then he usually employs a canopy as an additional precaution. Biernacki thinks that ring-worm is readily air-borne. This also is the view held by Cates from a study of this disease in schools.[7]

Just as this is going to press an article by Rundle and Burton[8] has appeared reporting two years' experience with a hospital ward at Liverpool in which a variety of infectious and non-infectious cases were cared for without any attempt at air isolation. In all, 668 persons passed through the ward, of whom 69 had scarlet fever, 40 diphtheria, 37 measles, 38 varicella, 9 whooping cough and 215 erysipelas. There were only 2 cross infections, 1 of diphtheria and 1 of scarlet fever. These authors believe that in hospital wards the " danger of aerial infection is to be disregarded for practical purposes."

[1] Caiger, Rep. Metropol. Asylums Bd., 1907, 1908, 258; Med. Officer, 1910, V., 76.

[2] Thomson, Rep. Metropol. Asylums Bd., 1908, 261; Med. Officer, 1910, V, 197.

[3] Goodall, Rep. Metropol. Asylums Bd., 1910, 257.

[4] Gordon, Rep. on Health of Manchester, 1908, 154.

[5] Biernacki, The Nursing Times, 1908.

[6] Crookshank, Essays and Clinical Studies, Lond., 1911, 134.

[7] Cates, Pub. Health, Lond., 1910–11, 226.

[8] Rundle and Burton, Lancet, Lond., 1912, I, 720.

Typhus Fever not Air-Borne. — As will be shown in Chapter VIII, it is quite probable that typhus fever is transmitted by insects exclusively. But whether this is so or not, the successful management of this disease in the same wards with other patients in Edinburgh, in Liverpool and in Mexico City indicates that it is not an air-borne disease.

Pneumonic Plague. — The extensive outbreak of plague in Manchuria in 1910 attracted much attention, since rodents, while perhaps furnishing the original infection, played little part in the extension, as it seemed to be spread almost exclusively from person to person. Kitasato,[1] if reported correctly, concluded that the disease could not be air-borne but is caused "by coming in close contact with plague victims and by sputa." That droplet infection is of great importance in this type of the disease cannot be doubted and was amply demonstrated by Strong.[2] In a preliminary note he reports experiments in which 15 of 39 plates held in front of coughing patients were infected with virulent bacilli. He says that the air throughout the ward was infected, though the experiments, as reported, do not seem to furnish proof of this. Respirators are said to have been used successfully in avoiding infection by physicians and others in close contact with the patients. No real evidence, however, seems to have been advanced to show that the disease was air-borne other than by droplets.

Infection by Air not Impossible. — Since the development of bacteriology, evidence has been accumulating to show that the air as a vehicle of infection is of less importance than was formerly believed. Very little evidence has been found in support of the theory and much against it. It has been definitely proved that some diseases are not air-borne and the evidence against certain others is very strong. While the tendency is thus away from air infection we must

[1] Kitasato, U. S. Pub. Health and Mar. Hosp. Serv., Pub. Health Rep., 1911, XXVI, 567.

[2] Strong, J. Am. M. Ass., Chicago, 1911, LVII, 1270.

be on our guard lest our generalization carry us too far. It may be a fact that most diseases are not air-borne, and yet further investigation may show that certain other diseases concerning which we are still in doubt may be usually transmitted in this way.

Winslow has recently been making some interesting experiments in New York concerning the presence of living streptococci in dust. He finds that certain types of streptococci characteristic of human secretions are found in a viable condition in enormous numbers in both house and street dust, notwithstanding the fact, which also has been demonstrated, that these bacteria tend to die off with great rapidity when thrown off from the body. Several observers in different parts of the country have recently noted the presence of streptococci in outbreaks of severe sore throat, and Winslow asks whether it may not be possible that street dust as well as indoor dust may be a factor in the spread of this affection.

Infection by Air at Short Range. — Most of the discussion thus far has related in large part to alleged extension of disease through the air from apartment to apartment, or from house to house, or from hospital to adjoining districts. Transmission over such considerable distances might be rare or even impossible, and yet nevertheless the air might be the chief vehicle in ordinary institution or family infection. That it is believed to be so is indicated by the common regulation that a wet sheet shall be hung before the door of the sick-room to prevent the escape of germs, by the wearing of caps by visitors and the disinfection of inaccessible portions of the room. If we ask the reason for this universal belief in the importance of air-borne infection, we shall find that it is based entirely on theory, and that there is no clinical evidence at all to indicate that such a mode of infection is of any great importance. What evidence we have indicates rather that infection by means of the air is of comparatively little importance.

Reasons for Belief. — The real reasons why people generally attach so much importance to this mode of infection are, first, the hearty belief in the general theory of aerial infection which has prevailed from remote antiquity, and, secondly, because infection so often takes place when there has not been any known contact. Contact is the most certain and obvious mode of infection, and other modes should not be assumed without good reason. The burden of proof rests on those who make the assumption.

Air and Aseptic Surgery. — The history of aseptic surgery is very suggestive in connection with the theory of air-borne infection. Lister at first unquestionably considered the air to be the chief source of wound infection, and this view for awhile dominated surgical practice. Then gradually more and more attention was given to contact infection, contact with instruments, contact with the patient's own skin, contact with the operator's hands. As danger from these sources was more and more perfectly guarded against, surgery became more and more successful and aerial infection was less and less dreaded. A successful surgeon of my acquaintance tells me that he can operate with as little wound infection in a tenement house as in the best operating room. Ochsner[1] says, "Air infection is not impossible, but practically no wound infection is to be considered except from contact." Most surgeons at the present time consider aerial infection of very little importance. Nevertheless it has been shown, as we shall see, that the air, even of well-constructed operating rooms, contains considerable numbers of living pus-forming bacteria. Yet they are usually not numerous enough nor virulent enough to infect, and unless there is some other source of infection the wound heals aseptically. Pus-forming bacteria are quite resistant, and are by far the most numerous and ubiquitous of all disease germs and more likely to be found in the air, and the fact that they generally fail to infect should give pause to any claim that the much less numer-

[1] Ochsner, Clinical Surgery, Chicago, 1902, 26.

ous air-borne germs of other diseases are the chief source of infection.

Sewer Air and Bacteria. — In this connection the relation of sewer air to the transport of bacteria should be referred to. Winslow [1] in a very valuable paper gives a brief history of the theories on this subject, and shows how the former ideas as to the great danger to be apprehended from sewer air gradually gave way before increasing knowledge of bacteria, and particularly after it was determined that these organisms are not readily detached from moist surfaces. From that time it was generally believed that sewer air had little or nothing to do with the extension of the infectious diseases. The subject, however, was reopened by Andrewes [2] and Horrocks.[3] The latter showed that under natural conditions *B. prodigiosus* and also the bacillus of typhoid fever might be carried by the sewer air long distances and escape at manhole and soil-pipe openings. Lewis [4] also showed that sewage bacteria could be found in the air passing over a sewage farm, and also in that blowing at low tide over a beach where sewage was discharged. Winslow by a series of careful experiments confirmed the work of Horrocks, but went further and determined the number of bacteria that are transported in this way. He found, as have others, that mechanical splashing may produce a slight local infection of the air in immediate contact with the spray, but such infection extends for only a very short distance and persists for not more than a minute or two. A careful quantitative study of the air of nineteen different plumbing systems in various parts of Boston showed that very few sewage bacteria are found in such air. These bacteria were found only four times in 200 liters of air,

[1] Winslow, Rep. to San. Com. Nat. Ass. Master Plumbers, 1907–09; Abst. Am. J. Pub. Hyg., Bost., 1909, V, 640.

[2] Andrewes, Rep. Med. Off. Local Gov. Bd., Lond., 1906–07, XXXVI, 183, and 1907–08, XXXVII, 266.

[3] Horrocks, Pub. Health, Lond., 1907, XIX, 495.

[4] Lewis, Scot. M. & S. J., Edin., 1907, XX, 487.

and then in the presence of mechanical spraying of sewage at the point of collection. To illustrate the paucity of dangerous bacteria in sewer air he says:

"In a surface water of good quality, like that of New York City, the colon bacillus can almost invariably be isolated from ten cubic centimeters. This means a slight degree of intestinal pollution, but experience has shown that the chance of infection from such a water is but slight; and we drink it without serious alarm. If one were to breathe for 24 hours the undiluted air of a house-drainage system, at any point not immediately infected by mechanical splashing, it appears that less than fifty intestinal bacteria would be taken in; for the daily consumption of air is about 10,000 liters, and in 200 liters I obtained negative results from air of this sort. In drinking New York water twice as many colon bacilli are ingested every day, for 1000 cubic centimeters is a small amount for daily consumption. So there would be less danger of contracting disease from continually breathing the air of a vent pipe, or of a soil pipe, except where liquid is actually splashing, than from drinking New York water."

Anthrax.— Some time since, while considering this subject, it occurred to me that anthrax ought to be air-borne more often than any other disease. The spores are extremely resistant, and are found in great numbers in hair, wool, etc., and the manipulation of these materials is quite likely to raise a considerable amount of dust. If this be so, and if floating germs are carried to the alveoli of the lungs, as is alleged, the pulmonary type of this disease ought to be very common. Formerly this seems to have been the case. According to the report of the Local Government Board,[1] of thirty-two cases occurring in the woolen industry of Bradford during nine months, twenty-three were of the internal type. Since then great effort has been made to eliminate dust as much as possible from the woolen and other industries in which dry

[1] Rep. Med. Off. Local Gov. Bd., Lond., 1882–83, XII, 98

infected material is handled. As a consequence, as stated in the last report of the factory inspector which I have at hand,[1] of four hundred forty-four cases of industrial anthrax in England from 1899 to 1907 only twenty-one were of the pulmonary type, and all of these twenty-one were in the dusty woolen industry. The disease is not nearly so common in the United States, owing to the fact that less infected material is imported, but of fifteen cases in Philadelphia two only were internal. Even now, under the best conditions, there must be considerable infected dust caused by opening and separating the bales, and the comparative rarity of the pulmonary type of the disease indicates that it is not very easily air-borne, though it appears almost certain that some cases develop in this manner. Furthermore, it appears that this disease may be transmitted by the air even out of doors. Legge states that he has seen two horses infected by feeding where the dust from the blower of a wool-sorting room was discharged, and Silberschmidt[2] reported a similar infection of eight out of twenty-two horses near a hair factory at Zurich.

Slight Evidence that Disease is Air-borne. — It is thus seen that clinical and epidemiological evidence of the spread of contagious diseases through the medium of the air is scanty. No proof of extension through the external air is presented for any important disease except smallpox, and this is far from conclusive. I have never seen any good clinical evidence that diseases are air-borne, even indoors. On the contrary, there is much evidence that this mode of infection is not a common one. The reasons for the widespread belief in the transmission of disease through the air seem to be entirely theoretical, and to have been developed simply because no other satisfactory explanation was at hand. Let us now consider laboratory and experimental evidence.

[1] Report Chief Inspector of Factories and Workshops, 1904, 49; 1905, 49; 1906, 38; 1907, 56; also Legge, Lancet, Lond., 1905, I, 841.

[2] Silberschmidt, Ztschr. f. Hyg. u. Infectionskrankh., Leipz., 1896, XXI, 455.

Bacteria not given off from Moist Surfaces. — Among the many new conceptions which resulted from the study of bacteriology, one of the most novel was that, contrary to all previous ideas, bacteria are not given off from and are not readily detached from moist surfaces or liquids in a state of rest. This was first shown by Tyndall and has been confirmed by Nägeli,[1] Buchner,[2] Wernich,[3] Huhs [4] and others.

When this became known, numerous experiments were undertaken to determine whether the expired air was free from germs, as in accordance with the newly discovered facts it should be. Tyndall was the first to show that bacteria are not found in expired air, and Gotschlich [5] cites a dozen or so workers, all of whom obtained only negative results from an examination of the expired air. According to Flügge,[6] Cadéac and Malet, Grancher and Gennes, and Müller were unable to find tubercle bacilli in the ordinary expiration of phthisical patients, and these early observations have been amply confirmed by others.

It has been shown not only that air currents are incapable of removing bacteria from liquids but also that such currents do not remove them from the surfaces of solids. Most materials which contain pathogenic bacteria, such as culture media, saliva, mucus, pus, excreta, etc., present, when dry, a somewhat hard and often glazed surface, so that it is not surprising that exceedingly strong air currents, even of sixty meters per second, do not remove the contained germs. This,

[1] Nägeli, Die niederen Pilze, München, 1877, 107, Untersuchugen in die niederen Pilze, 1882.

[2] Nägeli u. Buchner, Sitzungsber. d. Bay. Akad. d. Wiss., München, 7 June, 1879.

[3] Wernich, Virchow's Arch. f. path. Anat. [etc.], Berl., 1880, LXXIX, 424.

[4] Huhs, Ztschr. f. Tuberk. u. Heilstättenw., Leipz., 1906, IX, 396.

[5] Gotschlich, Kolle u. Wassermann, Handbuch [etc.], Jena, 1902, I, 171.

[6] Flügge, Ztschr. f. Hyg. u. Infectionskrankh., Leipz., 1899, XXX, 107.

according to Gotschlich,[1] has been demonstrated by Nägeli, Buchner, Wernich, Hamburger and Stern, and Flügge. Gotschlich says that Honssell found it impossible to detach bacteria from infected clothing.

Infection in Dust. — So firmly was the theory of aerial infection intrenched in the minds of men, that search was made for some other means than the expired breath by which bacteria might get into the air. It was very early found that many bacteria could withstand drying for considerable periods of time, and it was at once suggested that material containing disease germs might become dry and pulverized, and that the resulting infective dust might readily be transported by currents of air. Indeed Koch[2] was one of the earliest, as well as one of the strongest, supporters of this view.

Resistance of Bacteria to Drying. — If dust is a vehicle for the transport of the germs of disease, and bacteria are air-borne on or in bits of dust, or float as separate particles, they must withstand a considerable amount of drying. That some species do retain their vitality and virulence after becoming quite thoroughly dry, has been demonstrated. Systematic studies of the effects of drying and of light on different disease-producing bacteria have been made, and almost every germ has been examined from this standpoint by men particularly interested in working out its biological characters. In some instances, as, for example, the tubercle bacillus, the experiments and observations are very numerous. In the chapter on fomites infection, the resistance of the different pathogenic organisms to dryness and to light was considered. While some species were shown to have very little resisting power, the germs surviving for a few hours or a few minutes only, others, like the bacilli of typhoid fever, diphtheria and

[1] Gotschlich, Kolle u. Wassermann, Handbuch [etc.], Jena, 1902, I, 170.

[2] Koch, Mit. a. d. k. Gesundheitsamte, 1884, II, Trans. Sydenham Soc. Pub., CXX.

tuberculosis, may, when dry, retain their vitality for months. In addition to the general knowledge of the resisting power of bacteria, which has been accumulating, special and systematic attempts have been made to determine directly the chances of infection by air-borne dust.

Studies on the Drying of Germs. — Among the earliest work of this kind was that by Germano.[1] He employed room dust and different kinds of earth, which after sterilization were inoculated with cultures of bacteria grown in various media. He found that generally the bacteria perished sooner in room dust than in other materials, and that bacteria which, like the typhoid bacillus, might survive for months even when dried on clothing or solid material, would speedily die in a very short time in dust. After a large number of experiments he concluded that cholera, plague, typhoid fever, influenza and gonorrhea could not be dust-borne; that under certain circumstances, with strong air currents, streptococcus and the germs of pneumonia and of diphtheria might be air-borne, and that, besides the spores of anthrax and tetanus, many of the pus organisms, meningococcus and the tubercle bacillus, might be transported in dust. It is suspected that he did not employ the true coccus of cerebro-spinal meningitis, for recent workers are agreed that this bacterium has very weak powers of resistance. His results with the pneumococcus also are surprising, as this too is rather feeble.

Neisser[2] in 1898 made a careful study of the strength of air currents necessary to move dust infected with various pathogenic bacteria. He showed that currents of from 1 to 4 mm. per second are sufficient to transport room dust, and it was chiefly with such currents that he worked. He used from twenty to thirty drops of an agar culture mixed with 30 c.c. of sterile dust. He drew dust through narrow tubes in a rather complicated apparatus, and it appears that

[1] Germano, Ztschr. f. Hyg. u. Infectionskrankh., Leipz., 1897, XXIV, 403; 1897, XXV, 439; 1897, XXVI, 66, 273.

[2] Neisser, Ueber Lauftstaub-Infection, Inaug. Dis., Breslau, 1898.

the conditions were too far removed from the natural to render the results of much value. Neisser's conclusions were that diphtheria, typhoid fever, plague, cholera, pneumonia, are not dust-borne diseases, but that spores, most of the pus organisms, tubercle bacilli, and the germs of cerebro-spinal meningitis may be so carried. It will be seen that to a large extent he agrees with Germano, but it is to be noted, however, that his tests, like those of Germano, were all culture tests, except those for tuberculosis, in which alone animal inoculations were made. Besides such systematic work as that of Germano and Neisser, much has been done in the study of special diseases by men particularly interested therein.

Drying of Typhoid Bacilli. — Firth and Horrocks [1] found that the typhoid bacillus would live for 23 days in sand dry enough to be blown by the wind. Harrison and Harrison,[2] working in India, recovered the organism after 118 hours when kept in diffused light in very dry dust. Aldridge [3] moistened sand with urine containing typhoid bacilli on three successive days, and dried it on the fourth day, and blew it with a bellows over sterile bouillon. He recovered the bacillus on the 1st, 4th and 9th day thereafter.

Horrocks [4] showed that the micrococcus of Mediterranean fever would survive in dry soil for about 3 weeks.

Drying of Diphtheria Bacilli. — Flügge [5] says that diphtheria bacilli perish when dry enough to be blown about in dust. This is confirmed by Pernice and Scagliosi and Reyes.[6] Reyes found they would live for 14 days in dry sand.

Drying of Plague Bacilli. — Tidswell,[7] experimenting with dust of various kinds, could not recover the bacillus of bu-

[1] Firth and Horrocks, Brit. M. J., Lond., 1902, II, 936, 1094.

[2] Harrison and Harrison, J. Roy. Army Med. Corps, Lond., 1904, II, 721.

[3] Aldridge, Indian M. Gaz., Calcutta, 1903, XXXVIII, 249.

[4] Horrocks, J. Roy. Army Med. Corps, Lond., 1905, V, 78.

[5] Flügge, Ztschr. f. Hyg. u. Infectionskrankh., Leipz., 1895, XVII, 401.

[6] Cited by Germano.

[7] Tidswell, Rep. on Plague in Queensland, 1902, 67.

bonic plague after 11 days when the dust was dried under natural conditions, and it usually died within 3 or 4 days. When dried very slowly it lived about twice as long. Rosenau[1] found that this bacillus did not live in dried bone dust over 6 days, and he did not recover it from dry and sterile garden soil after 1 day.

Drying of Tubercle Bacilli. — More attention has been given to the tubercle bacillus than to any other pathogenic organism. Besides other experiments referred to elsewhere in these pages it may be mentioned that Kirstein[2] experimented with various kinds of dust, and could not find living tubercle bacilli after 8 days. The dust was artificially infected and exposed to diffused light. He thinks droplet infection far more important than dust infection. Cadéac[3] was unable to reduce sputum to dust until it had been dried 10 to 12 days, while the tubercle bacilli had nearly died out on the 6th day. Even when pulverized sputum is injected into animals, tuberculosis rarely develops, and it must be still rarer as the result of inhalation. Sticher[4] also and Beninde[5] found it difficult to demonstrate living bacilli in dried and pulverized sputum under natural conditions. Nevertheless most observers do find living tubercle bacilli in dust, though usually with weakened virulence.

Drying of Cholera Spirilla. — According to Germano, cholera spirilla may sometimes survive in dust for 3 days, but oftentimes they die in 1 day. He says that Honssell was never able to obtain living spirilla from infected dust, though Uffelmann was able to do so for a short period.

[1] Rosenau, U. S. Pub. Health and Mar. Hosp. Serv. Hyg. Lab. Bull. No. 4, 1901.

[2] Kirstein, Ztschr. f. Hyg. u. Infectionskrankh., Leipz., 1905, L, 186.

[3] Cadéac, Lyon Méd., 1905, CV, 893; also Lyon Méd., 1908, CXI, 532.

[4] Sticher, Ztschr. f. Hyg. u. Infectionskrankh., Leipz., 1899, XXX, 163.

[5] Beninde, Ztschr. f. Hyg. u. Infectionskrankh., Leipz., 1899, XXX, 193.

William[1] believes that cholera cannot be a dust-borne disease.

Tubercle Bacilli in Dust. — Of more practical importance than experiments with artificially infected dust is the determination of the presence or absence of disease-producing bacteria in supposedly infected localities. The chief interest in such investigations has centered in tuberculosis. Cornet[2] has made a more extensive study than any one else of the natural distribution of tubercle bacilli in dust. He examined 147 specimens of dust collected from hospital wards, dispensaries, private houses, streets, etc. No bacilli were found in the street or in places not occupied by the tuberculous, and even in the environment of the consumptive germs were found only when the patient was careless in the disposal of sputum. Cornet's observations have been confirmed by Rembold, Krüger, Kastner, Ballinger, Kusterman, Le Noir and Camus and Enderlin, besides others elsewhere referred to. Gotschlich[3] examined one hundred and nineteen specimens of dust from streets and public places and was not able to demonstrate the presence of tubercle bacilli. While most observers have been unable to find the tubercle bacillus in street dust, it is said to have been found by Manfredi[4] and Schnirer.[5] Prausnitz[6] and Petri[7] obtained tubercle bacilli from the dust in railway carriages, and Bissell[8] found them in tramcars in Buffalo.

[1] William, Ztschr. f. Hyg. u. Infectionskrankh., Leipz., 1893, XV, 166.

[2] Cornet, Ztschr. f. Hyg. u. Infectionskrankh., Leipz., 1885, V, 98; Nothnagel's Encyclopedia of Pract. Med., Phila. & Lond., 1907, Tuberculosis, 85.

[3] Gotschlich, Die Verbreitung der Tuberkelbacillen in Staub von Räumen mit starkem Menschenverkehr, Inaug. Dis., Breslau, 1903.

[4] Manfredi, Jahresb. u. d. Fortschr. . . . d. path. Mik., Baumgarten, 1891, VII, 570.

[5] Schnirer, Wien. med. Presse, 1891, XXXII, 3.

[6] Prausnitz, Arch. f. Hyg., München u. Leipz., 1891, XII, 192.

[7] Petri, Arb. a. d. k. Gesund.-Amt., Berl., 1894, IX, 76.

[8] Bissell, N. York M. J., 1895, LXII, 783.

Some observers have not found the bacilli so numerous as did Cornet. Thus Hill,[1] following Cornet's methods, obtained virulent bacilli in but 5 of 496 swabbings from private houses where there were cases of the disease, and in 3 of 180 swabbings from hospital wards.

Heymann[2] has criticised Cornet's findings on the ground that the latter recovered the dust by means of moist swabs, thereby perhaps taking up many bacilli which were attached to the floor, table, etc., and which would not therefore have any part in air-borne infection. He does not find living bacilli so numerous in dust as did Cornet. Heymann in 120 tests found them only one-third as often, but Coats,[3] following Heymann's methods, was able by inoculation tests to demonstrate the presence of tubercle bacilli in 66 per cent of specimens of dust obtained from fourteen rooms occupied by tuberculous patients. On the whole, it appears that virulent tubercle bacilli are quite commonly found in the dust of rooms occupied by careless tuberculous patients.

In this connection may be mentioned an experiment of Heymann's in which he rubbed and shook a sputum-infected handkerchief, after two days' drying, in a closed box, and found floating bacilli after the lapse of an hour.

Meningococcus in Dust. — Jaeger[4] claimed to have found the meningococcus on the floor of barracks, and Netter[5] the pneumococcus in the dust of a sick-room four weeks after the case was removed, but from what is now known of the resistance of these bacteria this is highly improbable. Washbourn and Eyre[6] found the pneumococcus in dust from a ward and laboratory at Guy's Hospital, but failed to find it in

[1] Hill, Am. Pub. Health Ass. Rep., 1902, XXVIII, 209.

[2] Heymann, Ztschr. f. Hyg. u. Infectionskrankh., Leipz., 1901, XXXVIII, 21.

[3] Coats, Trans. Brit. Cong. on Tuberculosis, 1901, I, p. 88.

[4] Jaeger, Deutsche med. Wchnschr., 1899, XXV, 472.

[5] Netter, Compt. rend. Soc. de biol., Par., 1897, IV, 538.

[6] Washbourn and Eyre, Lancet, Lond., 1902, II, 1440.

street dust. Washbourn says that it has also been found in dust by Emmerich, Maximowitch and Netter.

Diphtheria Bacilli in Dust. — These bacilli have been found in the dust of a scarlet-fever ward,[1] and are said to have been found in a diphtheria ward by Richardiere and Tallemer,[2] but Schlichter [3] could not find them in a hospital in Vienna. Cobbett [4] exposed plates in a diphtheria ward, but could obtain no bacilli except when the plates had been touched by the fingers of the patients.

Dust and Other Diseases. — There has been much discussion of late in England about the necessity for disinfecting schoolrooms, and examination of school dust has shown the presence of colon bacilli [5] and the pus organisms.[6]

General Conclusions. — While these facts relating to the resistance of disease germs to drying, and their presence in supposedly infected localities, afford no definite information as to the danger to be apprehended from infection by air-borne dust, they do lead to some tentative conclusions. It is scarcely possible that gonorrhea, influenza, cerebro-spinal meningitis and pneumonia can be dust-borne. It is possible, perhaps, but highly improbable, that plague and cholera can be so borne. The bacteriological evidence indicates that the germ of typhoid fever, dysentery, Mediterranean fever, diphtheria, tuberculosis and suppuration may be carried by floating dust, and it is certainly possible for anthrax and other spores.

Danger from Dust Slight.—Bacteriology also teaches what is often forgotten, that pathogenic bacteria, with the exception of spores, die off quite rapidly when dried, and that the survivors usually have a weakened virulence. If in a

[1] Renney, Pub. Health, Lond., 1905, XVII, 706.
[2] Richardiere et Tallemer, Gaz. d. mal. enfant [etc.], Par., 1899, X.
[3] Schlichter, Arch. f. Kinderh., Stuttg., 1892, XIV, 129.
[4] Cobbett, J. Royal San. Inst., Lond., 1904, XXV, 405.
[5] Hewlett, Lancet, Lond., 1909, I, 741, 815, 889.
[6] Kerr, Med. Off. Educa., Lond., 1908, 31.

sick-room or hospital ward the germs of disease are scattered so freely on the floor or room contents that enough of them can survive drying and pulverization to float in the air and cause disease, the opportunities for contact infection with the comparatively fresh infective material must be very great, so great, it seems to me, that infection by air under such conditions must be very insignificant or entirely negligible as compared with infection by contact.

Droplet Infection. — Another way in which living bacteria may be carried by the air is in tiny floating particles of liquid. Flügge[1] was the first to call attention to the fact that during speaking, and especially during loud talking, coughing and sneezing, tiny droplets of saliva are thrown off from the mouth. Indeed such droplets may be readily seen in the proper light, and it hardly needed special experiment to prove their existence. Nevertheless, Flügge[2] and Laschtschenko,[3] by infecting the mouth with *B. prodigiosus*, showed that germ-carrying droplets are, during coughing, borne to a distance of nine meters in front of the mouth. These droplet experiments have been repeated with confirmatory results by Goldie, Esmarch, B. Fränkel, Möller, Hübner, Weismayr and Königer, and the last mentioned has shown that the droplets may be found two meters behind the person coughing.[4] Goldie showed that in fourteen per cent of the cases tubercle bacilli could be caught on plates after a single act of coughing. Every patient examined at one time or another gave positive results. No bacilli were found, even as near as six inches, during deep breathing, but after coughing they could be recovered from all parts of the room.

[1] Flügge, Ztschr. f. Hyg. u. Infectionskrankh., Leipz., 1897, XXV, 179.

[2] Flügge, Ztsch. f. Hyg. u. Infectionskrankh., Leipz., 1899, XXX, 107.

[3] Laschtschenko, Ztschr. f. Hyg. u. Infectionskrankh., Leipz., 1899, XXX, 125.

[4] Königer, Ztschr. f. Hyg. u. Infectionskrankh., Leipz., 1900, XXXIV, 119.

Amount of Droplet Infection. — Since it has been shown by Flügge that droplets from speaking may float for from five to six hours, and be transported by air currents of only one mm. per second, it is not surprising that they should be carried such distances. Nor is it surprising that Hutchinson[1] was able to prove that a fine spray of a culture of *B. prodigiosus* was carried fifty-five meters along a corridor, and up two flights of stairs, and also a considerable distance out of doors. Others have shown that the bacteria of the mouth may be carried by the air during speaking over a large room or hall.[2] Leon[3] showed that in speaking three hundred words 250,000 bacteria were thrown off from the mouth, and Ziesché[4] found over 20,000 tubercle bacilli on a plate 324 sq. cm. exposed for half an hour. But it has further been shown by Kirstein[5] and Königer[6] and Laschtschenko[7] that the size of the droplets and the distance they can be carried depend to a large extent upon whether the liquid is thin and watery or a thick mucus. Hence we should expect that droplets of thick sputum would not be carried nearly so far as droplets of more liquid saliva, and according to Goldie[8] droplets of the saliva rarely carry bacilli but only the droplets of sputum.

Quantitative Experiments.—Since the above was written Winslow and Robinson[9] have published a very interesting

[1] Hutchinson, Ztschr. f. Hyg. u. Infectionskrankh., Leipz., 1901, XXXVI, 223.

[2] Gordon, Rep. Med. Off. Local Gov. Bd., Lond., 1902–03, XXXII, 421.

[3] Leon, Arch. f. klin. Chir., Berl., 1903–04, LXXII, 904.

[4] Ziesché, Ztschr. f. Hyg. u. Infectionskrankh, Leipz., 1907, XLVII, 50.

[5] Kirstein, Ztschr. f. Hyg. u. Infectionskrankh., Leipz., 1900, XXXV, 123.

[6] Königer, Ztschr. f. Hyg. u. Infectionskrankh., Leipz., 1900, XXXIV, 119.

[7] Laschtschenko, Ztschr. f. Hyg. u. Infectionskrankh., Leipz., 1899, XXX, 125.

[8] Goldie, Canadian Pract. & Rev., Toronto, 1899, XXIV, 433.

[9] Winslow and Robinson, Jour. Infect. Dis., Chicago, 1910, VII, 17.

paper on this subject giving an excellent résumé of previous investigations. They repeat the experiments of some of the European writers, and like them they find that if the mouth of a speaker is infected with a specific germ, as *B. prodigiosus*, agar plates exposed in different parts of the room show numerous colonies of the bacillus. They also, by the exposure of plates in the room with the speaker, recovered Gordon's *Streptococcus salivarius*, which is a normal inhabitant of the mouth. The authors emphasize the distinction noted by others between the larger droplets of mouth spray which contain the most bacteria and which settle out of the air in the space of a few feet from the mouth and the smaller droplets which float for a longer time and may pass to some distance from the speaker, and which alone may be considered as properly constituting an infection of the air. The chief interest in their studies attaches to their quantitative work carried out on the lines devised by Winslow for his investigations of sewer air. Out of 140 liters of air taken at various points in the room immediately after 10 to 50 minutes' loud speaking by a person whose mouth was infected with *B. prodigiosus*, the bacillus was found seven times. Of 74 liters examined for *Streptococcus salivarius* none were found to contain this normal inhabitant of the mouth. The authors consider that an artificial infection of the mouth may give too high an index of air contamination, while the normal germs of the mouth may be thrown off in smaller numbers than are the disease germs from sick persons. The authors conclude that these experiments furnish "no basis for a belief that tuberculosis or any other disease is contracted to an appreciable extent through the inspired air" and are "in harmony with the conviction now generally gaining ground that aerial infection of any sort is a minor factor in the spread of zymotic disease."

Lepra Bacilli. — Schäffer [1] was able to recover bacilli from a leprous patient by holding cover glasses a short distance in front of the face while the patient was speaking and coughing.

[1] Schäffer, Arch. f. Dermat. u. Syph., Wien, 1898, XLIV, 159.

Pneumococcus. — Wood [1] found that pneumococci did not retain their vitality in floating droplets over one hour, and not half an hour in diffused light.

Influenza Bacilli. — According to Gotschlich,[2] droplets containing influenza bacilli will float for five hours. Very little has been done to demonstrate the existence of infected droplets in any other diseases.

Bacteria found in Air. — Having shown that bacteria may float in the air on particles of dust and in droplets of liquid, we must next inquire whether pathogenic germs have actually been found in the air. Graham-Smith[3] examined the air of the House of Commons for pathogenic bacteria with negative results, as did Andrewes[4] and Gordon[5] the air in the streets of London. Little light is thrown on our present problem by these and similar negative tests of outdoor air or of air away from the vicinity of the sick. Far more interest and value attach to the examination of air in the vicinity of cases of infectious sickness.

Tubercle Bacilli in Air. — Heymann[6] was able to recover virulent tubercle bacilli from the air of a small chamber in which was placed a coughing tuberculous patient. Similar results were obtained by Laschtschenko.[7] Corbett[8] recovered acid-fast bacilli from the ventilating shaft of a hospital, but made no inoculation tests. Klein[9] infected guinea pigs by exposure in the vent shaft of Brompton Hospital. According

[1] Wood, J. Exper. M., N. Y., 1905, VII, 592.

[2] Gotschlich, Kolle u. Wassermann, Handbuch [etc.], Jena, 1902, I, 175.

[3] Graham-Smith, J. Hyg., Cambridge, 1903, III, 498.

[4] Andrewes, Rep. Med. Off. Local Gov. Bd., Lond., 1906–07, XXXVI, 187.

[5] Gordon, Rep. Med. Off. Local Gov. Bd., Lond., 1902–03, XXXII, 421.

[6] Heymann, Ztschr. f. Hyg. u. Infectionskrankh., Leipz., 1901, XXXVIII, 21.

[7] Laschtschenko, Ztschr. f. Hyg. u. Infectionskrankh., Leipz., 1899, XXX.

[8] Corbett, St. Paul M. J., St. Paul, Minn., 1904, VI, 735.

[9] Stevenson and Murphy, Hygiene and Public Health, II, 212.

to Cornet and Meyer,[1] Williams, Celli and Guarnieri, Wehde, and Baumgarten have examined air for tubercle bacilli with negative results. Recently Le Noir and Camus[2] demonstrated by inoculation tubercle bacilli in the dust of a hospital ward, but they could not obtain them by the filtration of even 53,000 liters of the air. Viewing the human nose as a filter, they took swabbings from the nose of physicians and attendants of phthisical patients, but could not demonstrate tubercle bacilli by inoculation, though they found them in the nose of the patients themselves. Cornet considers that the germs are so sparsely distributed that one ought not to expect to obtain them by the filtration of even 1000 liters of air. He says that the finding of tubercle bacilli in settled dust has as much bearing on air infection as finding it in the air and is a much easier operation. It does not appear that Cornet is correct in his contention that the examination of dust is of more practical importance than the examination of air. The examination of dust can throw no light on the number of bacteria floating in the air at any one time, and as Winslow in his work on sewer air previously referred to has so clearly pointed out, a quantitative examination of the floating bacteria is necessary if we wish to determine the real danger from the inhalation of the air. No such enumeration of tubercle bacilli seems to have been made, and the difficulty of finding them suggests that they are not very numerous, even in the vicinity of patients, and that perhaps the air of a room is not always dangerous to breathe even if tubercle bacilli can be found in the settled dust.

Pus-forming Bacteria in Air. — Numerous observers are referred to by Gotschlich,[3] Friedrich[4] and Noeggerath[5] as

[1] Cornet and Meyer, Kolle u. Wassermann, Handbuch [etc.], Jena, 1903, II, 143.

[2] Le Noir and Camus, Comp. rend. Soc. de biol., Par., 1908, LXV, 464, 622; Ann d'hyg. et de méd. colon., Par., 1908, 4 s., IX, 74.

[3] Gotschlich, Kolle u. Wassermann, Handbuch [etc.], Jena, 1902, I, 176.

[4] Friedrich, Arch. f. klin. Chir., Berl., 1898, LVII, 288.

[5] Noeggerath, Deutsche Ztschr. f. Chir., Leipz., 1900–01, LVIII, 277.

having found various pus-forming bacteria in the wards and operating rooms of the hospitals. Among more recent American writers may be mentioned Robb,[1] Rosenow,[2] Monks [3] and Harrington.[4] The latter found that Petri dishes exposed in an operating room in Boston always contained pus organisms. The maximum was 131 per square inch per hour. Gordon [5] found staphylococci in an operating room in England, also in a barber's shop, and they have been demonstrated in the air by Hamilton.[6] Gordon could not find them in the open air, but they have been found in the air of streets by others.[7]

Other Bacteria in Air. — Concornotti [8] reports that he found pneumonia germs in the air of the Hygienic Institute of Cagliari.

Beck [9] found swine plague bacilli in the air of a laboratory where experiments with that germ were being carried on.

Bruce [10] could not find the germ of Mediterranean fever in air-borne dust in Malta.

Actual Danger of Infection by Air. — Pathogenic bacteria may withstand drying and the pulverization of the dried material, and they may be actually found floating in the air, yet they may not after all be dangerous, either because they have wholly or partially lost their virulence, or because they are too few in number, or for some other unknown reason.

Little Infection of Wounds by Air. — It has been shown that notwithstanding the presence of considerable numbers

[1] Robb, Am. J. Obst., N. Y., 1909, LX, 451.
[2] Rosenow, Am. J. Obst., N. Y., 1904, L, 762.
[3] Monks, Ann. Surg., Phila., 1904, XL, 466.
[4] Harrington, Ann. Surg., Phila., 1904, XL, 475.
[5] Gordon, Rep. Med. Off. Local Gov. Bd., Lond., 1904–05, XXXIV, 387.
[6] Hamilton, J. Am. M. Ass., Chicago, 1905, XLIV, 1108.
[7] Newman, Bacteriology and the Pub. Health, Lond., 1904, 78.
[8] Concornotti, Centrlbl. f. Bakteriol. [etc.], Jena, 1899, XXVI, 492.
[9] Beck, Jahresb. u. d. Fortschr. . . . d. path. Mik., Baumgarten, 1891, VII, 567.
[10] Nature, Lond., 1908, LXXVIII, 40.

of bacteria in the air of operating rooms, the aerial infection of wounds is of no practical importance. One reason for this failure to infect has been shown by Friedrich[1] and Noeggerath.[2] The conclusion of these authors is that drying and exposure to light so weaken the bacteria that they are not able to withstand the actively hostile influences of the tissues of the human body, though they may be able slowly to vegetate on the more favorable culture media of the laboratory. This lowering of virulence by drying and exposure to light may be of great practical moment in preventing infection by air. So also, though other pathogenic bacteria may be demonstrated in the air, it may be that they are usually too few in number to infect.

Experiments with Tuberculosis. — The experiment of Bernheim,[3] in which he was not able to infect animals with mouth spray over 25 cm. from the mouth, but was able to collect tubercle bacilli on agar plates at the distance of a meter, is most suggestive of the importance of the number of bacteria as a factor in infection. The proper way to determine the infectivity of the air is by animal experiment or, better still, by carefully conducted observations on human beings. Except in tuberculosis very few experiments of this kind have been made. Much, however, has been done with that disease.

Tappeiner[4] had, even before the discovery of the tubercle bacillus, shown that tuberculosis could be produced in dogs by causing them to breathe dry and pulverized tuberculous sputum. Bertheau, Veraguth, Weichselbaum and Frerich, like Tappeiner, succeeded in infecting animals by causing them to inhale pulverized sputum containing tubercle bacilli, while Koch, Cornet, Gebhardt and Preyss accomplished the

[1] Friedrich, Arch. f. klin. Chir., Berl., 1898, LVII, 288.
[2] Noeggerath, Deutsche Ztschr. f. Chir., Leipz., 1900–01, LVIII, 277.
[3] Bernheim, Clinique, Brux., 1905, XIX, 346.
[4] Tappeiner, Virchow's Arch. f. path. Anat. [etc.], Berl., 1880, LXXXII, 353.

same results by the use of dried bacilli obtained from cultures. More recently Cornet [1] reports a still more striking experiment. In a room of seventy-six cubic meters capacity, 48 guinea pigs were exposed in cages at various heights above the floor. Sputum was placed on a carpet, and after it was dry the carpet was shaken so that the dust rose up in clouds. This was repeated on four days. The result was that 47 of the 48 animals developed tuberculosis within two months. Kuss [2] carried on experiments very similar to those of Cornet and with similar results. Köhlisch,[3] while admitting that tuberculosis may be caused by the inhalation of dust, claims that his experiment shows that enormously larger quantities must be inhaled than are necessary when a spray is employed. While *B. prodigiosus* is not pathogenic, it has been used by various workers for studying the penetration of bacteria into the respiratory tract. Nenninger,[4] using both infected dust and a sprayed culture, found that the germs were quickly carried to the smallest bronchioles.

Dust Infection Questioned. — The contention that pulmonary tuberculosis may be caused by the inhalation of dust containing tubercle bacilli was not to go unchallenged. Sirena and Pernice, de Toma, Celli and Guarnieri, and Cadéac and Malet were unsuccessful in their attempts to produce the disease in this way. But perhaps Flügge[5] more than any other has cast discredit on this theory of the origin of pulmonary tuberculosis. He was unable to induce infection by causing animals to inhale tuberculous dust, and states that the dust is not carried to the alveoli. He also developed the theory of droplet infection, which has been received with much

[1] Cornet, Verhandl. d. Berl. med. Gesellsch., 1899, XXX, 2 Th., 91.

[2] Kuss, Sixth Internat. Cong. on Tuberc., Wash., 1908, I, 101.

[3] Köhlisch, Ztschr. f. Hyg. u. Infectionskrankh., Leipz., 1908, LX, 508.

[4] Nenninger, Ztschr. f. Hyg. u. Infectionskrankh., Leipz., 1901, XXXVIII, 94.

[5] Flügge, Ztschr. f. Hyg. u. Infectionskrankh., Leipz., 1899, XXX, 107.

favor, and did much to break down the almost universal view that dust is the chief vehicle of infection in this disease. Again when Koch in 1901 by his pronunciamento, that human tuberculosis is never caused by the milk of tuberculous animals, stimulated a great number of workers to attempt to prove the contrary, evidence began to accumulate that tuberculous infection of the lungs might be brought about in various ways, and facts came to light which told against the view that direct infection by means of dust is the only manner in which pulmonary tuberculosis can be caused.

Dust versus Droplets. — According to the school of Flügge, infection by droplets is much more likely to take place than infection by dust, and his pupils have demonstrated the presence of the bacilli in the lungs immediately after inhalation. Findel,[1] working in his laboratory, has shown that the inhalation of even so small a number as 62 germs is sufficient to cause the disease, and he asserts that several million times as many bacteria are necessary to infect when taken by the stomach. Laschtschenko[2] and Heymann,[3] working under the direction of Flügge, were able to infect guinea pigs with tuberculosis by causing them to breath directly in front of the mouth of phthisical patients while the latter were coughing. The pigs were not infected when distant over one meter. Flügge[4] himself infected 6 of 25 guinea pigs in this manner, holding them distant from twenty to forty-five cm. from the mouth of the patient. Pfeiffer and Friedberger[5] sprayed guinea pigs with a culture containing 35,000 tubercle bacilli to

[1] Findel, Ztschr. f. Hyg. u. Infectionskrankh., Leipz., 1907, LVII, 104.

[2] Laschtschenko, Ztschr. f. Hyg. u. Infectionskrankh., Leipz., 1899, XXX, 125.

[3] Heymann, Ztschr. f. Hyg. u. Infectionskrankh., Leipz., 1899, XXX, 139.

[4] Flügge, Ztschr. f. Hyg. u. Infectionskrankh., Leipz., 1899, XXX, 107.

[5] Pfeiffer and Friedberger, Deutsche med. Wchnschr., 1907, XXXIII, 1577.

the c.c. The animals were held for ten minutes at a distance of eight to twenty cm. in such a manner that their bodies were perfectly protected. Those held at the greater distance did not contract tuberculosis, but the others developed what appeared to be primary tuberculosis of the lungs. Bartel and Neumann,[1] after spraying guinea pigs with tubercle bacilli, found the germs immediately in mouth, throat and lungs. Bernheim[2] infected guinea pigs at the distance of not over twenty-five cm., but he was able to collect tubercle bacilli on agar plates at the distance of one meter from the mouth. So also Kuss and Lobstein,[3] carrying out very careful inhalation experiments with a sprayed culture of tubercle bacilli, very easily and constantly developed pulmonary disease. Kovács,[4] after inhalation experiments with tubercle bacilli, could immediately recover them from the lungs. But he thinks that they may also pass from the mouth to the lungs via the cervical and bronchial glands. Cobbett,[5] employing sprays both of *B. prodigiosus* and of the tubercle bacillus, reports that the bacteria are carried to the periphery of the lungs by the inspired air.

The Inhalation of Bacteria. — On the other hand, Hewlett and Thompson[6] found that inhaled bacteria were not carried even as far as the trachea, as Hildebrandt[7] had found before. Hartl and Herrmann[8] showed that inhaled germs decreased very rapidly back from the nose, and they consider that the upper passages are frequently the place of entrance for the infection, and that bacteria are rarely carried by the air to

[1] Bartel and Neumann, Wien. klin. Wchnschr., 1906, XIX, 167, 213.

[2] Bernheim, Clinique, Brux., 1905, XIX, 346.

[3] Kuss and Lobstein, Bull. méd., Paris, 1907, XXI, 821.

[4] Kovács, Beitr. z. path. Anat. u. z. allg. Path., Jena, 1906, XL, 281.

[5] Brit. M. J., Lond., 1909, II, 867.

[6] Hewlett and Thompson, Lancet, Lond., 1896, I, 86.

[7] Hildebrandt, Beitr. z. path. Anat. u. z. allg. Path., Jena, 1887, II, 411.

[8] Hartl and Herrmann, Wien. klin. Wchnschr., 1905, XVIII, 798.

the lungs. Vallée[1] carried on spray experiments without result, and Calmette and Guérin,[2] in a few experiments made with infected dust, did not find that the bacilli reached the alveoli. Weleminsky[3] could find no bacilli in the lungs of guinea pigs immediately after they had been subjected to inhalation experiments.

Lack of Agreement among Investigators. — Thus it is seen that the school of Cornet claims that pulmonary tuberculosis is almost always caused by the passage of infected dust to the alveoli, and that infected droplets are of little moment; while Flügge and his pupils attempt to show that dust rarely reaches the alveoli but that the inhalation of droplets is the easiest method of causing the disease. The unprejudiced reader must conclude that infection in either way is possible, but the conditions of the experiments are so far removed from the natural that there must be much hesitation before assuming that this work indicates in any degree the common mode of infection in human beings.

Bacilli may pass from Stomach to Lungs. — It is commonly assumed that because pulmonary tuberculosis begins in the apices of the lungs the bacilli must be carried directly to the alveoli by the inspired air. Moreover most pathologists consider that evidence points to the alveolar surface as the starting point of the disease, and that the relative age of the lesions in the lungs and the glands indicates that it is primarily a pulmonary disease. The writer is not competent to discuss the findings of the pathologists, but there are a large number of careful observers who believe on pathological and experimental evidence that the bacilli which cause pulmonary tuberculosis may find their way through the lymph and the blood from any part of the alimentary tract to the lungs. Some pathologists believe that the disease begins in the capillaries rather than in the alveoli. Calmette and

[1] Vallée, Ann. d. l'Inst. Pasteur, 1905, XIX, 619.
[2] Calmette and Guérin, Ann. de l'Inst. Pasteur, 1905, XIX, 601.
[3] Weleminsky, Berl. klin. Wchnschr., 1905, XLII, 743.

Guérin[1] say that primary tubercle of the lungs always begins in the capillaries, and never in the alveoli, and Aufrecht[2] from his pathological studies comes to the same conclusion.

Even pulmonary anthracosis may be caused by the ingestion of particles of carbon. Vansteenburgh and Grysez[3] caused animals to breath air loaded with soot from a smoky lamp, and though the nose was filled with soot, none was found in lungs or even trachea. If the experiment was prolonged, carbon appeared in the lungs, but not if the esophagus was tied. When one bronchus was occluded, the carbon appeared in the parenchyma of the lung just the same, provided the esophagus was open. Whitla[4] fed animals with carbon and bacilli, and both were found in the lungs in from four to twenty-four hours. Feeding was done with a tube, with great care to prevent inhalation. Hutchens[5] fed guinea pigs with coal dust, and also injected it into the abdomen, and found it in the lungs in three days. Grober,[6] after injecting India ink into the tonsils, was able to find the pigment in the lungs in a short time. He thought that he could trace a continuous lymphatic route from the tonsils to the costal pleura, whence the particles passed directly to the parietal pleura and the lungs. But such a connection has been denied by Beitzke,[7] Wood[8] and others.

Schultze[9] denies that pulmonary anthracosis can be pro-

[1] Calmette and Guérin, Ann. de l'Inst. Pasteur, 1906, XX, 609.

[2] Aufrecht, Deutsches Arch. f. klin. Med., Leipz., 1908, XCIV, 308.

[3] Vansteenburgh and Grysez, Ann. de l'Inst. Pasteur, 1905, XIX, 787.

[4] Whitla, Brit. M. J., Lond., 1908, II, 61.

[5] Cited by Oliver, Brit. M. J., Lond., 1908, II, 481.

[6] Grober, Die Tonsillen als Eintrittspforten für Krankheitserreger, Abdruck aus dem klin. Jahrb., Berl., 1905, XIV, 547.

[7] Beitzke, Virchow's Arch. f. path. Anat. [etc.], Berl., 1906, CLXXXIV, 1; Berl. klin. Wchnschr., 1908, XLV, 1235.

[8] Wood, Rep. Henry Phipps Inst. Study . . . Tuberculosis, Phila., 1906, IV, 163.

[9] Schultze, München med. Wchnschr., 1906, LIII, 1702.

duced by feeding, as is claimed by the French experimenters, and insists that during the feeding some inhalation takes place, and that if the animals are fed through a gastric fistula with adequate precautions, the fragments are not carried to the lungs.

A large number of workers have certainly demonstrated that pulmonary tuberculosis may be caused by infection through different portions of the alimentary canal.

The work of Calmette and Guérin[1] shows that tubercle bacilli are speedily carried from the intestines to the lungs.

Schroeder and Cotton[2] have shown that pulmonary disease develops no matter in what part of the body tubercle bacilli are inoculated, and in Bulletin 88 they have shown that marked pulmonary invasion occurs constantly in hogs fed on tuberculous material. So also Ravenel[3] has recovered tubercle bacilli from the lungs within a few hours after placing them in the stomach by celiotomy. Beitzke[4] in a review of the subject states that Schlossmann and St. Engel[5] found the bacilli in the lungs six hours after injection into the stomach by laparotomy, as did also L. Rabinowitsch, and that the latter and also Uffenheimer, Bacharach, and Stein and Orth found them after injection into the intestine. Ficker, he says, could not do this with adult dogs or cats, and Herrmann could not with monkeys. Vallée,[6] Calmette and Guérin,[1] Bonome[7] and Arloing[8] also have demonstrated pulmonary infection

[1] Calmette and Guérin, Ann. de l'Inst. Pasteur, 1905, XIX, 601; 1906, XX, 353, 609.

[2] Schroeder and Cotton, U. S. Dept. Agric. Bu. An. Ind. Bull. No. 86 and No. 93.

[3] Ravenel, Cleveland M. J., 1909, VIII, 179.

[4] Beitzke, Berl. klin. Wchnschr., 1908, XLV, 1235.

[5] Schlossmann and St. Engel, Deutsche med. Wchnschr., 1906, XXXII, 1070.

[6] Vallée, Ann. de l'Inst. Pasteur, 1905, XIX, 619.

[7] Bonome, Gazz. d. osp., Milano, 1907, XXVIII, Nos. 37–84, abstract in J. Am. M. Ass., Chicago, 1907, XLIX, 888.

[8] Arloing, Sixth Internat. Cong. on Tuberc., Wash., 1908, IV, 666.

via the alimentary tract, and very many of the experiments have shown that the bacilli easily pass through the intestinal wall without leaving a trace of their passage, so that the absence of lesion of the alimentary tract is no proof that infection has not taken place through it.

Unnatural Conditions of Experiment. — Although there has been, as is here shown, a vast amount of experimental work on infection with tuberculosis, there has been very little in which the conditions at all approached the natural. Usually there is an excessive amount of exposure, or an excessive number of germs in spray or dust. Thus in Cornet's notable experiment, where 47 of 48 guinea pigs were infected by breathing dust, the carpet had been smeared with large quantities of sputum, and it was forcibly beaten so that clouds of dust rose up directly in front of the animals. It is surprising that so few have thought it worth while to see how infection takes place in animals kept under conditions as nearly as possible like those under which human beings live.

Infection in Laboratory. — Animals kept in laboratories in company with others that have been purposely infected rarely contract the disease. Koch[1] in his original paper says that among the hundreds of animals so kept the disease did not develop for three or four months, and then only exceptionally. He reports autopsies on 17 guinea pigs and 8 rabbits thus naturally infected, which showed in all cases a pulmonary tuberculosis resembling that which occurs in man. But apparently no effort was made to determine whether infection was by the air, by the food, or by contact through the hands of attendants, though this laboratory infection has been urged as evidence that the disease is air-borne. Of many hundreds of guinea pigs confined in a room with various tuberculous animals in the Department of Agriculture Experiment Station at Washington, only one contracted tuber-

[1] Koch, Mit. a. d. k. Gesund.-Amt., 1884, II, Trans. Sydenham Soc. Pub., CXV, 129.

culosis, and that was in a cage with several infected animals.[1] In laboratories floating bacteria are not likely to be very numerous, owing to the cleanliness practiced and the fact that most of the laboratory animals do not excrete many bacilli.

Experiments under Natural Conditions. Tuberculosis. — Schroeder and Cotton[2] experimented under more natural conditions. Seven cows were exposed in adjoining stalls to 3 tuberculous animals, and all but 1 of them contracted the disease. As all but 2 were moved about from stall to stall, exchanging with the infected animals, infection may readily have been by contact. At the same time 100 guinea pigs were exposed in the stalls, one half in cages below the mangers where food could sift through from the mangers, and one half on the walls. The exposure lasted several months, and only 1 of the pigs, in a cage under the manger, became infected. In a subsequent experiment 35 guinea pigs were exposed for one hundred and thirty-five days on the walls of the stalls. Two developed generalized tuberculosis. Of 42 animals kept for fifty-one days under the manger of infected cows, 6 developed a more or less generalized type of the disease. There was no direct evidence that tubercle bacilli were in the air of the stalls, but as the infecting animals were excreting large numbers of bacilli, there is little doubt of it. There is no record that contact infection from the hands of attendants was strictly guarded against, and it may be that the 2 out of 135 guinea pigs, and the 2 cows supposed to have succumbed to air-borne infection, were really infected by contact. Swenson, quoted by Aufrecht, exposed five calves in a stable with tuberculous cows in such a manner as to preclude contact infection, and they all developed the disease, as Swenson thought, by dust infection. Klein[3]

[1] U. S. Dept. Agric., Rep. Bu. An. Ind., Wash., 1906, XXIII, 31.

[2] Schroeder and Cotton, U. S. Dept. Agric., Rep. Bu. An. Ind., Wash., 1903, XX, 61; 1904, XXI, 44, reprinted as Circ. No. 83.

[3] Stevenson and Murphy, Treatise on Hygiene and Public Health, Lond., 1893–96, II, 212.

exposed guinea pigs in the vent shaft of the Brompton Hospital, and most of them contracted tuberculosis.

Experiments in Tuberculosis Houses.—Bartel and Spieler,[1] realizing that most experiments are under unnatural conditions, exposed 12 guinea pigs in cages in a house occupied by tuberculous patients, and allowed 16 to run at large and be handled by the children. The exposure was from two to three weeks, and of the 12 cage pigs 3 developed tuberculosis, and of the 16 free pigs 10 developed tuberculosis of various glands and other organs. No statement is made that care was taken to prevent contact or mouth-spray infection of the animals in the cages. These authors[2] exposed 8 guinea pigs, running free, in a house where the tuberculous patient was taking fairly good care of the sputum. Only 1 of the guinea pigs developed tuberculosis.

At my suggestion Dr. M. S. Packard of Providence carried on an experiment for the health department of that city on the mode of infection of guinea pigs under natural conditions. A fairly clean laborer's house was chosen, where there was a consumptive whose sputum contained large numbers of bacilli, and who was taking no care whatever in regard to its disposal. Thirty-six small guinea pigs were exposed in cages placed in a dark place in the room in which the patient usually sat. The cages were much crowded. Of the animals, 16 were fed and cared for by the consumptive, and the others by an employee of the department free from disease. These latter animals were locked in a box covered with wire netting, fourteen meshes to the inch. There could be no question of contact infection for these pigs. The exposure was from February 11, 1908, to May 14. All but 21 of the animals died of non-tuberculous disease, or were starved or killed by rats after removal from the house. Of the 11 surviving animals exposed to air infection alone, 8 were

[1] Bartel and Spieler, Wien. klin. Wchnschr., 1905, XVIII, 218.

[2] Festschr. enthalt. Arb. u. Tuberk. . . . VI Internat. Tuberk. Konf. [etc.], Wien u. Leipz., 1907, 71.

shown to be tuberculous and 3 not tuberculous. Of the other lot, 7 were shown to be tuberculous and 3 not. It seems impossible that the test animals could have been infected otherwise than through the air. That it was mouth spray rather than dust infection seems likely, for the patient took much interest in the animals, and was often seen with his face close to the netting, talking to them, and coughing at them only a few inches distant. The guinea pigs were purchased, but I was unable to learn that they had ever been exposed to the disease.

Since writing the above I note that Le Noir and Camus[1] have undertaken a similar experiment. They exposed guinea pigs in cages in a ward for phthisical patients. Four pigs were placed in a cage on the floor and the patients fed these. One of them developed tuberculosis. Five pigs were kept for six weeks in a cage on the floor but protected so that the patients could not reach them. One of these also developed tuberculosis. Another pig with three little ones was placed in a cage near the ceiling so that they had to be fed from a ladder. One of the little ones died of an intercurrent affection, but the other two contracted tuberculosis.

Since it is claimed by the majority of those interested in tuberculosis that the disease is spread chiefly by means of dust, it is highly desirable that a sufficient number of well-conducted experiments under truly natural conditions be made to determine how important this mode of infection really is.

Except for tuberculosis very little animal experimentation has been done to determine whether diseases are air-borne. One reason for this, of course, is that so many of the commoner diseases affecting human beings are not easily contagious for the lower animals.

Experiments with Mediterranean Fever. — Horrocks,[2] experimenting with monkeys, could cause Mediterranean

[1] Le Noir and Camus, Presse méd., Par., 1909, XVII, 761.

[2] Horrocks, Report of Royal Commission on Malta Fever.

fever by making the animals inhale dust artificially infected with large numbers of *M. melitensis*, but he was not successful with dust naturally infected with urine, though the organism of this disease is very resistant to drying. Monkeys kept in cages near infected animals did not contract the disease, unless there was actual contact with infected material, i.e., there was no air-borne infection. Epidemiological evidence is against this being a dust disease, for it prevails far less during the dry than during the wet season. That it is in reality exclusively milk-borne seems now to have been demonstrated.

Experiments with Anthrax. — Büchner [1] was the first to attempt to infect animals by making them breathe dried anthrax bacilli or spores. He easily succeeded in thus causing primary pulmonary disease. Müskatblüth [2] showed that the spores would readily pass the lungs without causing local disease. Morse, Hildebrandt, Tschistovitsch and Gramatschikoff [3] could not cause the disease by inhalation even when the spray was sent directly into the trachea. Baumgarten[4] believes that these various experiments show that infection takes place by the tonsils rather than directly by the lungs.

Experiments with Plague. — Bubonic plague is often considered an air-borne disease, but the experiments of the present Indian Plague Commission[5] have shown that this is not the case. Both monkeys and guinea pigs have in considerable numbers been put in flea-proof cages, but exposed freely to the air, and the cages placed in dwellings known to be infected, and in no instance did they contract the disease. In other instances the animals were exposed freely to the air, but

[1] Büchner, Centrlbl. f. Bakteriol. [etc.], Jena, 1890, VII, 733; VIII, 1.

[2] Müskatblüth, Centrlbl. f. Bakteriol. [etc.], Jena, 1887, I, 321.

[3] Cited by Sobernheim in Kolle u. Wassermann Handbuch [etc.], Jena, 1903, II, 49.

[4] Lehrbuch der Pathologischen Mycologie, Braunschweig, 1890.

[5] Journal Hygiene, 1905, 835; 1906, 445–471; 1907, 432, 835, 979.

were protected from fleas by "tangle-foot," with like results. These experiments were made at various times and places, but the animals never succumbed to air-borne infection. In all instances control animals not protected from fleas usually contracted the disease.

Conclusions. — After the foregoing survey of the subject we are, I think, justified in the following conclusions:

1. The theory of the aerial transmission of disease was developed as the most reasonable way of explaining the phenomena of infection.

2. Contact infection with carriers and missed cases affords a better explanation of the phenomena.

3. The best medical thought has been steadily restricting the supposed sphere of aerial transmission.

4. Only a few authorities now assert that disease is carried by the atmosphere outside of dwellings, and this assertion is made only in regard to smallpox.

5. Bacteriology teaches that former ideas in regard to the manner in which diseases may be air-borne are entirely erroneous; that most diseases are not likely to be dust-borne, and they are spray-borne only for two or three feet, a phenomenon which after all resembles contact infection more than it does aerial infection as ordinarily understood. Tuberculosis is more likely to be air-borne than is any other common disease.

6. Surgeons at first developed aseptic surgery on the theory that air infection was of the highest importance. They have gradually learned to pay less attention to it, until at present some of the best surgeons consider it a negligible factor.

7. Animal experimentation indicates that tuberculosis and anthrax may be air-borne, and that plague and some other diseases are not.

8. Pathology has not determined, as is sometimes alleged, that even pulmonary consumption is an air-borne disease.

9. There is no good clinical evidence that the common diseases are air-borne.

10. There is considerable clinical evidence that scarlet fever, diphtheria, smallpox, measles, whooping cough, typhoid fever and plague are not easily transmissible through the air.

11. Scarlet fever and diphtheria can be cared for in the same ward with other diseases without extension, if cleanliness be maintained and infection by contact avoided.

In reviewing the subject of air infection it becomes evident that our knowledge is still far too scanty, and that the available evidence is far from conclusive. Yet it is of the greatest practical importance that we should know definitely just what danger there is of air-borne infection and in what diseases it is to be feared. Infection by air, if it does take place, as is commonly believed, is so difficult to avoid or guard against, and so universal in its action, that it discourages effort to avoid other sources of danger. If the sick-room is filled with floating contagium, of what use is it to make much of an effort to guard against contact infection? If it should prove, as I firmly believe, that contact infection is the chief way in which the contagious diseases spread, an exaggerated idea of the importance of air-borne infection is most mischievous. It is impossible, as I know from experience, to teach people to avoid contact infection while they are firmly convinced that the air is the chief vehicle of infection.

While it is not possible at present to state with exactness the part played by aerial infection in the transmission of the different infectious diseases, we are by the evidence forced to the conclusion that the current ideas in regard to the importance of infection by air are unwarranted. Without denying the possibility of such infection, it may be fairly affirmed that there is no evidence that it is an appreciable factor in the maintenance of most of our common contagious diseases. We are warranted, then, in discarding it as a working hypothesis and devoting our chief attention to the prevention of contact infection. It will be a great relief to most persons to be freed from the specter of infected air, a specter which has pursued the race from the time of Hippocrates, and we may rest assured that if people can as a consequence be better taught to practice strict personal cleanliness, they will be led to do that which will more than anything else prevent aerial infection also, if that should in the end be proved to be of more importance than now appears.

CHAPTER VII.

INFECTION BY FOOD AND DRINK.

Infection by Water.

Broad Street Well.—From time immemorial water has been believed to be the bearer of disease, but it is only since the middle of the nineteenth century that the subject has been scientifically studied. One of the first instances of a clear-cut demonstration of the causation of sickness by infected water was that of the now famous Broad Street well, so ably studied by Snow.[1] During the outbreak of cholera in London in 1854 there was an enormous concentration of cases in a very limited area just east of Regent Street, there having been reported, during a period of about six weeks, over 600 fatal cases. A careful study of the site, soil, subsoil, streets, density and character of population, dwellings, yards, closets, cesspools, vaults, drains, conditions of cleanliness and atmospheric conditions, revealed nothing of interest. But a study of the water supply discovered most interesting facts. Nearly all of the cases were nearer a certain public pump in Broad Street than any other well, and most of them gave a definite history of getting water from this pump. Of the very few cases (ten at the time of the investigation) outside of the area supplied by this pump, half were known to drink water from Broad Street. There were also several cases of cholera in distant parts of London in persons who drank water from this well. In the workhouse with 535 inmates, in the midst of this district, but with its own well, there were only 5 deaths, less than one-tenth the rate in the neighborhood, and

[1] Sedgwick, The Principles of Sanitary Science and the Public Health, New York, 1902, 170.

in a brewery with 70 employees and using its own well there was not a single case. It was also shown that a privy vault and cesspool in the adjoining house discharged through a leaky drain which ran within two feet of the well. There were 4 fatal cases of cholera in this house at the time of the outbreak and obscure earlier cases which were not unlikely cholera also.

North Boston Well. — In the United States the outbreak of typhoid fever at North Boston, N. Y., in 1843, referred to by Flint in his popular text-books, did much to call attention to drinking water as a factor in the spread of disease. A young man from Massachusetts went to the hamlet sick with typhoid fever, and died there. He lodged at the tavern where there was a well of water used by 6 of the neighboring families. One near-by family and 2 distant families did not use the water and had no illness. In the other families which did use the water there were 28 cases with 10 deaths.[1]

Recent Studies. — Such striking demonstration in a few instances of the spread of disease through the medium of drinking water led to unwarranted generalization, and during the last half of the nineteenth century it was the common belief of health officials and medical men that infected water was the chief factor in the causation of typhoid fever and cholera, and that it was of great importance in malaria, yellow fever, dysentery, diarrhea, and was perhaps of moment in all the "zymotic" diseases. The discovery of the specific organisms of these diseases, and the application of more scientific methods to their study, has of late shown that water, while a factor of very great importance, is not so important as was at one time supposed. Let us consider its relation to specific diseases.

Typhoid Outbreaks. — For dwellers in temperate regions typhoid fever is the most important water-borne disease. The demands of modern civilization require for the constantly increasing urban population a pipe-distributed municipal

[1] Am. Pub. Health Ass. Rep., 1873, I, 167.

supply which in numerous instances must be taken from streams or lakes more or less contaminated with sewage. The plentiful use of water rendered possible by a municipal supply produces a large amount of sewage, which in the past has usually discharged into the nearest watercourse, thus carrying danger to any other community which might become a user of the water. From what is known of the life history of the typhoid bacillus it is not surprising that in some cities great explosive outbreaks of the disease have been caused by a temporary pollution, and other cities, owing to continuous pollution of their source of supply, have suffered from a continuous high death rate from this disease. The former class of outbreaks, while in the aggregate less destructive, are most impressive lessons for the public and have been exceedingly instructive to the epidemiologist. The demonstration of a water-borne outbreak depends primarily upon statistics. If there is an excess of typhoid fever among the users of a certain water over the neighboring population living under the same conditions but using a different water, and if other sources, as food and milk, are excluded, the outbreak is probably water-borne. The more closely the users and non-users of the water are commingled, and the greater the difference in the incidence of the disease upon them, the more certain is the demonstration. During the outbreak in Scranton, 1906–07,[1] there were four separate sections of the city not supplied from the infected reservoir in which there was very little typhoid, and most of the cases which did occur in these districts were shown to have used the infected water in other places, or to have been subject to contact infection. In Paris,[2] owing to partial failure of the good supply, the impure Seine water was turned on to one *arrondissement* after another, with the result that a well-defined epidemic followed in each instance. In Philadelphia the gradual introduction of filtered water has resulted in a decrease in typhoid

[1] Wainwright, N. York M. J., 1907, LXXXV, 1027.
[2] Jordon, J. Am. M. Ass., Chicago, 1907, XLVIII, 1669.

fever, limited to those districts to which the water has been supplied.

These water-borne outbreaks are usually explosive in character and are frequently of short duration. An inspection of the supply not rarely shows that the feces of typhoid cases have entered the water shortly before the outbreak. Such outbreaks are apt to occur in the spring when the freshets wash the surface of the ground into the streams. The bacilli have rarely been found in the incriminated water.

While studying this subject in 1888,[1] I was able to find thirteen recorded instances of the recovery of typhoid bacilli from water which had presumably been the cause of an outbreak of the disease. In the outbreak in Providence in that year Prudden and Ernst reported finding the bacilli in house filters. Methods of identifying the bacillus at that time were, however, not entirely satisfactory, and it is not certain that the bacteria isolated were really typhoid bacilli. By better methods the germs have since been occasionally found in infected waters,[2] but as might be expected, it is more often from wells than from rivers or lakes. According to Gotschlich,[3] typhoid-fever germs have been identified in drinking water by the agglutination test only four times. Since then, however, they have been isolated by Wesbrook[4] from the Mississippi water at Minneapolis, and by Fox from the reservoir which was the source of the Scranton outbreak.[5] The bacillus isolated by Wesbrook was used for years as a test organism in his laboratory and also by Harris at Johns Hopkins. Anderson and Hutchings and Wheeler, as will be referred to, determined the presence of typhoid bacilli in ice presumed to be the cause of the disease.

[1] Chapin, Boston M. & S. J., 1889, CXX, 604.

[2] J. Mass. Ass. Bds. Health, Bost., 1904, XIV, 66.

[3] Gotschlich, Kolle u. Wassermann, Handbuch [etc.], Jena, 1903, I, 191.

[4] Wesbrook, Brit. M. J., 1897, II, 1774.

[5] Rep. St. Bd. Health, Penn., 1907, 410.

Temporary Typhoid Infection. — These explosive and temporary outbreaks of typhoid fever among the users of municipal supplies are sometimes due to an accidental pollution with sewage, but are more often due to the overflow of privies, or the placing of the discharges of typhoid patients on the ground where they can be washed into the streams. In our lake cities they have sometimes resulted from the wind temporarily blowing the sewage of the city towards the intake of the waterworks,[1] or the dumping of dredged mud near the intake.[2] Outbreaks are sometimes due to the careless temporary use of polluted water, owing to failure of the good supply, as at Newburyport,[3] or the accidental sucking in of polluted water owing to some derangement of valves or other mechanism, as in Lowell,[4] Baraboo and Millinocket.[5]

Continuous Typhoid Infection. — When considerable amounts of sewage are discharged into a stream or lake, the water, owing to the prevalence of typhoid fever, must be continuously charged with the bacilli. The users of the water under such circumstances generally suffer from a continuously high death rate from this disease. Among cities which have so suffered may be mentioned Chicago, Pittsburg, Cincinnati, St. Louis, Philadelphia, Newark and Albany. The unenviable position of many Pennsylvania cities in this respect is well set forth by Morris.[6] Among European cities which have had a bad water supply are Berlin, Hamburg, Paris, Frankfurt, Altona, Breslau and Zurich. Under these circumstances the typhoid rate may, while remaining high, vary considerably. Sometimes the incidence of the disease may reach enormous proportions, as in Chicago

[1] Whipple, Typhoid Fever, New York, 1908, 167–168.

[2] Whipple, Typhoid Fever, New York, 1908, 167; also U. S. Geol. Survey, Wash., Water Supply and Irrigation Papers, No. 194, 138.

[3] Rep. St. Bd. Health, Mass., 1892, 701.

[4] Whipple, Typhoid Fever, New York, 1908, 174.

[5] Whipple, Typhoid Fever, New York, 1908, 178–179.

[6] Morris, Sanitation, Phila., August, 1904, 47.

in 1891, when it was 173.8 per 100,000, and in Pittsburg in 1900, when it was 144.2. Sometimes epidemic waves of the disease can be followed down a river from one municipality to another, as in the Merrimac, Kennebec and Hudson.[1]

Cities with Infected Water. — The connection between an excessive typhoid death rate and the sewage contamination of municipal water supplies is thus shown by a large amount of epidemiological evidence, but it is even more certainly demonstrated by the improvement which almost always follows when a pure water is substituted for the impure. Formerly typhoid fever was very common in English cities, but now the disease is far less prevalent, due in large measure to the almost universal use of clean water. Many continental cities present marked illustrations of the decrease in typhoid fever, due to improvement in water supply. Among such may be mentioned Paris, Berlin, Altona, Hamburg, Zurich, Breslau and Frankfurt. The United States also presents numerous examples, as Lawrence, Lowell, Albany, Buffalo, Newark, Jersey City, Cleveland, Chicago and Philadelphia. (For more detailed information see Whipple, "Typhoid Fever;" Fuertes, "Water and Public Health;" Hazen, "The Filtration of Public Water Supplies;" and Hazen, "Pure Water and How to Get It.") It has in one or two instances happened that the purification of a polluted water supply has not resulted in any very marked diminution in the typhoid death rate. This was so at Youngstown, Ohio, and notably at Washington.[2] At Youngstown the disease was shown to be spread chiefly by contact, or by the use of infected wells. The conditions at Washington are not so well understood, and a special commission [3] has been able to find no very definite cause for the disease. Levy and Freeman[4] after a very careful study

[1] Whipple, Typhoid Fever, New York, 1908, 149, 154, 236.

[2] Whipple, Typhoid Fever, New York, 1908, 248.

[3] U. S. Pub. Health & Mar. Hosp. Serv., Hyg. Lab., Bull. Nos. 35, 44 and 51.

[4] Levy and Freeman, Old Dominion J. M. & S., 1908, VII, 315.

of conditions in Washington and Richmond, conclude that Washington must be put in the category of southern cities in which an excessive typhoid-fever rate depends chiefly on climatic conditions operating more or less directly, and that perhaps to a considerable extent the disease depends on the presence of flies. However that may be, Washington affords a practically unique example among large cities of a mistake in attributing the excess of typhoid fever to the pollution of the water supply.

Amount of Sickness Due to Water. — To how great an extent pollution of public water supplies is responsible for the excessive typhoid mortality in the United States it is difficult to determine. Whipple[1] says that the average typhoid death rate in American cities is about 35 per 100,000, while cities with a good water supply average not over 20. He would thus attribute to the pollution of public water supplies about 40 per cent of the typhoid fever of the cities of the United States. We must remember, however, that an excess of typhoid fever in a city with a questionable water supply is not always due to the water, as witness Washington and Youngstown, and Dr. H. W. Hill writes me that Duluth is another example. But a majority of the people of this country live beyond the reach of municipal water supplies, and typhoid fever is even more prevalent among this rural population. So that if the whole country is considered, it appears that 10 or 15 per cent, rather than 40 per cent, of our typhoid fever is the proper proportion to attribute to the infection of municipal supplies.

Amount Due to Wells. — Doubtless the majority of the inhabitants of the United States obtain their drinking water from wells. Formerly polluted wells were believed to be the chief source of typhoid fever. This was particularly so while Murchison's "pythogenic" theory of the origin of the disease prevailed. When wells were a principal source of supply in cities where privy vaults and cesspools abounded, probably

[1] Whipple, Typhoid Fever, New York, 1908, 132.

they were often the source of typhoid fever. With the substitution of municipal pipe-supplies, the well has become a factor of comparatively little moment in city typhoid fever. As it now appears that the bacillus of this disease does not survive long in soil or water, and that each case must have some connection with a previous case of human typhoid infection, it seems improbable that country wells, largely isolated as they must be from danger of indiscriminate human contamination, play an important part in the propagation of the disease. This is the view held by Hill, who has had a large experience in the study of this disease in Minnesota. He states, however, that sometimes in loose coarse gravel, or in seamy shale and limestone formations, wells may become infected from sources of pollution situated at long distances, and have then been known to be the cause of much sickness.

Instances of Infected Wells. — That wells have actually been the source of typhoid fever there is much evidence. Instances of outbreaks due to infected wells at Basingstoke, England, Newport, R. I., and Trenton are narrated by Whipple,[1] and a dozen or more instances in England are referred to by Poore,[2] and some of the 179 milk outbreaks of typhoid fever tabulated in "Milk and Its Relation to the Public Health"[3] were due to infection of the milk by water from a contaminated well. Outbreaks due to well water continue to be reported from time to time. During twenty-five years no instance of typhoid fever from infected well water has come under my personal notice except at a summer hotel on the shore of the bay, in which case the well was probably infected by a broken drainpipe near by. An interesting case was noted in Washington a few years since.[4] Typhoid fever occurred in four houses on a certain street, all supplied from

[1] Whipple, Typhoid Fever, New York, 1908, 183–188.

[2] Poore, The Earth in Relation to the Preservation and Destruction of Bacteria, Lond., 1902, 135.

[3] U.S. Pub. Health & Mar. Hosp. Serv., Hyg. Lab. Bull. No. 41, 50.

[4] District of Columbia, Report of Health Officer, 1903, 29.

wells. A little further up the street there had previously been some cases, the feces from which had been thrown into a privy box after what was probably only partial disinfection with carbolic acid. At any rate carbolic acid could be tasted in the water in the wells below. While in this instance the infecting material probably percolated through the soil, as it did also in the outbreak at Trenton, Whipple states:[1] "Sandy soil is a good filtering material, and when a well in such soil stands at the center of a circle twenty-five or fifty feet in radius in which there are no privies, cesspools, sink wastes, or other sources of contamination, the water can usually be depended upon as fit for domestic use,—provided, of course, that the top of the well is properly guarded against surface wash." Sometimes, as in the Trenton incident, the infecting material passes a considerable distance apparently through channels or crevices. The writer once knew of a well which became polluted (though without causing sickness) from a privy 300 feet distant, after there had been much blasting near by, which presumably opened seams in the somewhat slaty rock. As Whipple says, most wells which have been the cause of typhoid outbreaks have been contaminated from the top.

Infected Springs. — Springs are essentially natural wells, and there is no reason why they should not occasionally be contaminated. A typhoid outbreak caused by spring water occurred at Mount Savage, Md., in 1904,[2] another at Springfield, Mass.,[3] one at Northampton, Mass.,[4] one at Ridgway, Penn.,[5] and two others in Maryland.[6]

Typhoid Fever from Bathing. — It has been suggested from time to time that typhoid fever may result from bathing

[1] Whipple, Typhoid Fever, New York, 1908, 85.
[2] Whipple, Typhoid Fever, New York, 1908, 188.
[3] Rep. Bd. Health, Springfield, 1903, 16.
[4] Rep. St. Bd. Health, Mass., 1900, 844.
[5] Rep. St. Bd. Health, Penn., 1907, 927.
[6] J. Am. M. Ass., Chicago, 1905, XLIV, 595.

in water containing typhoid bacilli, the infection presumably being due to the accidental swallowing of some of the water. Reece [1] has recently reported an outbreak, presumably due to this cause, at the naval recruiting station at Walmer. The swimming tank was infected with sewage containing typhoid excreta, and the earlier cases seemed to be closely connected with the use of the tank. From the report, however, it does not appear that contact infection outside the tank could be rigidly excluded.

Cholera from Water. — Cholera was early shown to be a water-borne disease. The longevity of the spirillum in water is probably not so great as that of the typhoid bacillus, but it is sufficient to permit of the disease being easily transmitted in this manner. Whenever the excreta of human beings infected with cholera gain access to cisterns, wells, streams or other sources of drinking water, cholera is pretty sure to follow. The cholera-infected Broad Street well in London has been referred to, and although for many years the views of health officials were somewhat colored by the miasm theory of Pettenkofer, the transmission of the disease by water was kept in mind, and many outbreaks due to this cause were reported. Radcliffe, Simon and others [2] showed that infected water played a large part in the outbreaks of cholera in London in 1848–49, 1853–54 and 1866. Shakespeare in his very valuable Report on Cholera in Europe and India [3] gives numerous instances of water-borne cholera infection, as from wells at several places in France (pp. 76–81), and from municipal supplies in Genoa and Naples (p. 151). In Spain many towns and villages suffered from water-borne outbreaks, caused often, doubtless, by the universal custom of washing soiled linen in running streams. According to Shakespeare, water plays an important part in the spread of cholera in

[1] Rep. Med. Off. Loc. Gov. Bd., 1908–09, XXXVIII, 90.

[2] Sedgwick, Principles of Sanitary Science and the Public Health, New York, 1902, 182.

[3] U. S. Government Printing Office, 1890.

India, and Koch[1] reported finding the spirilla in a tank used as a village water supply. A number of instances of the finding of cholera spirilla in water that was presumably the cause of the disease are noted by Kolle.[2] Cases are recorded of explosive outbreaks of cholera on shipboard, probably due to infected water.[3] The most striking instance of the transmission of cholera by water is the celebrated outbreak in Hamburg and Altona in 1892. These two municipalities form practically one city, though each has its own water supply. In the outbreak Hamburg, which used unfiltered and polluted Elbe water, suffered severely, while Altona, the water for which was filtered, was almost exempt. The line of demarcation between the two water supplies could be recognized by the incidence of the disease. Our officers in the Philippines attribute great importance to water as a vehicle for the diffusion of cholera, particularly in the villages and smaller towns, where the streams are used for washing clothes and for sewers and at the same time as sources of domestic supply. The municipal supply of Manila has been kept free from infection during the last outbreaks, though wells have to some extent been the cause of sickness. Woodruff[4] states that in one town a spring supplied part of the people, who were quite free from the disease, which nearly decimated those using the river, and in those towns where the people had well-protected rain-water cisterns they were quite immune. While we are not in a position to determine the relative importance of water in the causation of cholera, it appears certain that it is a factor of great consequence, and that people using a sewage-polluted water are, on the advent of cholera, liable to suffer from severe epidemics of the disease.

Dysentery from Water.—The bacillus of dysentery is found in the discharges from the bowels, and has about the same

[1] Koch, Brit. M. J., Lond., 1884, II, 403, 453.
[2] Kolle u. Wassermann, Handbuch [etc.], Jena, I, 191; III, 61.
[3] Wendt, Asiatic Cholera, New York, 1885, 113.
[4] Woodruff, J. Am. M. Ass., 1905, XLV, 1160.

resistance as the typhoid bacillus, so that we should expect this form of dysentery to spread in much the same way as typhoid fever does, and that infected water would prove a factor of importance. Shiga[1] reports outbreaks in Japan from the use of well and river water. Eldridge[2] states that dysentery is a rural disease in Japan, and the use of human feces as a fertilizer, and the frequency of the infection of the numerous small streams and wells, renders it preëminently a water-borne disease.

Little is heard about water-borne outbreaks of dysentery in England or the eastern United States, and it is highly probable that such are not very common. Dr. H. W. Hill reports four such outbreaks in Minnesota, three of which are briefly referred to in the report of the Minnesota state board of health for 1911. At Hibbing in 1907 about 2000 out of 8000 persons were attacked, although only 5 deaths occurred. The infection was probably caused by workmen going down into the well to make repairs. After the institution of the hypochlorite treatment of the water the outbreak abruptly ceased. At St. Peter there were outbreaks in 1908 and in 1909. Both were due to a polluted river water overflowing into a reservoir. At the Agricultural College a deep well was infected by the backing up of a sewer, and almost every person who drank the water developed dysentery. At Mankato, Minn., there was an outbreak of 405 cases of typhoid fever due to sewage leaking into the well which supplied the town. Preceding the typhoid cases there were 4000 to 6000 cases of diarrhea and dysentery, nearly half the population, the first cases appearing June 25, immediately after the infection of the water and lasting until early in July.[3]

There is every reason to believe that dysentery amebæ

[1] Shiga, Mod. Med. [Osler], Phila. & N. Y., 1907, II, 781.

[2] Eldridge, U. S. Pub. Health & Mar. Hosp. Serv., Pub. Health Rep., 1900, 1.

[3] J. Infect. Dis., Chicago, 1911, IX, 410.

are carried in water. Musgrave and Clegg[1] claim to have found the amebæ in the water supply of Manila, but there is some doubt as to the pathogenicity of the forms studied by them. Allan[2] reported a small outbreak of amebic dysentery in North Carolina, due to an infected well.

Diarrhea from Water. — Reincke[3] states that infantile diarrhea was greatly lessened after the improvement in the water supply of Hamburg. Sir Shirley F. Murphy, Seaton and Newsholme in the discussion of the paper took issue with its writer as to the part played by water in the causation of this disease. Sedgwick[4] says that there is no doubt that drinking water is the ready vehicle of dysentery and diarrhea. He refers to the Ninth Report of the Medical Officer of the Privy Council, London, 1867, p. 16, and to his own investigations as to the excessive prevalence of typhoid fever and diarrhea in Burlington owing to the sewage contamination of the water supply.[5] Sedgwick also, in the paper mentioned on another page, quotes freely from Reincke's various writings to show that well-defined outbreaks of diarrheal disease have occurred in Altona, Hamburg and Berlin in connection with defective working of the filters or with unusual pollution of the water supply due to other causes.

Water in Relation to Seasonal Distribution of Diarrhea.— In an article just published, McLaughlin[6] attributes very considerable importance to water supplies in the causation of infantile diarrheas. He recognizes the fact that these diarrheas may include at times much typhoid fever and much dysentery, and perhaps other varieties of intestinal

[1] Bull. 18, Bu. Gov. Lab., P. I., 93; Rep. Bd. Health, P. I., 1904–5, 10.

[2] Allan, J. Am. M. Ass., Chicago, 1909, LIII, 1561.

[3] Reincke, Trans. Epidemiol. Soc., Lond., 1904, n. s., XXIII, 135.

[4] Sedgwick, Principles of Sanitary Science and the Public Health, New York, 1902, 217.

[5] J. N. Eng. Water Works Ass., X, 167.

[6] Pub. Health Rep., U. S. Pub. Health and Mar. Hosp. Serv., Wash., 1912, XXVII, 579.

infection. He also admits that many factors other than the water supply are often of far more importance than is the water. He bases his contention as to the danger from water on an excessive prevalence of diarrheal diseases in the winter months, alleging that while ignorance, poverty and "unsanitary conditions" may cause an enormous excess in summer, in towns with pure water, they do not cause such an excess in the winter. He gives some striking illustrations of communities with a grossly polluted water supply which have an excess of winter diarrhea as well as of winter typhoid fever. Among these may be mentioned Niagara Falls and Cohoes, N. Y., and Escanaba and Marquette, Mich. The evidence from the larger cities of Cleveland, Chicago, Milwaukee and Pittsburg is not so convincing. It is true that these do show a very considerable excess of winter diarrhea and that the curves for the three lake cities are strikingly parallel, but if this winter diarrhea is really the result of and proof of dangerous pollution of the water we should expect a correspondingly great excess of typhoid fever in these cities; yet the typhoid death rate in all of them is below the average. Indeed there is no very marked parallelism between typhoid fever and diarrhea either in different cities or in the same city at different seasons. In some of McLaughlin's tables the curves of winter diarrhea and winter typhoid fever correspond exactly and in others they are months apart. While on guard not to attribute too much importance to water as a source of diarrhea we must admit that McLaughlin has presented new evidence to show that water is at times a factor to be reckoned with.

The Mills-Reincke Phenomenon. — In 1893 Mills of Lawrence, Mass., and Reincke of Hamburg, Germany, noted that the purification of the water supplies of their respective towns was followed by a decrease in the general death rate as well as in the death rate from typhoid fever. Hazen later called attention to these facts, which he found to hold true for other American cities, and he was in accord with the first-named observers in attributing the decrease to the improvement in the water and maintained that where one death from typhoid could be prevented by improving the water supply two or three deaths from other causes would be prevented by the improvement. Sedgwick and McNutt,[1] in an elaborate paper, have presented a large amount of material which they believe establishes the fact of the phenomenon and also indicates which diseases are chiefly affected by the water supply. The authors consider that their data show that an improvement in a poor water supply may be expected not only to reduce the death rate from typhoid fever but to decrease infant mortality and the death rate from gastro-intestinal disturbance and from tuberculosis and pneumonia. It has been suggested that these changes may be due to the removal of disease germs from the water, or to increased bodily resistance due to better water, or to both. As to the explanation, however, Sedgwick and McNutt offer no opinion.

Water Purification and the General Death Rate. — According to the theory under discussion the purification of a polluted water supply causes a fall in the general death rate below that due to the diminution of typhoid fever. This decrease certainly took place in Lawrence and Lowell, but the deaths in a city during a year are due to a great number of diseases, and the prevalence of each disease and each death from that disease are due to the joint action of very many causes. To attribute a change in the death rate to any one cause is extremely dangerous and in the past has led to most serious errors. It can be seen from the diagram shown by Sedgwick and McNutt that in both the cities under consideration there had been a considerable rise in the death rate just previous to changes in the water supply and that a considerable part of the increase was due to pneumonia as was also a considerable part of the decrease. Changes equally as great in the mortality from

[1] Sedgwick and McNutt, J. Infect. Dis., Chicago, 1910, VII, 489.

pneumonia and in the general death rate have occurred in Albany, as shown in Sedgwick and McNutt's diagram, and doubtless in other cities, entirely independent of changes in the water supply, and such changes may as well be assumed to be due to variation in the prevalence of influenza or to some other cause as to changes in the water supply. That two cities close together had a decrease in the death rate, in large part due to decrease in respiratory diseases, at the same time that the water supply was changed might well be due to chance. It is suggestive that the change was most marked in the two cities in the same year although the water in Lowell was only partially improved in that year. It may also be noted that the decline in the death rate in Albany started from a maximum in 1892, the year before the maximum in the Massachusetts cities, and that this maximum coincided, as in Massachusetts, with a maximum mortality from respiratory diseases. The rate of decrease in total mortality and in respiratory mortality was not as great after filtration as before, and it was about as great as the decline in Lawrence and Lowell which was supposed to be due to water.

Water Purification and Diarrhea. — The infant death rate, in which the diarrheal diseases play an important part, has been shown to have the closest sort of relation to kinds of food and methods of feeding and to vary enormously in different sections of the same city and among different classes residing in the same section. A body of statistics, far more voluminous than are marshalled in support of the Mills-Reincke theory, indicates that very great reduction can readily be made in the infant death rate by better feeding and other care. Yet we are asked to believe that the diarrheal deaths in Hamburg were cut in half by the change in the water. One cannot help thinking either that the old water supply was specifically infected with the germs of diarrhea, which is not the case in most English and American cities, or else that the changes in population and in sanitation, after the great cholera outbreak, produced in themselves great changes in the diarrheal death rate. Indeed, the writer has been informed by a well-known scientific man, then residing in Hamburg, that the cholera outbreak, by its destruction of life, and consequent changes in the population, profoundly modified mortality rates. If we turn to Sedgwick and McNutt's diagram for Lawrence we see no change in the diarrheal death rate between the 7 years before and the 7 years after filtration. In Lowell the diarrheal death rate did decline decidedly after the improvement in the water. In Albany the decrease began before the improvement in the water and continued at about the same rate afterwards.

Water Purification and Tuberculosis. — As shown by Sedgwick and McNutt, pulmonary tuberculosis had been declining for many years in Lawrence and Lowell, as it had in most cities, and the diagrams indicate a retarded rather than an accelerated decline after the improvement in the water. The authors, in order to show the alleged effect of the water improvement, are obliged to compare these cities with Manchester, which they assume differs from Lowell and Lawrence chiefly in having a good water supply, and which they consider a " normal " city for their purpose. Compared with Manchester, Lawrence shows a greater decrease by 30 deaths and Lowell by 68. While the authors state that the age, sex, occupation and nationality of the population of the three cities is substantially the same, it would appear rather risky to assume that all the conditions affecting health are the same. Cities show great variation as regards their mortality, even when the figures are corrected for age and sex, and would doubtless do so if corrected for nationality and occupation. One of the most difficult problems in vital statistics is to make correct deductions from a comparison of the death rate of different cities, particularly in such a disease as tuberculosis. A theorem which depends upon a comparison made as above seems to require further study. In Albany following filtration there was no apparent change in the steady decrease in tuberculosis which had been going on for several years. Notwithstanding the efforts that have been made by some to show by statistics that the decline in tuberculosis has been due to sewerage, and by others that it is dependent on the segregation of advanced cases, and by still others that it is the result of the recent popular propaganda, and now by the supporters of the Mills-Reincke theory that it is dependent in a very appreciable measure on improvement in water supplies, I cannot see that the evidence presented along any of these lines is sufficient to warrant official action or definite predictions. We know less about the causation of tuberculosis than about almost any other infectious disease.

Water Purification and Pneumonia. — While Sedgwick and McNutt say with reference to diphtheria that "the mixed character of the title and the highly epidemic character" of the disease render no conclusions possible, they believe that valid deductions can be drawn from a study of pneumonia. This disease group has, however, during the last 25 years, shown marked epidemicity, due, I believe, in large part, to the effect of influenza. There was in New England a notable increase of pneumonia in the early nineties followed by a decline and then another increase a few years later, though the curves have varied somewhat in different cities. There was a sudden drop in pneumonia mortality in Lawrence after filtration and a slight increase in Lowell, but for the reason given no deduction is permissible as to the influence of the water.

Results of Purification in Providence. — An excellent sand filter was installed in Providence in January, 1906. There was an appreciable decrease in the amount of typhoid fever but it is doubtful if it was dependent on filtration. There was not very much change in the general death rate in Providence following filtration, though it was slightly higher in the 2 years after filtration was begun than it was in the 2 years before filtration. Tuberculosis, which had been declining for many years, exhibited a somewhat retarded decline after 1906. Pneumonia after 1905 showed a decided increase over the preceding 10 years, though there was little change during the 3 years before filtration and the 2 years after. Diarrheal diseases had been declining and reached a minimum in 1905, the year before filtration, followed by a considerable increase during the next 2 years. Certainly there is nothing in these figures to indicate that an improved water supply has caused a decrease in the diseases mentioned.

McLaughlin's Evidence concerning Mills-Reincke Phenomenon. — McLaughlin[1] has also given consideration to the Mills-Reincke theorem, and, as does the present writer, hesitates to make deductions from such a complicated phenomenon as changes in the general death rate. He prefers to study single diseases, and considers, in the paper cited, infantile diarrhea. His argument as to the effect on the diarrheal death rate by improving the water supply is based on the causative connection between water and diarrhea which he seeks to establish as referred to above. He also gives tables of deaths in four cities which have recently wholly or to a large extent changed their water supplies, namely Cincinnati, Columbus, Pittsburg and Philadelphia. All have shown a very great decrease in the death rate from typhoid fever. In Cincinnati and Columbus there was no decrease in diarrhea; in Philadelphia it was very slight, but in Pittsburg it was quite noticeable. This maintenance of the diarrheal death rate is rather remarkable in view of the direct efforts that have been made during the last few years to decrease infant mortality. The figures for pneumonia are not given by McLaughlin. Tuberculosis decreased in the four cities, but the decrease had been going on for some time as in most cities.

[1] Pub. Health Rep., U. S. Pub. Health and Mar. Hosp. Serv., Wash., 1912, XXVLI, 597.

Conclusion concerning the Theorem. — No attempt is here made to disprove the reality of the Mills-Reincke phenomenon but only to call attention to certain difficulties in accepting it. It is a question of great importance which ought to receive extended study. A number of important cities have recently improved their water supplies with a corresponding decrease in typhoid fever. The effect upon other diseases should be carefully examined. At present it seems unwise to consider the proposition demonstrated and to promise a lowering of the general death rate as a result of the purification of water supplies.

Malaria from Water. — Until recently malaria has been believed to be transmitted by means of drinking water. Numerous instances were reported, such as that of the ship *Argo*, in which it was supposed that the evidence pointed conclusively to this mode of transmission. The discovery of the part played by the mosquito in the causation of this disease led to a more critical consideration of the alleged evidence in support of its water-borne character, and most of this evidence was found to be worthless, or in the few instances in which water still seemed to be at fault it appeared probable that the water served as a breeding place for mosquitoes, and did not directly cause disease by its ingestion.

There was nothing in the earlier demonstrated facts of the transmission of the disease by insects to preclude the possibility of its transmission by water, and indeed Laveran and Manson thought this not improbable. Celli [1] attempted to demonstrate this in various ways by administering water from the most malarious regions of Italy to human beings, daily, up to a month. He failed completely, as, according to Craig,[2] have all other experimenters, except Ross in one instance, which, however, from the conditions of the experiment, was far from conclusive. Celli considers the fact that

[1] Celli, Malaria, Lond., 1900, 94.

[2] Craig, The Malarial Fevers, New York, 1909, 82.

large numbers of railway employees and others living in intensely malarious regions around Rome use an unquestionably pure aqueduct water, but are yet frequently attacked by malaria, is corroborative evidence that water cannot be an important vehicle of the disease. But probably the best evidence we have that drinking water plays no part in the causation of malaria is the fact that preventive measures all over the world, directed solely against the mosquito and with no reference to the water theory, have resulted in an enormous decrease and in some places in the eradication of the disease.

Yellow Fever from Water. — Yellow fever also was formerly believed to be at times water-borne, but, as in malaria, the epidemiological evidence therefor will not stand criticism. The success of the preventive measures directed solely against the mosquito indicates that drinking water has no part in the diffusion of this disease.

Worms in Water. — The eggs and young of some of the parasitic worms are often swallowed in drinking water, and the *Ankylostoma* and *Bilharzia*, and others probably, enter the skin from water in which they are contained, but the consideration of the diseases caused by them is outside the scope of this essay.

Conclusions. — Among the diseases which may be transmitted by water, typhoid fever is doubtless by far the most important in Europe and North America at the present time. When water-borne disease is mentioned, typhoid fever comes first to mind. Yet there are those who think that the role of water in this disease has been exaggerated,[1] and it is doubtless true that in Europe, and even in this country, recent improvements in water supplies have greatly diminished this disease, but there are still a great many communities drinking polluted water and having a consequently high typhoid death rate. It is probably true that other fecal-borne diseases such as the diarrheal group

[1] Houston, J. State M. Lond., 1912, XX, 21, 92.

are transmitted through the medium of water. Asiatic cholera too may cause great devastation through infection of water supplies, but for a number of years the western world has been remarkably free from this disease. Typhoid fever is, however, such a common and serious disease, causing probably 25,000 deaths annually in the United States, as well as an enormous amount of disability at the most useful period of life, that it is worth while to make large expenditures for its prevention. Such expenditures are to be still further encouraged, since it is certain that the means taken to prevent the diffusion of typhoid fever by water will also prevent the spread of cholera and bacillary dysentery.

Protection of Water Supplies. — In the three diseases just mentioned the sole source of infection of water is the excreta of persons infected with the specific germs. If these excreta can be kept out of drinking water, or if the germs can be removed from it after it is infected, the problem is solved, and this can be done at a not prohibitive expense. For a full and practical consideration of the means for obtaining a pure water supply reference should be had to such works as Hazen's "The Filtration of Public Water Supplies" and "Pure Water and How to Get It." Suffice it to say here that pure water may be obtained by securing a clean source or by adopting some method of purification.

Domestic Wells. — The larger part of our population obtains its drinking water from shallow wells, and it is usually neither difficult nor expensive so to locate them that they will not receive drainage from privies or sink drains, and so to protect them that they will not receive surface washings. The federal Department of Agriculture and the state and local boards of health should do and are doing much to instruct farmers and villagers concerning the location and protection of wells.

Municipal Supplies. — As regards municipal supplies it is desirable if possible that the water be uncontaminated. This may be secured by drawing from deep wells, or seeking a source in a sparsely inhabited region. Some cities, as Liverpool, Boston and New York, have spent large sums to bring clean water from long distances. Other cities, notably Chicago, have secured good water by the construction of expensive works to remove sewage from the watershed. Many cities, when there is only a limited danger of pollution, accomplish much by a continuous patrol of the watershed and the removal of minor sources of pollution under general or special nuisance laws. In many states this duty of protection has been laid upon the state boards of health, and in some instances coöperation between states becomes necessary.

Purification of Water. — Unfortunately it often happens that it is physically impossible for a municipality to obtain a sufficient supply of water which is not subject to dangerous pollution. Purification then becomes a necessity, and owing to the labors of a long line of chemists, engineers and bacteriologists, several efficient and economical methods for accomplishing this have been developed. First among these is filtration. There are various methods of filtration, applicable to different waters and different localities, and it is the business of specialists to devise the best system for each city confronted by the problem. Efficient filtration will remove over 99 per cent of the contained bacteria, but cannot be relied upon to remove amebæ. Hence filtration will not protect against amebic dysentery, but it will protect against the bacillary form and against typhoid fever and cholera. That it is efficient against typhoid fever is shown by the experience of London, Berlin, Zurich, Hamburg, Lawrence, Albany, Paterson, Philadelphia and many other cities, and the removal of cholera spirilla was beautifully shown by the experience of Altona in 1893. The storage of water rapidly removes bacteria by sedimentation and through the death of the organisms, and is often a useful adjunct to filtration, notably so in the case of some of the London water companies. The boiling of water is an effectual means of destroying dangerous bacteria, and as a domestic measure it is sometimes extremely useful.

The use of hypochlorite of lime (commercial bleaching powder) has within a short time come into use for the purpose of sterilizing municipal water supplies. While this method of protection had been used in England as a temporary expedient, its first use as a permanent method of treatment seems to have been by Leal, at Boonton, N. J., in 1908.[1] A high degree of safety seems to be secured at a low cost. The subject has been investigated also by Clark and Gage,[2] Phelps, Park, Pratt and others. The process has been used at East Providence, R. I., Poughkeepsie, Chicago and other places.[3]

Infection by Ice.

Danger Exaggerated. — The use of ice from polluted sources has always been viewed with some alarm, and when it became known from the work of Prudden[4] and others that the bacilli of typhoid fever live for some months when frozen into ice, the alarm was believed to be well founded. But further researches (see page 10) have shown that in the freezing of ice under normal conditions a large proportion of the bacteria in the ice are frozen out, and those that remain tend to die off quite rapidly, somewhat as they do in water. Hence theoretically little danger is to be apprehended from the use of ice cut from water considerably polluted, even so polluted that if the water itself were used it would probably cause disease. There is very little epidemiological evidence that ice has been the cause of sickness. The literature relating to the subject was collected by Sedgwick and

[1] Leal, Fuller, Johnson, Papers read at the 29th Annual Convention of the American Water Works Association, 1909.

[2] J. N. Eng. Water Works Ass., 1909, XXII, 302.

[3] Discussion of a paper by Phelps at a recent meeting of the Boston Society of Civil Engineers, Abst. Eng. Rec., 1910, XLI, 80.

[4] Prudden, Med. Rec., N. Y., 1887, XXXI, 341.

Winslow[1] in 1902. An outbreak the exact nature of which was not determined occurred at Rye Beach, N. H., in 1875, due presumably to the use of ice from a pond grossly polluted with decaying vegetable matter. A single case of typhoid fever in Connecticut appeared to be due to the use of specifically infected ice. Alleged outbreaks of typhoid fever and dysentery in the United States, and of typhoid fever in Evesham, England, and Rennes, France, were also noted by the above-named authors, but the evidence was far from conclusive. More recently Hutchings and Wheeler[2] report an outbreak of typhoid fever in a hospital at Ogdensburg, N. Y. Many were attacked, and the disease was suspected to be due to the use of ice. An examination of the ice in the ice house showed that some of it contained visible dirt from which colon and typhoid bacilli were isolated. A certain lot of ice harvested the winter before began to be used on September 26. Eight cases of typhoid fever developed from October 2 to 5 and subsequent cases followed until some time in November, involving in all 39 persons. The earliest cases had a temperature of 104° and 105° on the first day. An examination of the ice in the ice house showed that it contained visible dirt from which colon and typhoid bacilli were isolated, the latter determined by agglutination. Dr. H. W. Hill[3] suggests that the evidence in this case is far from conclusive, because 6 days is a very short period of incubation, and for 8 cases to develop in 9 days would be still more unusual, and to have the cases, after so short an incubation, develop a temperature of 104° and 105° on the first day is even more remarkable. Hill thinks that this indicates an infection before the use of the ice, and he calls attention to the fact that typhoid outbreaks in hospitals

[1] Sedgwick and Winslow, Mem. Am. Acad. Arts & Sc., 1902, XII, No. 5, 472.

[2] Hutchings and Wheeler, Am. J. M. Sc., Phila., 1903, n. s., CXXVI, 680.

[3] Hill, Address, National Ice Association of Amercia, N. York, 1910.

for the insane due to other causes are by no means rare. If typhoid bacilli really survived in the ice he says that it would indicate a persistence of a month over what has ever been observed in experiments. At Batangas in the Philippines [1] an outbreak of bacillary dysentery at the army post was said to be due to contaminated artificial ice, but no data were given. Park, in the paper cited below, refers to a small outbreak of typhoid fever due to ice cut from a pond where sewage flowed onto ice already formed and then became frozen. Anderson [2] reports an outbreak at Lexington, Va., possibly due to artificial ice made from spring water polluted with typhoid excreta, from which water he isolated typhoid bacilli, proved to be such by cultural and agglutination tests. Hamer [3] refers to a possible instance of ice-borne typhoid in London in 1898. Judging from the small number and indefinite character of these reports, it appears that there is little direct evidence of danger from ice. In the outbreak reported by Anderson and in the one in the Philippines the ice was artificial. With such artificial ice the danger must be very much greater than in the case of natural ice, for in the former the bacilli are not excluded during the process of freezing and little time is allowed for their natural death in the ice. The one noted instance of infection by natural ice which has seemed most conclusive has been shown by Hill to have no significance. There is on the other hand strong epidemiological evidence that ice is not a factor of much moment in the causation of disease. Hundreds of thousands of tons of ice are cut from sewage-polluted waters in the United States, but sickness does not appear to follow the use of this ice in drinking water. Park [4] has studied this point in New York City, where four-fifths of the ice is cut from the markedly

[1] Rep. Bu. Health, P. I., 1908–9, 54.
[2] Anderson, Med. Rec., N. Y., 1908, LXXIV, 909.
[3] Hamer, Rep. Med. Off. Health, Lond., 1904, Appendix I.
[4] Park, J. Am. M. Ass., Chicago, 1907, XLIX, 731.

contaminated Hudson River. Vast quantities of this ice are used in drinking water, and if it is the bearer of typhoid fever there should begin a noticeable increase of the disease when the use of the new ice commences in March, and this increase should continue during April and May. During the ten years studied by Park no such increase was noted, and no outbreak occurred which could be attributed to ice.

Infection by Milk.

Character of Outbreaks. — It has long been known that some of the common contagious diseases of human beings may be transmitted by means of milk. The only diseases that are definitely known to be so carried are typhoid fever, scarlet fever and diphtheria. There is no reason why dysentery and cholera, and perhaps other diseases, should not be transmitted in the same way, but no evidence of it has come to my knowledge, except that referred to by Kober,[1] who states that McNamara in Calcutta, in 1872, traced an outbreak of cholera to an infected dairy. Outbreaks of the above diseases have been reported from time to time, and have been studied by Hart, Kober and others, but the latest tabulation and the fullest consideration of the subject are to be found in Bulletin 56, Hygienic Laboratory, United States Public Health and Marine Hospital Service, 1909. Milk outbreaks of these diseases have an explosive character, such as is shown by water-borne outbreaks of typhoid fever. In scarlet fever and diphtheria the explosive character is owing to the shorter incubation of these diseases, more pronounced than it is in typhoid fever. A milk outbreak is determined to be such from the presence of an excessive number of cases on a particular milk supply which cannot be accounted for in any other way. From three to five cases within a few days on a route covered by one wagon in a city with an average typhoid death rate is highly suspicious, and in most

[1] Kober, J. Am. M. Ass., Chicago, 1907, XLIX, 1091.

instances proves to be the beginning of an outbreak. The more the customers of a dealer are scattered, the stronger is the evidence. Care must be taken to exclude all other sources, such as neighborhood or family contact, water, ice, shellfish or other foods. Milk outbreaks often prevail more extensively among the well-to-do, owing to their greater consumption of milk, and a typhoid milk outbreak usually shows a high percentage of children attacked. Often the source of infection can be found. In only two instances reported by Konradi [1] and Shoemaker [2] has the typhoid bacillus been isolated from milk, and in only four instances has the diphtheria bacillus been recovered.[3]

Number of Outbreaks. — The number of outbreaks pretty definitely traced to milk is quite large. Trask, in the Hygienic Laboratory Bulletin referred to, tabulated 179 outbreaks of typhoid fever, 51 of scarlet fever, 23 of diphtheria and 7 of sore throat. Besides these Hart reported 51 of typhoid fever, and Busey and Kober 86 of typhoid fever, 59 of scarlet fever, 21 of diphtheria, making in all 316 outbreaks of typhoid fever, 125 of scarlet fever, 51 of diphtheria and 7 of sore throat. In these are not included the 90 outbreaks tabulated by Caroe. This is certainly an impressive aggregate, but it must be remembered that these records cover a period of perhaps half a century. To determine within any degree of accuracy how large a part milk plays in the spread of these diseases is difficult, but it seems to me that the tendency at the present time is to exaggerate its importance. Schüder [4] found that of 640 outbreaks of typhoid fever 462 were caused by water and 110 by milk, but it is highly improbable that cases caused respectively by water and by milk

[1] Konradi, Centralbl. f. Bakteriol. [etc.], Jena, I Abt. Orig., XL, 31.

[2] Shoemaker, J. Am. M. Ass., Chicago, 1907, XLVIII, 1748.

[3] Nuttall and Graham-Smith, The Bacteriology of Diphtheria, Cambridge, 1908, 326.

[4] Schüder, Ztschr. f. Hyg. u. Infectionskrankh., Leipz., 1901, XXXVIII, 343.

occur in any such ratio in the United States. Most of the water-borne typhoid fever does not occur in outbreaks, but is due to the continuous pollution of municipal supplies. Milk-borne typhoid fever, on the other hand, probably does occur chiefly in the form of outbreaks. During the last four years, in Providence, 155 of the 600 milk dealers have had one or more cases of typhoid fever on their routes. In only 9 instances have there been more than 2 cases on a single route within a week. Investigation promptly showed that in 3 instances the groups of cases were due to personal contact, and in the other 6 instances an unmistakable milk outbreak developed. It is true that some epidemiologists assume that a considerablo number of sporadic cases are due to milk, but the evidence appears to be the other way. I think that a study of the distribution of typhoid cases on milk routes in Washington, as shown in diagrams in bulletins 35, 44 and 52 of the Hygienic Laboratory, United States Public Health and Marine Hospital Service, bears out my contention that outbreaks of typhoid fever due to milk are not likely to escape notice if the cases are daily tabulated according to milk supply. Furthermore, these charts show that there is little excess of typhoid fever on individual milk supplies except in those instances where there is a noticeable outbreak.

Fewer Outbreaks in Large Cities. — It is also to be noted that very few outbreaks are reported from the large cities like New York, Chicago and Philadelphia, due perhaps to the fact that the chemical and bacteriological changes in the milk resulting from the long haul necessary for such cities are unfavorable for the typhoid bacillus. In the country, milk outbreaks are not likely to be a factor of moment, as large milk routes are not common. It is in the medium-sized and smaller cities and villages that most of the milk outbreaks are reported. It will be noted that though scores of outbreaks of typhoid fever may occur each year, they do not include more than a small fraction of the total typhoid fever.

It may be claimed that only a small proportion of the milk-borne outbreaks are recognized as such, but I cannot think that this is so in the English cities and the better class of American cities. In Providence during the last twenty-five years there have been nine outbreaks of typhoid fever, including 363 cases, or about 8 per cent of the total occurring during that time. But the typhoid death rate in Providence is below the average, so that 8 per cent in Providence would probably be equivalent to not over 4 per cent in the average American city with its polluted water supply and numerous privy vaults. In only a few cities have Trask, Hart, and Busey and Kober been able to find records of more than two, or more rarely three, outbreaks; yet we can scarcely believe that milk outbreaks could have, except rarely, escaped detection in the English cities, or in such cities as Boston, Worcester, Springfield, Rochester, Baltimore, Philadelphia and New York.

Amount of Typhoid Fever Due to Milk. — The city of Washington is reported as showing an excessive amount of milk-borne typhoid fever.[1] In 1906, 79, or 9 per cent, of the 866 cases investigated by the commission, were traced to milk; in 1907, 31, or 5 per cent, of 635 cases investigated; and in 1908, 54, or 8 per cent, of 679 cases. According to figures furnished by Dr. Woodward, Health Officer of Washington, the number of typhoid cases due to milk during the three years was 139, which gives a percentage of 4.6. The commission considers that 10 per cent of the typhoid fever in Washington is due to milk. These percentages, however, seem to me unfair, as doubtless all the outbreaks were reported, and the percentages should, from the standpoint of the present consideration, be based on the total number of cases reported in the city, and not on the cases studied and of known origin. This gives a percentage, as above stated, of 4.6 of the typhoid fever in Washington during the three years 1906–08 as due to milk-borne typhoid. The importance and value of the

[1] U. S. Pub. Health & Mar. Hosp. Serv., Hyg. Lab., Bull. No. 35, 59; No. 44, 46; No. 52, 100.

reports on typhoid fever in Washington have, as it appears, given a rather exaggerated importance to the danger from milk. That there was a certain amount of typhoid fever in Washington due to milk, during the three years in question, is no reason for assuming a similar percentage of milk-borne typhoid fever for the other cities of the country. Trask was able to find during the years 1903–07 about 1900 cases in the United States traced to milk. During this period there were in the registration area 57,023 deaths, and the total number in the whole country must have been at least double, or 114,000. The fatality is probably not over 10 per cent, so that there must have been at least 1,000,000 cases. Nineteen hundred is 0.19 per cent, which is very different from the 10 per cent now commonly assumed as due to milk. I do not of course believe that all the milk outbreaks were reported, but the number would have to be increased fifty-fold to equal 10 per cent, and it can scarcely be believed that 98 per cent of all milk outbreaks fail of recognition.

Scarlet Fever and Diphtheria. — Scarlet fever and diphtheria are certainly much more rarely transmitted by means of milk than is typhoid fever. Although the percentage of typhoid fever, scarlet fever and diphtheria due to milk is small, the danger is a real one and the aggregate of cases not inconsiderable, and their occurrence should, if possible, be guarded against.

Animal Sources. — The infection of milk with the above diseases is almost invariably from human sources. There is no evidence to show that cows may be infected with the bacillus of typhoid fever, and the contamination of the milk by drinking sewage-polluted water does not occur. Scarlet fever also does not appear to be an animal disease. Power and Klein in England believed that they had found the cause of milk-borne outbreaks of scarlet fever in the sickness of the cows supplying the milk. These findings have not been substantiated, and the micrococcus which Klein believed was the cause of the disease has not been accepted as such by bacteriologists. While many of the lower animals may be successfully inoculated with diphtheria, the disease does not appear often to occur spontaneously among them. Nevertheless two milk-borne outbreaks have been traced to diphtheria of the cows' udder. One of these was reported by Dean and Todd[1] and the other by Ashby.[2]

Human Sources. — Besides the bacteriological evidence that milk rarely acquires its infection of these diseases from animals, we have the direct evidence that in a considerable number of outbreaks the milk is known to have been handled by persons sick with the disease or carrying its organisms. Trask [3] says that in 113 of the 179 outbreaks of typhoid fever reported by him an infected person was found to have handled the milk, and in only 4 instances was the infection reported to have come from polluted water used in washing utensils, and in 4 others to the use of milk bottles from infected houses. In 35 of the 57 scarlet-fever outbreaks an infected person was found to have handled the milk, and 3 others were due to the use of bottles from infected houses. Of the 23 diphtheria outbreaks, 18 were traced to handlers of the milk. A study of the details of milk outbreaks shows that in a large proportion the infecting case was not recognized as such, that the symptoms were mild or atypical, that infection occurred during the incipient stage, or that the person was merely a carrier. Infection may occur at any time during the handling of milk, from the beginning of milking until the milk is delivered to the consumer, and it may also be caused by those who take care of the pails, cans, bottles, strainers, drums, etc. Outbreaks are believed to have been caused by the tasting of milk by infected dealers, and in the instance reported by Shoemaker [4] a convalescent patient was in the habit of start-

[1] Dean and Todd, J. Hyg., Cambridge, 1902, II, 194.

[2] Ashby, Pub. Health, Lond., 1906–07, XIX, 145.

[3] Trask, U. S. Pub. Health & Mar. Hosp. Serv., Hyg. Lab., Bull. No. 41, 25 et seq.

[4] Shoemaker, J. Am. M. Ass., Chicago, 1907, LXVIII, 1748.

ing a siphon from the milk drum by sucking the tube. It is also believed by many that flies are an important factor in the contamination of milk.

Protection of Milk. — There are various ways in which the danger from infected milk may be avoided.

First. If all recognized cases of the diseases just considered are promptly reported, and proper measures of isolation are insisted on, there will be a considerable decrease in the amount of milk-borne infection. When such a disease occurs in the family of a milk producer or dealer the patient should usually be removed from the premises, and the vessels, etc., if possibly infected, should be disinfected. The greatest difficulty is encountered in the management of convalescents, and particularly carriers, and it is the view of most health officers that the latter should be permanently excluded from the milk business. Unfortunately there are many mild cases of contagious disease which are never recognized and are not likely to be. Moreover, persons in the incipient stage are quite likely to transmit the disease, and we cannot hope for much earlier recognition than we now have. Hence for the prevention of outbreaks from these unknown sources we must rely on other methods.

Second. It is possible to reduce the chances of infection by insisting on cleaner methods in handling milk and requiring the sterilization of all vessels, particularly of bottles. If all handlers would wash their hands, and keep their hands out of the milk and out of the vessels, there would be no milk outbreaks. But we can hope for no very radical improvement as regards the cleanliness of milkers, farm hands and peddlers.

Third. The pasteurization of the milk by the dealer before delivery would also decrease to a large extent the amount of milk-borne disease, for a study of outbreaks shows that in a large proportion the infection of the milk takes place on the farm. But there is also considerable risk of contamination in the hands of the dealer after pasteurization. For this reason much attention has been devoted to the problem of pasteurization in bottles so that the milk may with certainty be delivered to the consumer free from infection. Pasteurization of beer in bottles has long been practiced by brewers, and investigators[1] and milk dealers have adapted the methods of brewers to the treatment of milk and some large milk dealers are now delivering milk prepared in this way.

Fourth. In the absence of pasteurization by the dealer, doubtless the most successful way of preventing milk-borne disease at the present time is for the public to consume no milk except that which has been pasteurized or scalded in the house. Many object to the trouble and do not like the taste of heated milk, so that this practice is not likely to become universal. Moreover outbreaks have occurred, as at Bristol,[2] where milk pasteurized in an institution had been afterwards infected by a maid.

It therefore seems that while it is possible materially to lessen by the above methods the amount of milk-borne disease, we cannot hope at present entirely to do away with the danger of milk-borne outbreaks of the diseases we have been considering.

Ice Cream. — As milk is so frequently the bearer of disease, it is not surprising that outbreaks have at times been attributed to food products derived from milk. Thus Soper[3] reported an outbreak due to the use of cream on breakfast food, and one of the outbreaks reported by Trask was due to whipped cream. Sedgwick and Winslow[4] collected records of four outbreaks of typhoid fever due to the use of ice cream, and another has been reported by Barras.[5]

[1] North, Med. Rec., N. York, 1911, LXXX, 111.

[2] Davies and Walker, Proc. Roy. Soc. Med., Lond., 1808, Epidemiol. Sec., 175.

[3] Soper, J. Mass. Ass. Bds. Health, Bost., 1904, XIV, 68.

[4] Sedgwick and Winslow, Mem. Am. Acad. Arts & Sc., 1902, XII, No. 5, 475.

[5] Barras, Lancet, Lond., 1904, II, 1281.

A quite remarkable ice-cream outbreak of typhoid fever occurred in Eccles and Manchester in November, 1910, involving 108 cases.[1] The makers and sellers of the ice cream were two Italians in a tenement house in Manchester. Professor Delépine, who investigated the outbreak bacteriologically, was of the opinion that the ice cream must have been so grossly infected as only to be explained by a multiplication of the bacilli in the materials used after they had been heated and before freezing. Of the 13 persons living in the house with the Italians there were 6 whose blood gave a positive Widal reaction. No examination of their excreta appears to have been made.

Buchan[2] refers to an outbreak of scarlet fever due to ice pudding and reported by Buchanan in 1875. He also notes two outbreaks due to the infection of ice cream with *B. enteritidis* (Gaertner). Buchan made many examinations of market ice cream in Birmingham and suggested a bacteriological standard for ice cream and a set of excellent rules for its manufacture.

Another typhoid outbreak due to ice cream has recently been reported from Fort Sill, Okla., where 20 cases were due to eating ice cream from the neighboring town of Lawton.[3]

Butter. — While it has been shown that pathogenic bacilli may live for some time in butter, only one outbreak seems to have been reported as arising from the use of this substance. This is probably due partly to the fact that the germs must die off pretty rapidly, leaving perhaps only a few survivors, and partly to the difficulty of tracing an outbreak to such a source.

An outbreak of diphtheria at Lewiston, Minn., was believed to have been caused by eating infected butter. There had been no diphtheria in the place until a boy re-

[1] Rep. Med. Off. Local Gov. Bd., Lond., 1910–11, XL, 18.

[2] Buchan, J. Hyg., Cambridge, 1910, X, 93.

[3] Rep. Surg. Gen. Army, Wash., 1909–10, 45.

turned from the "Twin Cities" after an attack of diphtheria. The milk from the farm where he lived was sent to a creamery and every family in the place, in which there was diphtheria, was found to have used butter from this creamery. Experiments showed that diphtheria bacilli can live in butter for a month.[1]

Epidemic Sore Throat or Tonsillitis. — According to Winslow[2] outbreaks of what is often called septic sore throat have many times been reported in England and have been shown to be associated with particular milk supplies. Some of these outbreaks more or less resemble scarlet fever or include some cases of typical scarlet fever. In others there is no reason to consider the infection of a scarlet-fever nature. Winslow, without a systematic search of the literature, was able to find 12 outbreaks of this character. In 4 of these outbreaks there was no evidence whatever as to the original source of the disease. In 4 others there was a dubious connection with some disease in cows. At Glasgow and Colchester, Winslow thinks that there was fairly strong evidence connecting the outbreaks with an inflammatory condition of the cow's udder. At Rothesay probability pointed to human infection and at Working there had been both human quinsy and bovine udder inflammation on the farm. Another outbreak[3] occurred in Christiania in 1908 and it was not determined whether it had a bovine or human origin.

Sore Throat in Boston. — The first recorded American outbreak occurred in Boston in 1911 and was reported by Winslow as above. In Boston and the adjoining towns of Brookline and Cambridge there were, during a short period in May, probably not far from 2000 cases, of which 48 proved fatal and many more were quite severe. Many of

[1] Rep. State Bd. Health, Minn., 1911, 203.

[2] Winslow, J. Infect. Dis., Chicago, 1912, X, 73.

[3] Norsk Mag. f. Lagevidenskahen, 1908, LXIX, 585, 811: Ref. J. M. Ass., Chicago, 1912, LVIII.

the cases developed abscesses, and not a few general septic infection, as has been the case in European outbreaks. The outbreak was quite clearly traced to milk and cream supplied by the Deerfoot Farm Dairy in Southboro. This dairy and the farms supplying it were under the constant supervision of a trained bacteriologist and the cows were frequently inspected by a veterinary physician; the milk received as little handling as possible and indeed everything was done to deliver milk of a high bacterial standard and free from infection. It seemed improbable that there was any udder disease among the cows which could have given rise to the trouble. The farms supplying the milk are largely located some distance from Boston in Southboro and to some extent in the adjoining towns of Westboro, Framingham and Marlboro. As shown by the investigations of Winslow there was a marked prevalence of the same disease in the towns of Marlboro, Southboro and Hudson all through April and May. In these towns the disease appeared to pass by contact from person to person in prosedemic fashion, just as diphtheria ordinarily does, except that there was marked and sudden excess in Marlboro and Southboro in May, coincident with the Boston outbreak. In both these towns much Deerfoot milk is sold, but none in Hudson, where there was no May exacerbation. Winslow is of the opinion that the milk in some way became infected from cases or carriers, though no such infection could be demonstrated. As streptococci were isolated from the internal organs of fatal cases these were thought to be the infecting organisms. Other outbreaks have been reported from Baltimore [1] and Chicago.[2]

Views concerning Tuberculosis. — Of all the animal diseases which are transmissible to man tuberculosis has received the most attention. After many years of discussion

[1] J. Am. M. Ass., Chicago, 1912, LVIII, 1109.

[2] Miller and Capps, J. Am. M. Ass., Chicago, 1912, LVIII, 1111.

and investigation there is now general agreement that while the two types of tubercle bacilli, human and bovine, are distinct and quite permanent, they are reciprocally infective, though not to the same degree. That human beings may become infected with tuberculosis derived from cattle is now generally admitted, but there is as yet no general agreement as to the amount of such infection, though present views are not so divergent as those of a few years ago. The question of the mode of infection in tuberculosis and the source of the bacilli is so largely dependent on pathological evidence that it is very difficult for one who is not a pathologist properly to weigh the evidence. Yet in view of the lack of agreement among pathologists it becomes necessary for the health officer, who must take definite action to combat the disease, to attempt to arrive at some sort of conclusion. It seems fair, from the evidence thus far available, to draw the following conclusions:

Bovine Bacillus may infect Man. — First. The bovine type of bacillus is capable of causing infection in human beings. This is shown by the successful inoculation of human beings with bovine virus. A considerable number of cases of the accidental inoculation of veterinarians and laboratory workers while manipulating animals dead with tuberculosis have been reported by Pfeiffer, Tscherning, Naughton, Coppez, Priester, Hartzell, Grothan, Jadasohn, Ravenel, de Jong,[1] Salmon [2] and others. In most cases the lesion was local, and some have argued that this is strong evidence of weakened virulence for man. The finding of the bovine type of the bacillus in human beings is generally considered as furnishing a more certain demonstration of the latter's susceptibility to the disease. As will be again referred to, the German and British commissions, and various Americans, have

[1] Moss, Johns Hopkins Hosp. Bull., 1909, XX, 39; Cornet, Nothnagel's Encyclopedia of Practical Medicine, Phila. & Lond., 1907, Tuberculosis, 77.

[2] U. S. Dept. Agric., Bu. An. Ind., Bull. No. 33, 16.

found the bovine bacillus in from 16 to 25 per cent of the cases studied. These facts, while demonstrating the susceptibility of human beings to the bovine form of the disease, do not indicate definitely to what extent the bovine type prevails in man, as the cases examined were usually specially selected.

Feeding Experiments. — Second. Tuberculosis may be produced experimentally in animals by the ingestion of material containing tubercle bacilli. Milk known to be infected with tubercle bacilli has been in numerous instances fed to guinea pigs, rabbits, dogs, calves, swine and monkeys, and has caused fatal tuberculosis in them. This has been demonstrated by a large number of workers in all parts of the world. A good summary of previous experiments is given by Mohler,[1] who himself produced tuberculosis by feeding guinea pigs with milk from tuberculous cows. Subsequent experiments by the Bureau of Animal Industry[2] show that while guinea pigs are with difficulty infected by feeding, hogs are very easily infected, the primary infection apparently occurring in the submaxillary glands, the lungs usually becoming secondarily infected.[3] That the ingestion of tuberculous material, especially milk from creameries, is the chief cause of tuberculosis in swine, is the opinion of the officers of this department and of Ravenel and Russell.[4] The more recent work of Calmette and the French school, while not always including direct experiments with milk, show that material containing tubercle bacilli, introduced in any way into the stomach or intestines, results in the production of tuberculosis, and even the pupils of Flügge admit that the ingestion of a sufficient number of bacilli will cause the disease, though it is produced, they say, much more easily by inoculation or inhalation. It

[1] Mohler, U. S. Dept. Agric., Bu. An. Ind., Bull. No. 44, 13.

[2] U. S. Dept. Agric., Bu. An. Ind., Circ. 83, Bull. Nos. 86, 88, 93.

[3] Bull. No. 88, 46.

[4] Ravenel and Russell, Am. Pub. Health Ass. Rep., 1906, XXXII, Pt. I, 139.

is also generally admitted that bacilli may be absorbed through the intestines without leaving any lesion. While some pathologists think that it is usually possible to determine the route of infection by the age and character of the lesions, other equally good men do not consider that any very reliable conclusions can be arrived at in this manner. Under these circumstances it appears that we cannot as yet appeal to the pathologists for a definite decision as to the mode of infection in this disease, and we may be permitted to assume that a large amount of tuberculosis *may* be due to infection through one part or another of the alimentary canal.[1]

Tubercle Bacilli in Milk. — Third. Tubercle bacilli are frequently found in cows' milk. It was formerly believed that tubercle bacilli do not occur in cows' milk unless the udder is diseased. Nevertheless various observers from time to time have reported finding the bacilli although no udder disease was evident. Finally Schroeder and Cotton[2] showed that frequently the feces of cattle contain large numbers of tubercle bacilli, although the animals present no visible symptoms of disease. They furthermore showed that the pollution of milk with infected feces is the most common source of tubercle bacilli found in milk. As from 3 to 50 per cent of the cattle in different parts of the United States react to tuberculin, and probably 25 per cent of the cattle in Great Britain are infected, it is not surprising that market milk in these countries is frequently found to contain tubercle bacilli in sufficient numbers to cause the death of test animals. Anderson[3] gives a résumé of the literature of the subject. Among the percentages of infected milk referred to are, in Copenhagen, 14.3 per cent; Boston, 21 per cent and 40 per cent; Liverpool, 5.2 per cent from city dairies, 13.4 per cent from

[1] For other references to the causation of tuberculosis through the alimentary canal see p. 255.

[2] Schroeder and Cotton, U. S. Dept. Agric., Bu. An. Ind., Bull. No. 99.

[3] Anderson, U. S. Pub. Health and Mar. Hosp. Serv., Hyg. Lab., Bull. No. 41, 163.

country dairies, though later,[1] owing to the efforts of the authorities in eradicating the disease, the percentage in city dairies was 1.4 per cent and in country dairies was 7 per cent; Genoa, 9 per cent; London, 22 per cent; and Berlin, 28 per cent. Recently of 620 samples of milk consigned to London, 61, or 11.6 per cent, were found to contain tubercle bacilli.[2] Anderson found 6.72 per cent of 223 samples of market milk in Washington to contain virulent tubercle bacilli. Hess[3] found virulent tubercle bacilli in 16 per cent of 107 samples of New York market milk (not bottled). He thinks the reason that his percentages are higher than those of Anderson is the employment of more test animals and the injection of the cream as well as the milk. He also found virulent tubercle bacilli in one of eight samples of commercially "pasteurized" milk. In Manchester, England, 7.7 per cent of 542 samples of milk were found to be infected.[4]

Danger Less than Supposed. — There seems to be no doubt that a large part of the milk consumed in Europe and the United States contains tubercle bacilli in numbers sufficient to cause the disease in test animals. It also seems to be certain that in the lower animals at least, particularly in young individuals, the ingestion of this tuberculous milk will cause not only tuberculosis of the alimentary canal, but will produce pulmonary disease and generalized tuberculosis also. It is probable that the ingestion of such milk by human beings will produce similar results. There is, however, considerable variation in different kinds of animals as regards their susceptibility to this sort of infection. Even in animals as susceptible to the disease as are guinea pigs, infection by the ingestion of milk under normal conditions is not very easy. Thus Schroeder and Cotton[5] fed 132 guinea pigs with tuber-

[1] Rep. on Health of Liverpool, 1906, 189.

[2] Rep. Med. Off. Health, Lond., 1908, 60.

[3] Hess, Sixth Internat. Cong. on Tuberc., Wash., 1908, IV, 523.

[4] Rep. on Health of Manchester, 1906, 187.

[5] Schroeder and Cotton, U. S. Dept. Agric., Bu. An. Ind., Circ. No. 83.

culous milk on the average for forty-seven days, and only 1, which was fed for 357 days, contracted the disease. This was only 0.76 per cent. At the same time 14.28 per cent of the guinea pigs exposed in the mangers of the cows from which the milk was obtained developed tuberculosis. Dr. Veranus Moore writes me that he knows of a small village where most of the people received the milk from a herd of cattle that later was found to be extensively diseased; that is, about 77 per cent reacted to tuberculin and some 2 or 3 per cent showed the disease on physical examination, and a considerable percentage of the guinea pigs inoculated with the mixed milk from the herd died of tuberculosis. This community had used this milk for a number of years. After the facts as stated above were ascertained the condition was changed and up to this time there has not occurred a single case of recognized tuberculosis. Hess [1] examined 18 children who a year previous had been known to be consuming tuberculous milk. None of them showed any visible signs of tuberculosis, though 4 reacted to the tuberculin test. Of 100 children at Randalls Island, N. Y., fed on milk from tuberculous cows, none developed the disease.[2] A recent note,[3] which I have not had the opportunity to verify, gives the results of some observations made by Weber of the German Imperial Health Office on the use of tuberculous milk. From January, 1905, to April, 1908, 69 cows with tuberculosis of the udder were kept under observation, the milk from which was consumed raw by 360 persons, of whom 159 were children. Of these, 5, of whom 2 were between 1 and 2 years of age, were "indubitably infected with tuberculosis through the use of the milk." The children had taken the milk of these cows from one to one and a half years. In both cases the milk was used raw by all the members of the family, the parents and several children; all these

[1] Hess, J. Am. M. Ass., Chicago, 1909, LII, 1014.
[2] Park, Sixth Internat. Cong. on Tuberc., Wash., 1908, I, 156.
[3] J. Am. M. Ass., Chicago, 1910, LIX, 886.

people remained healthy. In the sick children there was merely an affection of the cervical glands in which tubercle bacilli of the *typus bovinus* were demonstrated by bacteriological tests. There were no other symptoms. Whitla,[1] however, reports an instance where of 150 children fed on milk known to be tuberculous, 15 contracted the disease.

Percentage Due to Bovine Infection. — It has thus far been shown merely that human beings *may* contract tuberculosis by drinking the milk of tuberculous animals. It remains to determine, if possible, how great this danger really is. Various attempts have been made to estimate this. It has been assumed by some that intestinal tuberculosis, and to some extent generalized tuberculosis without preponderant pulmonary involvement, is indicative of infection by ingesta, and presumably by milk. The fact that these types of the disease are more common in children, of whose diet milk forms a relatively large part, has been thought to lend color to this view. It is not improbable, however, that the different form which the disease presents in early life may be due to the characteristics of the age rather than to the mode of infection. Children certainly consume a relatively large amount of milk, but tuberculosis is not so common among them as among adults. In Providence only about 15 per cent of the tuberculosis is in children under five years of age, and only about 4 per cent of the tuberculosis death rate is attributed to abdominal tuberculosis. In the registration area of the United States abdominal tuberculosis accounts for about 3.5 per cent of all deaths from this disease. This form of tuberculosis appears to be much more common in England.[2] But careful observers find that contact with other cases is probably responsible for a large proportion of tuberculosis in children. Park [3] states that of 100 cases of glandular and bone tuberculosis in St. Mary's Hospital, New York, 44 per

[1] Whitla, Lancet, Lond., 1908, II, 135.

[2] Bovaird, Sixth Internat. Cong. on Tuberc., Wash., 1908, II, 446.

[3] Park, Sixth Internat. Cong. on Tuberc., Wash., 1908, I, 157.

cent had been in close contact with tuberculous cases. LaFetra[1] found 40.4 per cent of 131 cases of tuberculosis in infants, probably due to family infection. Comby [2] considers family infection of prime importance in the tuberculosis of children. Floyd and Bowditch [3] found that 679 of 1000 tuberculous children had been in contact with the disease in their homes. Approaching the subject in another way, they found signs of the disease in 66 per cent of 746 children living in tuberculous families among the poor. Miller and Woodruff[4] found the same true in 51 per cent of 150 children, and Sacks[5] in 53 per cent of 322 children.

While there seems to be no doubt that tubercle bacilli may remain latent in the body for some time, there are very few who accept von Behring's view that most human tuberculosis is acquired in childhood from drinking tuberculous cows' milk. As greatly discrediting von Behring's theory may be mentioned the investigations of Speck,[6] who found that of 8010 cases of tuberculosis only 27 per cent had been fed on cows' milk in infancy. Von Ruck[7] found that certainly not over 25 per cent, and possibly not over 10 per cent, had been brought up on cows' milk. Flick[8] obtained similar evidence at the Phipps Institute in Philadelphia. Heymann[9] says that in Christiania, where nearly all the infants are nursed, tuberculosis is more common than in Bavaria, where artificial feeding is very common, and that in Prague, where nearly all

[1] LaFetra, Sixth Internat. Cong. on Tuberc., Wash., 1908, II, 361.

[2] Comby, Sixth Internat. Cong. on Tuberc., Wash., 1908, II, 503.

[3] Floyd and Bowditch, Boston M. & S. J., 1908, CLIX, 783.

[4] Miller and Woodruff, Sixth Internat. Cong. on Tuberc., Wash., 1908, II, 487.

[5] Sacks, Sixth Internat. Cong. on Tuberc., Wash., 1908, II, 479.

[6] Speck, Ztschr. f. Hyg. u. Infectionskrankh., Leipz., 1904, XLVIII, 27.

[7] Von Ruck, J. Am. M. Ass., Chicago, 1905, XLIV, 1350.

[8] Flick, Report of Henry Phipps Inst. Study . . . Tuberculosis, Phila., 1906, IV, 49.

[9] Heymann, Ztschr. f. Hyg. u. Infectionskrankh., Leipz., 1904, XLVIII, 45.

babies are breast fed, the tuberculosis death rate is as high as in any city in Europe. I am inclined to the opinion that such epidemiological facts as we have indicate that children are more susceptible to the human than to the bovine type of the disease, and there seems to be as much clinical evidence that the tuberculosis of childhood is due to family infection as is the tuberculosis of adult life.

Instances of Milk Infection. — Instances are not rarely reported in which there is considerable evidence of the production of tuberculosis in children by the use of milk from tuberculous animals. One of the most convincing is that narrated by Adams of Aberdeen and summarized by Hess.[1] Two children of a farm laborer died of tuberculous meningitis in January and March of 1907. There was no known exposure to the disease except the use of milk from a cow with tuberculosis of the udder. Bacilli identical in type with those found in the cow were recovered from the cerebro-spinal fluid of one of the children. Most of the cases reported are not so convincing as this, and in many the evidence is decidedly weak and would not stand critical examination. The evidence afforded by these cases is not of much value, for though some of the cases are doubtless caused in the manner alleged, they merely indicate what is also suggested by animal experiments, —the possibility of human infection from milk. An estimation of the extent of this danger must be made in other ways.

Proportion of Human and Bovine Types. — Since the significance of Theobald Smith's discovery of the difference between the bovine and human types of the tubercle bacillus has been recognized, the relative frequency of the two types in human beings has been used as a measure of the importance of milk infection, for it is conceded that it is through milk almost exclusively that bovine tuberculosis is transmitted to human beings. Much care and labor are involved in the differentiation of the two types, but the number of observations made is considerable, among which those of the

[1] Hess, J. Am. M. Ass., Chicago, 1909, LII, 1015.

German and British commissions are notable. Moss[1] summarizes the cases previously reported. In all there had been 306 cases investigated, in 63, or about 20 per cent, of which bovine bacilli were found. But it must not be inferred from this that 20 per cent of all cases of human tuberculosis would present this type. With the exception of 54 cases in adults studied by the German commission, most of the cases have been children with the intestinal or glandular forms of the disease. In the 54 adults no bovine bacilli were found. The bovine type of bacillus has rarely been found in pulmonary tuberculosis, even among children. It may perhaps be inferred that 25 per cent of bone and glandular tuberculosis in children is due to the bovine bacillus. But Tendeloo[2] calls attention to the fact that if the bovine type of bacillus is a permanent one, — and unless it is these observations are of little value, — the above figures are probably misleading, for the bovine bacillus if permanent will be transmitted from man to man and does not always indicate a bovine origin. As only about 15 per cent of the tuberculosis in the United States is of the form in which the bovine bacillus is found, and as only about 25 per cent of the cases show this type of bacillus, we are justified, using the type as a test, in assuming that only about 5 per cent of our tuberculosis is derived from bovine sources. But this, while a small percentage, would amount to almost 2500 deaths annually in the registration area of the United States, — certainly a number which ought to be considered.

Epidemiological Evidence. — It seems to be a fact that tuberculosis, even those forms of the disease which are generally supposed to be caused by milk, is not appreciably less in those parts of the world where cows' milk is little used, or where it is usually sterilized, or where there is little tuberculosis among cattle. Kitasato[3] says that there is very little

[1] Moss, Johns Hopkins Hosp. Bull., 1909, XX, 39.

[2] Tendeloo, Sixth Internat. Cong. on Tuberc., Wash., 1908, I, 87.

[3] Kitasato, Ztschr. f. Hyg. u. Infectionskrankh., Leipz., 1904, XLVIII, 471.

tuberculosis among the cattle in Japan, and so few cows that the daily milk supply does not average 3 c.c. per capita, yet nearly 8 per cent of all deaths are due to tuberculosis, and in a series of autopsies 17 per cent of the tuberculosis cases were under eighteen years of age, and 10 per cent of the cases showed primary intestinal infection. Cobb says that substantially the same conditions prevail in China. According to Heymann[1] tuberculosis is very common in Greenland, where no cows' milk is used. Fisch[2] states that on the Gold Coast no milk is used, yet 12 per cent of the sick have tuberculosis. Tuberculosis prevails as extensively in Cuba as in the United States, but Dr. Guiteras tells me that milk is practically never used without scalding, and tuberculosis is comparatively rare among cattle. If, as appears from a study of the relative prevalence of the two types of bacilli, less than 5 per cent of all tuberculosis is due to cows' milk, the entire elimination of this factor would not, as, from the data furnished by Japan, Cuba, and other places, it appears that it does not, have any appreciable effect on the death rate from this disease. The total elimination of bovine tuberculosis, so far from "stamping out the great white plague," as some assert, would probably not make any noticeable difference in the tuberculosis death rate. Nevertheless it appears from present evidence that in the aggregate a large number of deaths are due to this cause, and if there is any practical method of reducing this cause of death, effort should be made to apply it.

Protection against Tuberculous Milk. — Various ways are suggested for eliminating this danger from milk. Among these is the heating of milk to a sufficient temperature to kill tubercle bacilli as well as typhoid bacilli and other pathogenic organisms. Some have urged compulsory pasteurization by dealers, and this practice is, without any legislation, making rapid progress in cities. But, as is shown by Hess in New

[1] Heymann, Ztschr. f. Hyg. u. Infectionskrankh., Leipz., 1904, XLVIII, 45.

[2] Fisch, Cor.-Bl. f. schweiz. Aerzte, 1904, XXXIV, 761.

York, commercial pasteurization does not always destroy tubercle bacilli, and the proposition that commercial pasteurization be under the control of health officials is a timely one. As has already been stated, there are objections to the compulsory pasteurization of all milk sold, hence the federal Department of Agriculture[1] has suggested a classification of market milk into —

First. Certified milk, which presumably would be free from danger and of high quality, and would be sold at a higher price to those who desired it.

Second. Inspected milk, which also should be from cows free from tuberculosis, but which would not show so low a bacterial count as the certified milk and which could be sold for not much if any more than the next class.

Third. All milk not produced under such rigid inspection should be pasteurized under municipal supervision.

There certainly is a tendency, without any compulsion, for municipal milk supplies to become classified in the way above indicated. Another way of removing the danger is for the consumer to heat the milk after it is received from the dealer. In this way each consumer can protect himself from the danger of contracting tuberculosis, typhoid fever and similar diseases. But most persons will not do this unless they are induced to do so by a slow process of education, and this education can scarcely be hastened without causing an unreasonable fear of milk, which will result in lessening the consumption of a cheap, digestible and nutritious article of food. It seems to me that what is needed is a better and more exact knowledge of the relations of milk to disease on the part of health officers and physicians, from which ought to follow a gradual education of the public, but without an alarmist propaganda, and then there will probably gradually develop a specialization in the milk business to meet the necessarily different needs of different people.

[1] U. S. Pub. Health & Mar. Hosp. Serv., Hyg. Lab., Bull. No. 41, 559.

Eradication of Bovine Tuberculosis. — Another way of dealing with the tuberculous milk problem is to strive to eradicate bovine tuberculosis, or at least to eliminate from herds of milch cows all animals in the active stage of the disease. This is urged by many, and has been and is being attempted. It is claimed by the federal and state departments of agriculture that the existence of bovine tuberculosis entails great loss upon the farmers, and if this is true, these departments should devise and urge means for eliminating the disease, but the expense should be borne by the farmers and not by the public. If, however, the restriction or elimination of bovine tuberculosis is urged as a public health measure, as it so often is, we should count well the cost before placing it upon the general taxpayer. We ought to have a finer sense of financial perspective in sanitary matters. The cost of efficient measures, if efficient measures have yet been devised, for eliminating bovine tuberculosis will be enormous, and we may well consider whether as good results from a public-health standpoint may not be secured, say by pasteurizing milk, and whether the money might not be expended in other ways with far greater results. It is very doubtful whether the expenditure of $100,000 a year for several years in a state like Massachusetts would really result in stamping out the disease in cattle; but consider how much such a sum would accomplish if spent in the establishment of dispensaries and the employment of district nurses, with perhaps $5000 to $10,000 used for further scientific study of the many unsolved problems connected with the causation, prevention and cure of the disease.

Tubercle Bacilli in Butter. — From what is known of the viability of the tubercle bacillus, there can be no doubt that it will live for some time in butter. Schroeder and Cotton[1] carefully investigated the subject and found virulent tubercle bacilli in butter after three months, and Trask[2] refers to a large

[1] Schroeder and Cotton, U. S. Dept. Agric., Bu. An. Ind., Circ. No. 127, 1898.

[2] Trask, J. Am. M. Ass., Chicago, 1908, LI, 1491.

number of similar observations. Cases of tuberculosis do not seem to have been traced to the consumption of such butter, and it is very unlikely that they would be traced even if they occurred. Owing to the small amounts of butter consumed, it is probable that very few cases of tuberculosis are caused in this way. Butterine also has been shown to be infected from the milk, fat and butter of which it is made.[1] Owing to the mode of making and the time occupied in curing cheese, virulent tubercle bacilli are probably rarely if ever found in it.[2]

Mediterranean Fever from Milk. — Mediterranean fever, which is an important disease around the shores of the Mediterranean, has been considered on a previous page, and reference made to the brilliant researches of Bruce, Horrocks and others, who determined that it is primarily a disease of goats, and only incidentally transmitted to man through the medium of milk. The obvious remedy is to avoid the use of goats' milk whenever these animals are known to be infected, and in the Malta garrison the disease has by this means been eliminated. It is rather surprising that in view of the known facts the United States Department of Agriculture should in 1905 have imported a large number of goats from Malta, but the importation resulted in a complete demonstration of the infectiousness of the milk, for quite a number of persons on the ship, and one in America, developed the fever as a result of drinking the milk. The goats have now all been killed.

Anthrax from Milk. — Experiments have shown that anthrax bacilli may be absorbed through the intestines, and they are found in the milk of diseased animals.[3] Instances of this mode of infection in man have been reported, but they are certainly very rare.[4]

[1] U. S. Dept. Agric., Rep. Bu. An. Ind., 1907, XXIV, 152.

[2] Harrison, U. S. Dept. Agric., Rep. Bu. An. Ind., 1902, XIX, 217.

[3] Horrocks, J. Roy. Army Med. Corps, Lond., 1908, XI, 46.

[4] Teacher, J. Comp. Path. & Therap., Edinb. & Lond., 1906, XIX, 225; Meyer, Deutsche med. Wchnschr., 1908, XXXIV, 108; J. Hyg., Cambridge, 1909, IX, 279, 315.

Foot-and-Mouth Disease. — Foot-and-mouth disease is said to be transmitted to human beings by means of milk, and according to Salmon such cases are frequently reported in European outbreaks,[1] but none occurred during the last outbreak in Massachusetts, perhaps owing to the fact that suitable precautions were taken. An instance of this sort of infection occurred near Boston in 1871.[2] Kober[3] refers to other instances of the transmission of foot-and-mouth disease by milk.

Rabies from Milk.—According to Kober,[4] Nocard proved experimentally that rabies could be conveyed in milk, and Burdach infected animals with the milk of a woman sick with the disease at the Pasteur Institute. Repetto[5] was able to kill rats by feeding them with rabies virus, and Remlinger[6] did the same. Dr. Austin Peters of Boston writes me that "Several times where cows have had rabies I have had milk taken from them and brought to the Harvard Medical School. Rabbits and guinea pigs inoculated with it have never developed rabies. From this I should say that there is very little danger of rabies being carried through the milk."

Other Animal Disease and Milk.—As regards actinomycosis, botryomycosis, tetanus, cowpox and many other animal diseases, little or nothing is known about their transmission by milk.

Diarrhea from Milk. — The diarrhea of infants is probably not a specific disease, but the group of disturbances which pass under this name are likely to be due to infection by a number of organisms, and perhaps to some extent to intoxication with the products of bacterial growth outside of the

[1] U. S. Dept. Agric., Rep. Bu. An. Ind., 1902, XIX, 405.

[2] Marion, J. Mass. Ass. Bds. Health, Bost., 1903, XIII, 11.

[3] Kober, Milk in Relation to Public Health, Senate Doc. No. 441, 57th Congress, First Session, 1902, 154.

[4] Kober, Idem, 157.

[5] Repetto, Compt. rend. Soc. biol., Paris, 1908, LXIV, 716; Abst. Am. J. Pub. Hyg., Bost., 1909, XIX, 426.

[6] Remlinger, Compt. rend. Soc. de biol. Par., 1908, LXV, 385.

body. Among the bacteria suspected of causing diarrhea are *B. coli*, *B. enteritidis sporogenes*, *B. enteritidis* (Gärtner), *B. dysenteriæ*, *B. paratyphosus* and *Streptococcus enteritidis*.

The summer diarrheas are confined principally to infantile life, the chief incidence falling on the last half of the first year. According to Newsholme[1] they are associated with a deficient rainfall, and their dependence upon a high temperature is particularly marked. A very large proportion of the deaths occur during the hot summer months, and the hotter the season, as a general thing, the higher the mortality. The relation between temperature and this disease is probably more or less indirect, and at present is not well understood. Another marked characteristic of the summer diarrheas is that they are intimately associated with the mode of feeding. Breast-fed infants are very little affected, while artificially fed infants suffer severely. As the artificial food of infants is chiefly cows' milk, and as these diseases appear to be of bacterial origin, and as the growth of bacteria in milk is enormously facilitated by hot summer weather, it is generally assumed that diarrhea is due to the growth of infective organisms in the milk. Some, however, doubt the validity of this assumption. Liefmann[2] considers that artificial feeding causes disturbances of digestion and nutrition, and that these lay the foundation and open the way for new and injurious factors. The latter are mostly bacterial, and the bacteria effect an entrance into the child's body in various ways, usually by contact infection, and not so often by milk as has been commonly supposed. He says that the use of sterilized milk is disappointing, which indicates that milk is not the chief vehicle of the infection.

Epidemiological Studies. — In 1901–02 a very valuable series of observations was undertaken in New York by Park and Holt, under the auspices of the Rockefeller Insti-

[1] Newsholme, Pub. Health, Lond., 1899–1900, XII, 139.

[2] Liefmann, Ztschr. f. Hyg. u. Infectionskrankh., Leipz., 1908–09, LXII, 199; Abst. Pub. Health, 1909, XXII, 430.

tute.[1] It appeared to these observers that lack of care in the feeding and general management of the babies had more to do with the development of diarrhea than had the character of the milk. It is true that exceptionally dirty store milk gave worse results than any other, but the users of this milk were poorer and dirtier and gave less intelligent care to their children. A rather limited number of children were fed on fairly good milk raw, and another group on the same milk pasteurized, other conditions being nearly the same. Those on pasteurized milk had much less diarrhea, but the authors state that a considerable percentage do quite as well on raw milk. Condensed milk was found to be associated with a large percentage of diarrheal cases. Intelligent care and feeding seem to the authors more important than the character of the milk. They also consider the infection of the milk in the home or store as a very important factor. Breast-fed babies are not immune to diarrhea, and Newsholme,[2] in a very careful study of the subject at Brighton, found that 6.6 per cent of the deaths from diarrhea were in breast-fed infants, who almost certainly could not have been infected by the milk. Newsholme pertinently asks why, if these cases were not due to milk, should it be assumed that all the artificially fed infants who succumbed to diarrhea met their death because of milk contamination. From a study of the kinds of milk used in Brighton it was found that more diarrhea was associated with the use of condensed milk than with that of any other. Similar results from the use of condensed milk were found by Richards in the neighboring city of Croydon,[3] and by Sandilands in Finsbury, London,[4] and their findings do not differ materially from those of Park and Holt. In the English cities a very good brand of condensed milk, viz. Nestles', was the one chiefly employed, and Sandilands found

[1] Med. News, N. Y., 1903, LXXXIII, 1066.
[2] Newsholme, J. Hyg., Cambridge, 1906, VI, 139.
[3] Rep. Med. Off. Health, Croydon, 1904, 1908.
[4] Sandilands, J. Hyg., Cambridge, 1906, VI, 77.

it very free from bacteria. He also states that this condensed milk is collected and put up in Switzerland in such a manner as to make infection during the process much less likely than in ordinary market milk. All the writers above referred to consider that these facts indicate that the infective material of infantile diarrhea gets into the milk and other food to a large extent in the home. Newsholme especially insists on this, and he attributes not a little to direct contact. Tompkins,[1] from a study of the very local distribution of the disease in Leicester, concluded that it must have its source in local conditions. Robertson and Niven, from a study of cases in their respective cities of Birmingham and Manchester, believe that the infection takes place in the city chiefly, either by direct infection or through the milk.

Explosive Outbreaks of Diarrhea. — Sometimes what appear to be explosive milk-borne outbreaks of diarrhea occur. Several such are referred to by Newman.[2] Recently a very interesting outbreak of this kind has been reported by Hay.[3] Various bacteria, such as *B. coli*, *B. enteritidis sporogenes* and *B. enteritidis* of Gärtner, have been isolated from the milk in such cases and also from the evacuations of the patients. It is uncertain whether such outbreaks have any connection with ordinary summer diarrhea, though that they have is the view of Delépine,[4] and he believes that the contamination of milk usually takes place at the farm.

Prevention of Diarrhea. — It appears, then, that we have very little accurate knowledge as to the causation of infantile diarrhea. It certainly has some intimate relation to the diet, but exactly what is not known. We do know, however, that the most efficient means we have of combating it is correct feeding. Breast feeding is far superior to anything else, but good success can be obtained with the careful and scientific

[1] Tompkins, Brit. M. J., Lond., 1889, II, 180.
[2] Newman, Infant Mortality, Lond., 1906, 170.
[3] Hay, Pub. Health, Lond., 1910, XXIII, 180.
[4] Delépine, J. Hyg., Cambridge, 1903, III, 89.

use of good cows' milk. Pasteurized milk appears to be better than dirty raw milk of high bacterial count, but there does not seem to be any definite connection between the disease and an increasing bacterial content. The longer milk remains exposed in shops and houses, the more dangerous it seems to be. Almost all who have had to do with modern milk stations, either those using pasteurized milk or those dispensing clean raw milk, agree that the larger part of the resulting good is due to the education of the mother in the care of her child. The chief thing, then, is to teach the mothers how to modify, keep and feed milk. It is of importance, too, that the mothers should be enabled to get fairly clean and fresh milk. In some cities it is doubtless necessary to establish milk stations for this purpose, which dispense either pasteurized milk, or preferably clean raw milk. In Providence stations were found to be unnecessary, as there is no part of the city in which it is not possible to get 18 to 24 hours' old milk with less than 50,000 bacteria per c.c., and a number of dealers furnish milk below 10,000. This milk is sold by the producer in glass bottles and at the ordinary market price. The milk is by no means equal to certified milk, but the observations of Park and Holt, and our experience in Providence, seem to show that milk of the grade above indicated is ordinarily as little likely to cause infantile diarrhea as is certified milk. Only a small amount of the milk supply of a city is used for feeding infants, and it seems unnecessary to insist on a high grade of expensive milk for all consumers. At present it is more economical to bring the existing good supplies to the knowledge of the mothers through physicians, the health department, district nurses and milk stations. In cities up to 200,000 or 300,000 it is probable that enough dealers can be found to supply the necessary demand for a good though not certified milk.

Infection by Meat.

Inspection of meat is considered by the public a matter of the greatest importance, but concerning many forms of meat infection we have little definite knowledge, and the danger of others has been greatly exaggerated, not only by the public, but also by physicians and health officials. Various animal parasites, such as tapeworms and trichinæ, are derived from the lower animals through the use of their flesh as food, but a consideration of these is beyond our present purpose. One of these animal parasites, the trichina, is quite common in pork, and a considerable number of deaths are caused by it each year.

Food Poisonings. — What are commonly called food poisonings, when resulting from eating meat, are due to two general causes. One class is the result of the action of various kinds of putrefactive organisms which infect the food after slaughter. These cases we need not consider. Another class results from infection of the flesh during the life of the animal, and is due, so far as known, to various members of the colon group, such as *B. paratyphosus*, *B. enteritidis* (Gärtner) and *B. morbificans*. In many instances this unwholesome meat is derived from diseased animals, usually showing some sort of enteritis or septic infection. That the infection is always derived from diseased animals seems unlikely, for several observers have found in healthy animals the bacteria which are believed to be the cause.[1] Savage,[2] however, was unable to isolate *B. enteritidis* (Gärtner) from the intestines of 23 healthy animals which he carefully studied. But from what is known of the relations of this group of bacteria to human beings we should expect to find them occasionally in healthy animals, convalescents and carriers. Unfortunately the toxins produced by these bacteria are not always de-

[1] Bolduan, Food Poisoning, New York, 1909, 33.

[2] Savage, Rep. Med. Off. of Local Gov. Bd., 1906–07, XXXVI, 253; 1907–08, XXXVII, 425.

stroyed by heat, so that while cooking may kill the bacteria, cooked meat, which has been the seat of bacterial growth, has been known to cause sharp outbreaks characterized by acute gastrointestinal symptoms. If living bacteria of this group are present, infection with them may result, causing a slow after development of symptoms somewhat akin to those of typhoid fever. The cooking of meat cannot be relied upon wholly to prevent sickness arising from this sort of food infection. Government inspection is suggested as the only method by which these diseases can be prevented. If, however, bacilli are found in healthy animals, it is questionable whether any amount of inspection would entirely eliminate the danger. How great the danger is it is difficult to determine. A good many outbreaks have been reported in Germany, aggregating thousands of cases, and reports come not rarely from England. No data are available for the United States. For several years I have been on the lookout for the reports of such cases in the medical press and in the "Index Medicus," and one year I employed a press-clipping bureau to secure cuttings from the lay press, but I have notes of scarcely more than a dozen outbreaks. Doubtless others occurred, but they cannot have been very numerous. A good many reports of instances of "ptomaïne poisoning" find their way into the newspapers, which prove on investigation to have no basis in fact.

Meat and Tuberculosis. — In the public mind the fear of contracting tuberculosis by eating meat is very considerable, and public sentiment is sufficient to support very stringent regulation of the sale of meat from diseased animals. Yet it does not appear that there is a single recorded instance of the transmission of disease in this way. And we should expect that if such were possible it would be exceedingly rare. Tubercle bacilli have their habitat in lungs, liver, intestines, glands and other viscera, and not usually in the muscle or fat. The tubercle bacillus is easily killed by heat, and very little of this class of food is eaten without cooking. Smoked beef and ham are occasionally eaten without cooking, but even then considerable time is consumed in the process of corning and smoking, and in the rare cases in which a few bacilli are contained in the meat they are likely to have lost most of their virulence. As for the viscera, if they are used at all for food they are generally pretty well cooked. Cornet states that Schottelius studied the use of meat from tuberculous animals in Würzburg, and could not find a case of the disease, although the meat was eaten in every form. It has been said that while tuberculosis has been decreasing the consumption of meat has been increasing; and this is certainly an indication that the use of meat cannot be a factor of any great moment in the causation of the disease. At the most it is scarcely possible for the disease to be derived from this source except in rare instances.

Conclusions. — The diseases which it is alleged may be transmitted by flesh foods are those caused by animal parasites, of which trichinosis is the most important, diseased conditions produced by the colon group of bacilli, and tuberculosis. The latter is a negligible quantity, the second group probably causes very few deaths in this country, while trichinosis is doubtless the most important disease transmitted in this manner.

Federal Control. — The federal government has instituted an expensive meat-inspection service, ostensibly to guard the health of the public, but as trichinosis, the most common and serious of the animal diseases, though it is very rare in man, is ignored, it is suspected that the system was instituted by Congress as the result of an ill-informed though popular demand. Filthy conditions in the slaughterhouses, and the killing of diseased animals, though their flesh may not be injurious to health, are shocking to the æsthetic sense and the public demands reform. Including the expense of inspection and the value of the meats condemned, the cost to the country is $5,000,000 or $6,000,000 per annum. It is true that the conditions of labor in the great packinghouses have been improved, and that cleanlier methods of handling meat have been enforced, but it is doubtful whether any sickness among consumers has been prevented. I cannot help thinking how much ultimate good might have accrued if a tenth of the sum spent in meat inspection had been devoted to the systematic study of the many unsolved problems of sanitation, such as, for instance, the danger from fomites, the part played by air in the spread of disease, the causes of the decline of tuberculosis and the mode of extension of the disease, the relation of food to health, the causes of infantile diarrhea, the relation of water supplies to the general health, or the meaning of bad air and its effect on health.

Infection by Shellfish.

Oysters. — Since oysters and other shellfish are often eaten raw, and often live in sewage-polluted waters, they might be suspected, and indeed were suspected by Sir Charles Cameron as long ago as 1880, of being the cause of typhoid fever, and in 1893 Thorne suggested that the sporadic cases of cholera which appeared here and there in England were due to the eating of raw shellfish infected at the mouth of the Humber. The first demonstration of the relation of shellfish to disease was by Conn.[1] He showed that 23 of 100 students who went to a certain banquet developed typhoid fever, probably as a result of eating oysters. Of those who did not eat raw oysters none were sick, and one man who did not go to the banquet ate oysters at the dealers' and also was sick. The oysters had been kept about 300 feet from a drain leading from a house where there was typhoid fever. Similar outbreaks have been reported by Chantemesse,[2] Mosny,[3] Chatin,[4]

[1] Conn, Rep. St. Bd. Health, Connect., 1895, 253; Med. Rec., N. Y., 1894, XLVI, 743.

[2] Chantemesse, Bull. Acad. de méd., Par., 1896, 3 s. XXXV, 588, 724.

[3] Mosny, Rev. d'hyg., 1900.

[4] Chatin, Semaine méd, 1897, XVII, 91.

Thresh and Wood,[1] a committee which studied the subject at Atlantic City,[2] Fraser,[3] Soper[4] and Morse.[5]

Clams, Mussels. — Clams as well as oysters have been believed to be the cause of outbreaks,[6] and where mussels and cockles are consumed raw in considerable quantities they are equally liable to carry the infecting organisms. Three outbreaks in Norwich, England, in 1908 were traced to mussels.[7] Mussels also were believed to be the cause of an outbreak of typhoid fever in North Ormsby,[8] and have been an important factor in the causation of typhoid fever in Belfast.

Shellfish in English Cities. — Not only have shellfish been shown to be the cause of marked outbreaks of illness, as just shown, but they are strongly believed by many, especially by English health officials, to be an important source of the ordinary "residual" typhoid fever occurring in cities. Newsholme[9] is especially insistent on this. A careful study of the matter in Brighton, where he was then health officer, showed that in 1894–96, of 189 reported cases of typhoid fever, 41 were imported, and of the 148 remaining, 51, or nearly 30 per cent, had eaten raw oysters or mussels within the incubation period of the disease. These shellfish all came from grounds which were contaminated with sewage. From 1894 to 1902, of 643 reported cases of typhoid fever, 158 were due to eating oysters and 80 to other shellfish, making in all about 37 per cent due to this cause. Similar observations and conclusions may be found in the reports of the health officers of Birmingham, Leicester, Southend, Manchester, London,

1 Thresh and Wood, Lancet, Lond., 1902, II, 1567.
2 Phila. M. J., 1902, X, 634.
3 Fraser, Lancet, Lond., 1903, I, 183.
4 Soper, Med. News, N. Y., 1905, LXXXVI, 241.
5 Morse, Rep. St. Bd. Health, Mass., 1900, 836.
6 Plowright, Brit. M. J., Lond., 1900, II, 681.
7 Rep. on Sanitary Condition of Norwich, 1908, 14.
8 The Medical Officer, 1909, II, 431.
9 Newsholme, J. San. Inst., Lond., XVII.

Portsmouth and other places. The typhoid death rate in English cities is low and health officials find it difficult to account for the origin of the cases. The pollution of shellfish with sewage is not uncommon around the English and Irish coasts.[1] A considerable percentage of the cases of typhoid fever are known to have eaten shellfish, often from polluted sources, within two to four weeks of the date of attack. Perhaps the assumption is justifiable that some of these cases at least are due to the shellfish. Typhoid fever has for some time been rather prevalent in Belfast, and a special commission was appointed for its investigation. This commission believes that the chief source of the disease is mussels and cockles, picked up by the poorer people along the sewage-polluted flats.[2] Mair[3] states that in Belfast it was impossible to make a satisfactory canvass of the number of mussel users, either among the general population or among the typhoid patients. He bases his conclusions as to the part played by mussels on a careful statistical study, and shows that the disease in Belfast has varied according to changes in the amount of mussels consumed. He also shows that Jews and the wealthier classes, who use no mussels, had little typhoid fever. Nash[4] states that at Southend 54 per cent of the typhoid-fever cases confessed to the eating of shellfish, while only 0.4 per cent of 501 sick with other diseases confessed to such eating. Since the consumption of raw shellfish has decreased, typhoid fever has decreased also. In Leicester,[5] 50 per cent of the typhoid cases ate mussels, but they were used in only 15 per cent of a small number of noninfected houses. Johnston[6] found that 25.8 per cent of 62 persons

[1] Rep. Med. Off. Loc. Gov. Bd., 1894–95, XXIV; Loc. Gov. Bd. for Ireland, Rep. on Shellfish Layings, 1904.

[2] U. S. Pub. Health & Mar. Hosp. Serv., Pub. Health Rep., Wash., 1908, XXIII, 995.

[3] Proc. Roy. Soc. Med., Lond., 1909, II, Epidem. Sect., 187.

[4] Nash, Pub. Health, Lond., 1903–05, XVI, 80.

[5] Rep. Med. Off. Health, Leicester, 1908, 31.

[6] Johnston, The Medical Officer, II, 1909, 431.

with typhoid fever had eaten shellfish, mussels and periwinkles within a short time of their illness, while of 827 other persons only 7.3 per cent had eaten them during the whole summer. In the United States, also, non-epidemic or "residual" typhoid has been attributed to the use of raw oysters, as in New York.[1] The chief reason for this seems to be that there is known to be a considerable consumption of sewage-infected oysters.[2] Most of the beds on which oysters are grown are free from dangerous pollution, but it is quite common to "fatten," i.e., freshen and swell them, in estuaries near sewer openings.

Danger Variable. — It seems reasonable to conclude that the danger from eating sewage-infected shellfish is a real one. Exactly how great it is, is difficult to determine. In England anywhere from 15 to 50 per cent of the disease in cities is attributed to eating raw mussels or oysters, but this is on the supposition that every typhoid patient who has recently eaten raw shellfish derived the disease from that source. In Providence raw oysters are very popular; they are consumed in restaurants in large numbers, and form a course in a large proportion of banquets and dinners. Many oysters are grown in the upper part of the bay, in water grossly contaminated with sewage, and in the water and in the oysters colon bacilli are found. Until within two or three years, numbers of oysters from clean water have been "fattened" near sewer openings, yet Providence has a typhoid death rate less than half that of the average American city. Oysters are not eaten to any extent in August, when typhoid fever begins to increase, and they are largely consumed in the winter and spring, when there is little of the disease. During the years 1902–05, of 263 typhoid-fever patients who

[1] Med. News, N. Y., 1904, LXXXIV, 325; 1905, LXXXV, 571.

[2] Report of U. S. Commissioner of Fisheries for year ending Jan. 30, 1904, Appendix, 189; Rep. Dept. Health, City of N. Y., 1904, I, 313; Rep. St. Bd. Health, New Jersey, 1904, 226; Rep. Dept. Health, Baltimore, 1907, 124.

replied definitely as to whether they had eaten oysters, only 26, or about 10 per cent, said that they had. Very few raw oysters are eaten by laboring people, but at present laboring people furnish fully their share of typhoid fever.

While the amount of typhoid fever due to the use of raw shellfish is not very great, this danger ought to be eliminated entirely, and state boards of health should have the authority to forbid the sale of shellfish from polluted waters.

Crawfish and Typhoid Fever. — Dr. Bissell of Buffalo wrote to me about an interesting local outbreak of typhoid fever which was at first suspected to be due to milk. But further investigation showed that it was confined chiefly to boys, and that these boys were in the habit of catching crawfish from a lake grossly polluted with sewage. After partially cooking the crawfish before an open fire in the field, the boys would eat them.

Infection by Fried Fish.

In 1900, Hamer[1] of London reported outbreaks of typhoid fever in Southwark, Lambert and Kensal-town which seemed to be confined in each case to the customers of certain fried-fish shops. While the sickness was believed to be due to the eating of fish, no conclusion was reached as to how the fish became infected. It is scarcely possible that infection of the fish before cooking should not be destroyed by the process, and yet it seems unlikely that handling by carriers after infection could cause such an outbreak.

Infection by Watercress.

In the summer of 1903 there was a very considerable outbreak of typhoid fever in Hackney, London.[2] This was very carefully investigated by Warry, and he eliminated all articles of food and drink as sources of the infection, except watercress. Of the 110 cases 55.3 per cent ate watercress which

[1] Hamer, Special Rep. to Med. Off. Health, Lond., 1900.

[2] Warry, Rep. Med. Off. Health, Lond., 1903, 35.

grew in sewage-polluted water. An inquiry showed that the incidence of the disease on watercress eaters was three times as great as upon those who did not eat it.

Infection by Celery.

Morse[1] reports an outbreak of typhoid fever due to the use of celery. There were 49 cases in an insane asylum. Nearly all of these belonged to the class of pay patients, to whom alone celery was served. Several other persons, however, had access to the celery and contracted the disease. There were no cases except four contact cases among non-users of celery. There had been typhoid fever in the institution some months before and the celery bed had received the hospital sewage. The disease developed soon after the celery came into use.

[1] Morse, Rep. St. Bd. Health, Mass., 1899, 761.

CHAPTER VIII.

INFECTION BY INSECTS.

Importance of Subject. — The subject-matter of this chapter is of the utmost importance in the practical work of preventive medicine, and it is of equal interest to the student of scientific epidemiology. Our actual knowledge of the insect carriers of disease has all been acquired during the last fifteen or twenty years, and marks as brilliant and successful an epoch in the history of medicine as did the phenomenal development of bacteriology in the years immediately preceding.

I hesitate very much to discuss the subject at all, as most of the diseases considered are essentially tropical, and of tropical diseases I have had no personal knowledge. But even we who dwell in temperate regions are likely to meet with isolated cases of tropical diseases, or to suffer from occasional invasions of yellow fever, bubonic plague and relapsing fever. In any event, it is important that both the student of preventive medicine and the health officer keep informed as to current progress in this line of research, and ever bear in mind the possibility that insects may play a part, at least, in the spread of those diseases with which he is more familiar.

Modes of Transmission. — There are various ways in which disease may be transmitted by insects. The most interesting and to us novel manner in which this happens is that the discovery of which we owe to Theobold Smith, in which the insect, as well as the higher animal, serves as the true host of the pathogenic organism which causes the disease. Most of the diseases transmitted in this way are probably caused by animal parasites, usually protozoa. As a rule, they propagate asexually only in man or the higher animals, but develop sexual forms in insects, which thus become, zoölogically considered, their true hosts, while man, if it be a human disease, is the intermediate host. The insects in such instances are sometimes called biological carriers. In other cases the parasites do not develop in the insect, which is then merely a mechanical carrier, as would be a lancet or a hypodermic syringe. The classification of insect-borne diseases is far from definite, owing to the present fragmentary condition of our knowledge. We will first consider those diseases which appear to be biologically carried by insects.

First Proof of Transmission by Insects. — Although there had previously been suggestions that disease might be transmitted by insects, the first definite proof was the demonstration in 1893 by Smith and Kilborne [1] of the development of *Piroplasma bigeminum* and the part played by ticks in the transmission of Texas cattle fever. This discovery did much to point out the lines on which experimental work should proceed. These authors demonstrated the presence of the *Piroplasma* in the blood of infected cattle and in the ticks which fed upon them. They also showed that the ticks transmit the germ through their eggs to their progeny. The new generation of infected ticks then become attached to cattle, and by their bites inoculate them and cause the disease. It was demonstrated that there could be no infection of the fields or fodder, either by the excreta of cattle or by dead ticks or ova. The living tick is necessary for the transmission of the disease, and doubtless the *Piroplasma* passes through definite phases of its development in the body of the tick. Smith and Kilborne showed not only that ticks transmit this disease, but also that it is transmitted only in this way. They furthermore showed that apparently healthy cattle might be carriers of the *Piroplasma*, and therefore in the presence of ticks could cause the spread of the disease. Texas

[1] Smith and Kilborne, U. S. Dept. Agric., Bu. An. Ind., Bull. 1, 1893.

cattle fever, though of immense economic importance in the cattle-raising industry, is not transmissible to human beings. The great importance of Smith and Kilborne's discovery, from our present point of view, is the encouragement it gave to the study of the transmission of human diseases by insect agencies. Koch has demonstrated a similar connection between ticks and a disease of cattle in German East Africa caused by another species of *Piroplasma*, — *P. parvum*. Nuttall and Graham-Smith [1] have investigated a similar disease in dogs, also transmitted by ticks, and have described the development of the parasite *P. canis*. Christophers also [2] has studied the development of this parasite. There appears to be no doubt that piroplasmosis of horses and sheep is transmitted by ticks.

Malaria.

Discovery of Insect Transmission. — While Nott,[3] King,[4] Laveran,[5] Koch and others had suggested, on epidemiological grounds, that this disease might be insect borne, it was not until 1895 that Ross,[6] stimulated by the work of Manson on filariasis, watched the development of the malarial parasite in mosquitoes which had been allowed to bite persons sick with the disease. As Manson had already shown that in filariasis it is only a particular species of mosquito which can serve as host for the filaria, Ross suspected that the same might be true of human malaria, and he finally determined that it was only in individuals of the genus *Anopheles* that the malarial parasite can develop. Ross [7] now turned

[1] Nuttall and Graham-Smith, J. Hyg., Cambridge, 1904, 1905, 1906, 1907.

[2] Christophers, Brit. M. J., Lond., 1907, II, 1333.

[3] Nott, N. Orl. M. & S. J., 1847–48, IV, 563.

[4] King, Tr. Philos. Soc., Wash., 1883.

[5] Laveran, Le Paludisme, Paris, 1891, 147.

[6] Ross, Abst. by Manson, Lancet, Lond., 1896, I, 831.

[7] Ross, Rep. on the Cultivation of *Proteosoma Labbé* in Grey Mosquitoes, Indian M. Gaz., Calcutta, 1898, XXXIII, 133, 401, 448.

to the study of the malaria of birds due to a *Proteosoma*, and he demonstrated that the disease could be transmitted from bird to bird by the bites of mosquitoes. The parasites of the disease are taken up with the blood by the insect in the act of biting, and after undergoing sexual multiplication, spread through the insect, and are found in the salivary gland, whence they are injected into the next bird bitten. Meanwhile Grassi in Italy had come to the conclusion, from a study of the distribution of different species of mosquitoes, that *Anopheles* was one of the forms likely to transmit the disease. Bignami had previously been unsuccessful in transmitting malaria by the bites of mosquitoes, chiefly because he experimented largely with *Culex* instead of *Anopheles*. Finally Grassi, Bignami and Bastianelli in 1899 caused malaria in human beings by allowing anopheles mosquitoes to bite them some days after they had bitten other individuals sick with malaria. To avoid the criticism that these experiments were carried on in Italy, an intensely malarial country, where natural infection could not be absolutely excluded, Patrick Manson[1] had a number of infected mosquitoes sent from Italy to England in 1900, and caused two men, Dr. Thurburn Manson and Mr. Warren, who had never been in a malarial region, to be bitten. Both men developed malaria in exactly eighteen days. In the same year Sambon and Low lived for three months in the most malarial section of the Roman Campagna, protecting themselves absolutely against the bites of mosquitoes, but taking no other precautions. They did not contract malaria, but of fifteen or sixteen police sent from Rome, who spent one night unprotected in the same place, every one developed the disease.[2]

Mosquito Sole Carrier of Malaria. — The observations and experiments above noted prove conclusively that malaria is transmitted by the bites of infected anopheles mosquitoes, but do not indicate whether or not it may be spread in other

[1] Patrick Manson, Brit. M. J., Lond., 1900, II, 949.
[2] Sambon and Low, Brit. M. J., Lond., 1900, II, 1679.

ways. It was Manon's theory at first that the malarial parasite is transmitted from adult to larvæ by means of the water in which the eggs are laid, and that this water is also the means of infecting human beings. He suggested that germs might be inhaled in dust from dried-up and infected pools. As regards transmission by water the experiments of Celli [1] and others have already been referred to, which indicate that such a mode of transference is highly improbable, and there is certainly no epidemiological evidence in its favor. That the plasmodium of malaria grows outside of the animal body is also improbable, for it has never been possible as yet to cultivate it in any way.[2] It has never been found in the water of malarial regions.[3] Even if there are sporelike forms resistant to drying, there is strong evidence that such are not airborne, for mosquito netting would in no way interfere with the free movement of particles small enough to be wafted by the air; but abundant evidence has shown that efficient screening against mosquitoes affords complete protection against this disease, even in the most intensely malarial regions. Moreover the success attending methods of prevention based on the mosquito theory point indubitably to the truth of the theory. Experimental, clinical and epidemiological evidence combine to demonstrate that malaria is a disease transmitted solely by the bites of infected mosquitoes. There are several forms of malarial fever, such as tertian, quartan, aestivo-autumnal, apparently caused by different species of *Plasmodium*, but there is no need here of considering these different forms and their relation one to another. Suffice it to say that the mosquito appears to be the true host of this parasite, and in its body it undergoes sexual reproduction. From eight to ten days after the mosquito is infected, its entire body, including its salivary gland, becomes infested with the so-called sporozoite forms, and when these are injected into human be-

[1] See chapter on Infection by Water.

[2] Craig, The Malarial Fevers, New York, 1909, 93.

[3] Craig, idem, 83.

ings they continue to undergo a vegetative or asexual proliferation, the successive phases of which give rise to the symptoms of the disease. It is believed that no vertebrate other than man serves as the host of the *Plasmodium*, and until recently it was thought that no mosquitoes except those belonging to the genus *Anopheles* could transmit the disease; but recent observations in the Philippines [1] indicate that a mosquito breeding in salt marshes, *Myzomyia ludlowii*, may become the host of the *Plasmodium*. But it is certain that almost always it is some species of *Anopheles* which is the carrier. Not all *Anopheles*, however, can serve as the host, for one of our common species in the northern United States, *A. punctipennis*, does not.[2]

Habits of Mosquitoes.—Mosquitoes develop only in water. The larval and pupal stages may occupy from eight days to a number of weeks, or the larvæ may even live all winter under the ice in northern regions, or retain their vitality for some time in the dried mud of the tropics. The mature insects usually live only a few weeks, but in northern regions hibernate during cold weather. The habits of life of the different species of *Anopheles* vary considerably, and should be carefully studied when measures for extermination are undertaken. Only the adult female bites, so she alone is the carrier of the disease. Anopheles usually bite at night. Gorgas[3] states that they do not usually fly above 100 yards, and that clearing and draining the area within this distance of houses affords great protection. Nevertheless it sometimes happens that under favorable conditions the insects may be carried a considerable distance by the wind. Craig[4] states that they may be borne even two and one-half miles.

Must be Many Mosquitoes. — Mosquitoes are not infected with the malarial parasite unless they bite infected human

[1] Banks, Philippine J. Sc. [B. Med.], 1908, III, 335.

[2] Hirschberg, Johns Hopkins Hosp. Bull., Balt., 1904, XV, 53.

[3] Gorgas, J. Am. M. Ass., Chicago, 1909, LII, 1967.

[4] Craig, The Malarial Fevers, New York, 1909, 69.

beings. The number of infected mosquitoes, then, varies with the number of infected persons to whom they have access. Craig[1] refers to the findings of himself and others as varying from 35 per cent to 0.6 per cent. For the spread of malaria it is necessary that there should be *Anopheles* and human beings infected with the parasites. But if the mosquitoes are not numerous and the cases of infection are not numerous, the chances of a mosquito becoming infected and then biting another victim after a proper interval are not great, so that it may happen that there may be mosquitoes and human infection without extension of the disease. Thus it is not known that cases of malaria have ever developed on the island of Rhode Island, but I have found a few *Anopheles* breeding there, and with the great numbers of summer visitors from all over the world, and many soldiers, and sailors of the navy, it is probable that the malarial parasite is frequently present on the island. These epidemiological facts led me for some time to suspect that the supposed mode of transmission of this disease above outlined did not contain the whole truth; but the directness and strength of the experimental proof, and, above all, the success of mosquito control in checking the disease render it certain that practically the only way in which malarial disease is caused is by the bites of mosquitoes. There are numberless interesting details connected with the life history and habits of the mosquito which are of great importance but which cannot be considered here. The way in which these habits explain the peculiarities in the development of malaria is well considered by Nuttall.[2]

Ways of Prevention. — There are several ways in which the spread of malarial disease may be checked.

First. Quinia. — The administration of the various salts of quinia prevents the development of the malarial parasite in the blood, and this drug is an extremely valuable remedy in the prevention and cure of malaria. Antitoxin and vaccines

[1] Craig, loc. cit., 74.

[2] Nuttall, Johns Hopkins Hosp. Rep., Balt., 1899, VIII, 78.

are of great value in the prevention and cure of certain of the infectious diseases, as diphtheria, typhoid fever and cholera, but they are of value chiefly to the individual. The difficulties attendant upon their administration are so great that they cannot be used except in rare instances to protect large bodies of people. The antitoxins, too, probably do not prevent the growth of the germs which are the cause of the disease, so that in a way their use, as for instance that of diphtheria antitoxin, may actually in some instances favor the spread of the disease, by preventing the development of symptoms when the bacilli are present, thus making a "carrier" instead of a "case," and carriers are always difficult to control. It is otherwise with quinia. This drug actually kills the *Plasmodium* or drives it out of the circulation and out of the way of the mosquito, and so not only protects the individual but prevents him from becoming a focus of infection. Quinia is not only universally used as a specific curative agent, but it is also employed in large quantities as a prophylactic, and its employment in this manner is considered a valuable means of fighting the disease, reducing as it does the number of foci of infection. Indeed Koch and some others claim that this is the only way in which malaria can be eradicated, as mosquito destruction is in many places impossible. All workers in this field employ quinia for this purpose, though there is considerable discussion as to its mode of administration, which varies from 15 grains every eight days, as used by Koch, to 3 grains daily, as advised by Gorgas. This subject is fully discussed by Craig,[1] who states that in the vast majority of instances $2\frac{1}{4}$ grains (0.15 grm.) daily is sufficient to prevent malarial infection. It is difficult to estimate the value of a particular prophylactic measure, for one measure is rarely used alone, but there is little doubt of the great efficiency of quinia in the fight against malaria. Craig states that at Camp Stotsenburg, in the Philippines, measures directed against mosquitoes had little result until supplemented by

[1] Craig, The Malarial Fevers, New York, 1909, 343.

the daily administration of quinia. Koch and his followers also report excellent results from the use of quinia alone. Celli,[1] while urging every method directed against the mosquito, considers that in Italy experience has shown that the daily administration of quinia has been the most effective measure in reducing the number of deaths from malaria, which have fallen steadily from 13,861 in 1901 to 4871 in 1906, during which year 20,723 kilos of quinia were sold.

Second. Isolation of Persons.—The attempt may be made to isolate the infected persons so that the mosquitoes may not pass from them to the healthy. This may be accomplished in various ways. In many tropical regions where the native population, or at least the native children, are always infected, the dwellings of the natives and the susceptible Europeans are separated a sufficient distance to escape the ordinary excursions of the mosquitoes.

Sometimes the patients, if few in number, are screened from mosquitoes in their own homes or are removed to screened hospitals. This is very commonly done with the imported cases which come to Havana,[2] and in Panama many malarial patients are treated in the screened hospitals. Others are cared for in their own well-screened houses.

To assist in this measure it is desirable to kill all mosquitoes in the house which may have bitten the patient before the disease was recognized or reported to the authorities. Gorgas considers sulphur dioxid the best for this, but as this cannot be used in an occupied room, pyrethrum may be burned, which so stupefies the insects that they may be easily swept up from the floor. Celli has given much study to this class of culicides and recommends one or two tablespoonfuls of a mixture of the unexpanded flowers of chrysanthemum and valerian root.

Third. Screening.—Effort should be made in all malarious regions to protect susceptible persons from the bites of mos-

[1] Quoted by Craig, The Malarial Fevers, New York, 1909, 345.
[2] Guiteras, J. Am. M. Ass., Chicago, 1909, LIII, 1165.

quitoes. The screening of the whole house is the most important step. Copper netting is the cheapest in the end, and it should, according to Craig, have 11 meshes to 2 cm. Gorgas says that it is necessary that houses should be screened by persons experienced in mosquito work, or openings are sure to be left. The experiments of Sambon and Low proved the efficacy of this method of prophylaxis, and Craig states that the screening of the houses of railway employees on certain Italian lines has been as effectual a method as the administration of quinia. Screening is carried on most extensively in the Canal Zone. Craig says that where screening is impossible the use of mosquito canopies over the beds at night is a very useful measure, and head nets and gloves for men obliged to be out at night are of much value. By the use of these methods the percentage of malaria among troops in Sardinia was reduced from 70 to 20, and in Formosa no malaria developed among 115 soldiers protected by netting, while of 717 not so protected 251 were attacked.

The removal of trees, vines and shrubs from the vicinity of dwellings is considered by Gorgas an important measure, as these serve as hiding places for the insects by day.[1]

A certain amount of protection may be secured by the application to the skin of substances annoying to the mosquito, or of ointment which mechanically interferes with biting. Oil of citronella or eucalyptus, and petroleum or cocoanut oil or vaseline, are used, but such applications are not by most writers considered of much value.

Fourth. Mosquito Prevention. — Theoretically the most effectual way to eradicate malaria is to prevent the growth of mosquitoes. While their complete destruction is not usually possible, its attempt must always take first rank in preventive measures. The fact that mosquitoes are a great nuisance, as well as carriers of disease, makes still more desirable their extermination wherever possible. Large sums, in certain parts of the United States, are being expended in fighting the

[1] Gorgas, J. Am. M. Ass., Chicago, 1909, LII, 1967.

salt-marsh mosquito, which is harmless so far as carrying disease is concerned.

Fifth. Draining. — When mosquitoes breed in pools and swamps, as they so often do, draining and filling must be done. If water cannot be entirely gotten rid of, the banks of streams, ponds and ditches must be straightened and deepened, and freed from vegetation, to remove hiding places for the larvæ and permit their destruction. Gorgas insists upon the importance of having this work done by men especially trained for it, and supervised by experts. Ordinary contractors and laborers are sure to overlook breeding places and to neglect important details of the work. Many species of *Anopheles* breed in cisterns or accidental receptacles of water near houses. Hence all such should either be removed or carefully screened.

Sixth. Oiling.— The growth of larvæ in water can be prevented by the application of crude petroleum or kerosene to the surface at the rate of an ounce to each 15 square feet of surface. Various poisonous substances may be added to the water, as hydrochloric acid, corrosive sublimate, formalin, chloride of lime and various aniline dyes. Some of the last named are strongly recommended by Celli, as they are harmless to the higher animals. The use of quicklime causes a glaze on the surface which is a protection, and sulphate of copper kills the algæ on which the mosquitoes live. Most fish are voracious feeders on the larvæ, and if pools and streams are supplied with fish, and kept free from weeds, mosquitoes cannot thrive. It is said that the introduction of a certain small fish into the streams of Barbados caused the extermination of mosquitoes.[1] According to Craig, the application of cultures of *Aspergillus niger* and *A. glaucus* destroys the larvæ.

Success of Measures. — There is probably scarcely a locality in which the application of a single prophylactic measure will be found effectual in "stamping out" malaria, and sometimes all methods combined fail to bring success. Thus at Mian Mir in India, according to Craig, the most

[1] Ballou, Nature, Lond., 1909, LXXX, 16.

careful draining and oiling were followed by very discouraging results. On the other hand, preventive measures have in many localities given wonderfully good results. The success of the work in Italy, as reported by Celli, has already been referred to. In Havana the deaths from malaria previous to the occupation by the United States averaged 350 per annum, rising to 1907 in 1898. The measures carried out by Gorgas to destroy the yellow-fever mosquitoes also practically eliminated the *Anopheles*, and the deaths now average only about 40, and three-fourths of these are, according to Kean,[1] due to infection contracted elsewhere. At Ismailia[2] the cases were reduced from 2284 in 1900 to 37 in 1905, chiefly by destroying the breeding places of mosquitoes. At Klang and Port Swettenham in the Federated Malay States 99 per cent of the mosquitoes were eliminated, with a corresponding decrease in malaria. Ross also refers to the successful reduction of malaria at Port Said, Durban, Hong Kong, Khartoum, and in Candia, St. Lucia, Greece and Algeria.[3]

Success in Panama. — To my mind the most wonderful success of all has been attained by Gorgas in the Panama Canal Zone. Here was a stretch of territory 45 miles long, intensely malarious, now occupied by a force of 44,000 persons, mostly foreigners. The rainfall is heavy, and the work of canal building alters in every direction the configuration of the land and the natural drainage. Malaria caused enormous losses during the French occupation and was second only to yellow fever in interrupting the work. Mosquitoes have been entirely eliminated from Colon, a town of 15,000 inhabitants, and the death rate from malaria among employees was only 1.34 per thousand in 1908, having been reduced from 5.57 in 1905. Considering the tremendous obstacles to be overcome, this success is certainly astonishing.[4]

[1] Kean, J. Am. M. Ass., 1909, LIII, 1166.
[2] Ross, Lancet, Lond., 1907, II, 879.
[3] Ross, Nature, Lond., 1909, LXXX, 415.
[4] Gorgas, J. Am. M. Ass., Chicago 1909, LII, 1967.

Yellow Fever.

History of Discovery. — Nott appears to have been the first (1848) to attribute to mosquitoes a rôle in the causation of yellow fever, but this was merely a suggestion which received little attention. According to Cruz,[1] Beauperthuy published on the 23d of May, 1854, in the *Official Gazette* of Cumana, Venezuela, an article which expounded with great clearness a mosquito theory of this disease. But to Finlay of Havana is due the credit for the first experimental work, a report of which was presented to the Royal Academy of Medical, Physical and Natural Sciences in Havana in 1882. Finlay continued to experiment and write until 1900, when the American Commission, consisting of Reed, Carroll, Agramonte and Lazear, undertook their investigations at Havana.[2] Finlay had come to the conclusion that *Culex fasciatus*, now *Stegomyia calopus*, was the species of mosquito which was likely to be involved in the transmission of the disease. After the occupation of Cuba by the United States in 1898, the war department undertook with great energy the extirpation of yellow fever from Havana. At that time the disease was believed to be essentially a filth disease, and the energy of the government was directed towards making Havana clean, and soon its "sanitary condition" vied with that of the very best cities in the United States. At the same time the most stringent measures of isolation, as isolation was at that time understood, were applied. But yellow fever refused to be stamped out, and in 1900 caused 1244 cases and 310 deaths, many of them among the "best people" in the cleanest parts of the city.[3] It was becoming evident that the old theories were not satisfactory, and the war department appointed the

[1] Cruz, U. S. Pub. Health & Mar. Hosp. Serv., Pub. Health Rep., Wash., 1909, XXIV, 1741.

[2] Lee, Am. Pub. Health Ass. Rep., 1905, XXX, 8.

[3] Series 4, Yellow Fever Pub., San. Dept., Havana, 1902, 10.

commission above referred to, which proceeded to Havana and in its earliest work put Finlay's mosquito theory to the test. They were not a little influenced to this step by the observations of Carter.[1] He had determined, from a study of the disease in isolated farmhouses, that from nine to sixteen days usually elapse, after the introduction of the disease, before the house can infect second cases. It was thought that this interval might depend upon a period of incubation in the mosquito. Owing to the hearty coöperation of General Wood, the governor, himself a medical man, every facility was accorded the commission, and inoculation experiments were made on volunteer human subjects, among whom was Lazear, a member of the commission. Of 11 persons bitten by mosquitoes which had some days before been allowed to feed on a yellow-fever patient, 2 developed the disease, one of whom was Lazear, who died as the result of the inoculation.[2] Carroll too was bitten and developed the disease. As critics suggested that natural infection could not be excluded, the experiments were repeated in November and December, 1900, under more convincing conditions, and 6 of 7 persons bitten developed typical yellow fever, and the transmission of the disease in this manner was demonstrated beyond question.[3] Later Guiteras [4] succeeded in inoculating 8 more persons, which made a total of 24 persons infected by the bites of mosquitoes. Of these 3 died, and the post-mortem examination demonstrated the lesions of yellow fever. The commission had by the direct transfer of blood shown that the infective agent exists in that fluid, even when filtered.[5] All the experimenters demonstrated that the mosquito could not transmit the disease until six to eighteen days after

[1] New Orleans M. & S. J., 1900, LII, 617.

[2] Am. Pub. Health Ass. Rep., 1900, XXVI, 37; Phila. M. J., 1900, VI, 790.

[3] Series 3, Yellow Fever Pub., San. Dept., Havana, 1902.

[4] Series 6, Yellow Fever Pub., San. Dept., Havana, 1902, 26.

[5] Am. Med., Phila., 1902, III, 301.

biting a yellow-fever patient, thus explaining the wonderfully accurate clinical observations of Carter. Although it has been shown that filtered blood contains the infective principle, thus far it has not been demonstrated by microscopical or cultural methods. It seems in the highest degree probable, from this very remarkable work, that the exciting agent of yellow fever closely resembles that of malaria, in that it is found in the blood, is taken up by a particular species of mosquito, develops in the mosquito during a period of some days, and is then transmitted to new subjects only by the subsequent bites of the insect.

Transmission by Fomites Disproved. — Belief in the infectiousness of the vomitus and excreta and in the important part played by fomites in the extension of the disease was so firmly fixed that it seemed necessary to test this theory by actual experiment. The commission for this purpose exposed a number of non-immune persons to the closest possible contact, during a period of two weeks, to bedding, clothing and other articles all grossly contaminated with supposedly infective material, but none of them contracted the disease. Later Guiteras, while carrying on his mosquito inoculations, incidentally exposed many non-immunes to fabrics that had been in close touch with yellow-fever cases, but with like negative results; and again Gorgas, at Las Animas Hospital in Havana, put the fomites theory to test in the most thorough manner by the exposure of non-immunes to close and continued contact.[1]

Even before these demonstrations, some acute observers, especially Carter,[2] had concluded from epidemiological studies that fomites played little part in the dissemination of this disease. Carter showed among other things that countless pieces of baggage, many of them certainly from infected houses in Cuba and Vera Cruz, had passed to northern ports without causing yellow fever in a single instance.

[1] Series 3, Yellow Fever Pub., San. Dept., Havana, 1902, 22.
[2] Carter, Med. News, N. Y., 1904, LXXXV, 878.

Transportation of Mosquitoes. — Theoretically there is no reason why infected mosquitoes might not occasionally be carried in baggage, but admission of baggage without disinfection, without any known instance of the development of yellow fever, shows that such a mode of transmission must be extremely rare. Even the carriage of infected mosquitoes in vessels must be unusual, though instances are recorded by Carter [1] and others. Grubbs [2] found *Stegomyia calopus* on three of sixty-five vessels entering the Gulf Quarantine Station. Souchon,[3] at New Orleans, found that 2.5 per cent of the mosquitoes caught on incoming steamers from Havana or the West Indies were *Stegomyia calopus*. Probably none of these were infected.

The rapid and brilliant demonstration of the true mode of extension of yellow fever was immediately followed by an equally rapid and brilliant application of the new knowledge. Two months after the termination of the commission's experiments, Gorgas was as energetically applying the new methods of yellow-fever control in Havana as he had previously devoted himself to cleansing the city, and within eight months the *Stegomyia calopus* had been nearly exterminated, and Havana was free from the disease for the first time in 150 years.

Habits of Yellow-fever Mosquito. — Different species of mosquitoes have different habits of life, and *Stegomyia calopus* is much more of a domestic mosquito than are the *Anopheles*. It prefers to breed in clean rain water, but will grow in any water that is not too muddy. It may even be found in cesspools and in gutters, but its favorite home is the rain-water cistern, barrel, jar or other container which is usually provided for every house. It seems to prefer dark, covered receptacles. The adult mosquito is rather feeble and rarely flies far.

[1] Carter, Med. Rec., N. Y., 1902, LXI, 441.

[2] Grubbs, Yellow Fever Institute, U. S. Pub. Health & Mar. Hosp. Serv., Bull. No. 11.

[3] Souchon, J. Am. M. Ass., Chicago, 1903, XL, 1647.

Preventive Measures. — The defensive measures against yellow fever must of course be somewhat like those directed against malaria, but differ in some important particulars. The most important of these is that there is no drug which will prevent and cure this disease as quinia does malaria. Another point of difference is that yellow fever is not nearly so widespread a disease as is malaria, and that it is an acute disease in which the patient remains infectious for only a short time. Among the measures directed against yellow fever are:

First. Quarantine. — While inland quarantine has never been successfully administered, maritime quarantine for yellow fever is certainly of value. The short period of incubation of the disease, the absence of chronic cases and the fact that it prevails in endemic form in only a few places which are in communication with the rest of the world chiefly by water, render it possible to intercept at the port of debarkation a goodly number of incoming cases. Quarantine, while often failing, has many times proved its value in the United States; and in Havana, after the disease was exterminated, it would certainly have many times been introduced from Vera Cruz and Colon, and indeed probably from New Orleans, if the careful inspection of incoming passengers had not been maintained by the department of health. The efficiency of quarantine is greatly increased if an agent is stationed at the port of embarkation, as is done at many ports by the United States Public Health Service.

Second. Screening of Houses and Cases. — Houses and their healthy inmates must be screened to protect them from infected mosquitoes, and cases must be screened to prevent mosquitoes from becoming infected. Extraordinary effort must be made to get control of every case. The harsh treatment formerly accorded these cases, the injury to property caused by disinfection and the loss to business by the old methods of quarantine put a premium on concealment; but there is much less tendency to hide cases now than formerly. When reported, the case is protected from mosquitoes either by efficient screening or, as is now usually done in Havana and the Canal Zone, by removing the patient to a well-screened hospital.

Third. Destruction of Mosquitoes. — Infected mosquitoes in the house occupied by the patient and in neighboring houses must be destroyed. Sulphur dioxid is the best culicide for this purpose, but pyrethrum powder may be burned while the room is occupied and the stupefied mosquitoes swept up, as in malaria.

Fourth. Prevention of their Growth. — The most important means of preventing yellow fever is to reduce the number of stegomyia mosquitoes to a minimum by destroying their breeding places in the same manner in which the breeding places of malarial mosquitoes are destroyed, by draining, filling, ditching and the use of petroleum and culicides in the water. As the stegomyia so often breeds in domestic receptacles which in the absence of a municipal water supply and sewers cannot be dispensed with, the efficient screening of these receptacles is an important part of sanitary work in the American tropics, and constant inspection is needed to see that the screening is maintained.

Success of Measures. — The phenomenal success of these measures in Havana has already been referred to, but the eradication of the disease in the Canal Zone is a still more remarkable achievement. Havana is a compactly built, well-drained city, and was under military rule. The Canal Zone is about forty-five miles long, with swamps and streams, many straggling villages and camps, a heavy rainfall, continuous high temperature, a constantly changing non-immune population, stupendous engineering works altering the configuration of the land, and a persistent yellow-fever infection for centuries. This disease had been the chief obstacle in the construction of the Panama railroad, and it was the chief obstacle to the French in their canal work. Their loss by death from this disease amounted probably to from 12 to 15 per cent per annum.[1] Sanitary work began on the isthmus in February, 1905, at which time yellow-fever cases were being constantly reported. The cases soon began to decrease, and within a year the disease was practically exterminated.[2] In Rio Janeiro the campaign against yellow fever began in April, 1903. The undertaking was expensive, as it always must be if it is to be successful. It required the expenditure of $1,650,000 a year and the employment of thirteen hundred men. Deaths from yellow fever, which had averaged twelve hundred a year for nearly forty years, decreased rapidly, as is shown by the following:

Year.	Deaths.
1903	584
1904	48
1905	289
1906	42
1907	39
1908	4
1909	0

In Vera Cruz, which was another stronghold of yellow fever, the disease has been almost eradicated by the employment of anti-mosquito measures.[3]

Filariasis.

First Parasite Studied in Insects. — While the infection of the blood of man with *Filaria bancrofti* is in most cases not accompanied by noticeable symptoms, it is of interest in this connection as being the first infection in which the parasite was proved to be taken up into and undergo metamorphosis in the body of an insect. This tiny worm is found swimming

[1] Gorgas, J. Am. M. Ass., Chicago, 1909, LIII, 597.

[2] Cruz, Pub. Health Rep., U. S. Pub. Health & Mar. Hosp. Serv., Wash., 1909, 1742.

[3] Liceaga, Am. Pub. Health Ass. Rep., 1905, XXXI, 284.

in vast numbers in the blood of those who are infected, but is found only at night. During the day it disappears from the peripheral circulation and is found only in the heart and lungs. When these larval forms are sucked up by the mosquito they increase rapidly in size and become more highly organized, and working their way to the proboscis of the insect, infect the next person bitten. The worms, now presenting sexual forms, reach the lymph ducts, where the eggs are laid and whence the young larvæ reach the blood current. It is now generally believed that injury to the worms in the lymph vessels causes obstruction of the latter and the development of tropical elephantiasis. *Culex fatigans* is probably the insect chiefly concerned in the spread of the infection. The disease has not been actually transmitted to man by the bites of infected mosquitoes, but the development of the worm in the mosquito was observed by Manson in 1878[1] and by Lewis in 1879.[2] A similar infection in dogs has been actually transmitted by means of mosquitoes.[3]

Sleeping Sickness.

Discovery of Trypanosome. — The trypanosome (*T. gambiensis*), which is the cause of sleeping sickness, was found in the blood of patients by Dutton and Todd in 1901. This disease is very widely distributed in Africa, and it is estimated to have caused over 100,000 deaths in Uganda during the six years from 1901–1907. This trypanosome is pathogenic for many of the lower animals, and in monkeys causes symptoms resembling those produced in man. Bruce and Nabarro[4] showed that the disease may be transmitted by insects, for in 1903 they succeeded in inoculating a monkey by allowing it to be bitten by tsetse flies (*Glossina palpalis*)

[1] Manson, Med. Times & Gaz., Lond., 1878, II, 731.

[2] Lewis, Quart. J. Micr. Sc., Lond., 1879, XIX, 245.

[3] Braun, The Animal Parasites of Man, 3d ed., New York, 1908, 285.

[4] Bruce and Nabarro, Rep. of Sleeping Sickness Commission, Roy. Soc., 1903, No. 1.

which had twenty-four to forty-eight hours previously bitten negroes suffering with the disease. While this much has been established with certainty, there are important points in the causation of the disease which are still under discussion.

While *Glossina palpalis* is known to transmit sleeping sickness, and the distribution of this fly in a large degree corresponds with the distribution of the disease, it is not certain whether it may not be carried by other species of tsetse flies, and perhaps by domestic insects and by mosquitoes,[1] and Koch[2] thinks it possible that it may be transmitted by the sexual act. Comparatively little is known about the breeding habits of the fly.

Does it infect Lower Animals?—There has also been much discussion as to whether the specific trypanosome of this disease naturally infects the lower animals. If they are generally affected, they become a vast reservoir from which the trypanosomes may be transferred to human beings by the fly, and the difficulties in the way of controlling the disease become enormous. Even the crocodile has been suggested by Koch as an important "reservoir." But Hodges[3] says that actual observation shows that no animal except the native dog, and that in only a few instances, has been found naturally infected. A cause of the uncertainty is a widespread distribution of several kinds of trypanosomes not easily distinguished from *T. gambiensis*.

Is it carried Mechanically?—Another question of importance, especially from a scientific standpoint, is whether the trypanosome passes through a cycle of development in the fly. It was at first supposed that this was the case, but later observations, especially those of Minchin,[4] seemed to indicate that this was not so. According to his observations flies are

[1] Bull. Soc. path. exot., Par., 1908, I.

[2] Koch, Deutsche med. Wchnschr., 1907, XXXIII, 1889.

[3] Cited in Supl. to Third Rep., Wellcome Research Lab., Khartoum, 1908, III, 172.

[4] Minchin, Quart. J. Micr. Sc., Lond., 1908, n. s., LII, 159.

infective at once after biting a subject, and the power to infect does not last over forty-eight hours. More recently, however, Bruce[1] has shown that the parasites do undergo developmental changes in the fly, and that flies do not infect until from 14 to 20 days have elapsed after feeding on a case. Kleine[2] also has demonstrated the same for other forms of trypanosomes. It is possible that the trypanosomes may be occasionally carried mechanically on the proboscis of the tsetse fly, in which case infection will take place at once, and also that the parasites pass through certain metamorphoses in the fly, thus permitting the flies to remain infective for some time.

Prevention of Sleeping Sickness. — The measures suggested for limiting sleeping sickness are:

First. Quarantine, or the prevention of the entrance of infected human beings into regions occupied by the fly. While this may be of value at times, it scarcely seems possible to an observer at this distance that it can be often employed effectually in Africa.

Second. The sick may be segregated and kept out of reach of the flies until the trypanosomes have disappeared from the blood.

Third. The removal of the entire population from the area occupied by the fly. The tsetse flies are found only from thirty to one hundred yards from water, so that if all settlements are removed this distance from rivers and lakes much will be done to prevent the spread of the disease.

Fourth. As trees and shrubs afford a hiding place for the flies, the thorough clearing of the land around villages and near landing places and shore market places has been found useful, just as similar clearing has been found to be an important means of controlling malaria in the Canal Zone at Panama.

[1] Bruce, Bull. of Sleeping Sickness Bu., 1909, Nos. 6 & 7.

[2] Kleine, Deutsche med. Wchnschr., 1909, XXXV, 924.

Fifth. The administration of atoxyl (anilin meta-arsenate) is believed by many to shorten the life of the parasite in the body, and if so, it becomes a valuable prophylactic measure, similar to the use of quinia in malarial affections.

Kala-azar.

Protozoan Discovered by Leishman. — Kala-azar, or dum-dum fever, occurs in various tropical countries, particularly in India. It runs a chronic course and is characterized by marked enlargement of the spleen. In 1900 Leishman discovered in splenic pulp, from a case of the disease, certain bodies the importance of which he did not appreciate, but later, in 1903, he concluded that they might be protozoa. The discovery was confirmed the same year by Donovan. These bodies are now recognized as protozoa, and are known as *Leishmania donovani,* and are probably the cause of the disease. Similar bodies were found by Wright of Boston in oriental sore, and by Nicolle and Cassuto in an infantile splenic disease in Tunis. Rogers, Patton and others have succeeded in growing the parasite in culture medium outside of the body, and both have also obtained evidence to show that the disease may be transmitted by the bedbug. Both Patton and Rogers have shown that a well-defined cycle of development takes place in the body of that insect, which renders it very probable that it is the intermediate host. Patton says, "There is no shadow of doubt that the bed-bug transmits the disease," but this has as yet not been definitely proved.[1] Further studies by Nicolle and others have shown that the dog can be inoculated with the type of the disease occurring in Tunis, and furthermore that the disease occurs spontaneously in dogs which are possibly the source of the human disease. In Tunis only children have so far been observed to be infected. The parasite at first was thought to be somewhat different from *L. infantum*

[1] Supplements to Third and Fourth Reps., Wellcome Research Lab., Khartoum, 1908, 95; 1911, 150.

but the two forms are now generally believed to be identical. Basile thinks the flea is the carrier, while Donovan suspects some species of *Connorrhinus*. The disease has recently been observed in Italy, Sicily, Malta and Portugal.[1]

Pellagra. — Although until recently the majority of writers have been inclined to attribute this disease to the consumption of spoiled maize, Sambon as early as 1905 seems to have suspected that it might be a true contagious disease transmitted by insects. Sambon considers that the topographical distribution of the disease in Italy corresponds closely with the distribution of a small biting fly, *Simulium reptans*. Other observers, as Alessandrini and Lavinder,[1] agree that it is a rural disease and even in the country has a "patchy" distribution as has malaria. Sambon and others have noted its prevalence along watercourses and its occurrence is confined to spring and autumn. Sambon thinks that *Simulium* is the carrier because it has the same geographical and seasonal distribution as pellagra and because it breeds in watercourses along which pellagra is found. The insect does not enter houses, which, according to Sambon, explains the limitation of the disease to out-of-door workers. It is the only insect which has the same distribution as pellagra.

Recently in South Carolina[2] the relation of pellagra to the *Simulium vittatum* has been noted. A similar relation has been reported in Kansas by Hunter.[3]

Opilacao or Canguary. — These names are in certain parts of Brazil applied to hook-worm disease, but in the region where it was studied by Chagas they are names of a quite fatal disease of children characterized by dropsy, glandular swellings and various nervous disturbances,

[1] Pub. Health Rep., U. S. Pub. Health and Mar. Hosp. Serv., 1911, XXVI, 1459.

[2] Pub. Health Rep., U. S. Pub. Health and Mar. Hosp. Serv., 1912, XXVII, 255.

[3] Hunter, J. Am. M. Ass., Chicago, 1912, LVIII, 547.

especially convulsions. Chagas found the disease to be characterized by the presence of a species of trypanosome named, by him, *Schizotrypanum cruzi*. This trypanosome is also found in various animals from which it is probably transmitted to man by a large biting bug, *Connorrhinus megistus*. The bugs only become infective on the eighth to tenth day after feeding.[1]

Pappataci Fever. — This fever, which much resembles dengue, occurs along the eastern coast of the Adriatic, in Malta and Crete and probably in India. Doerr in 1908 definitely proved that it is transmitted by a species of "sand fly," *Phlebotamus papatassi*. The cause of the disease is probably ultra-microscopic, as it is contained in the filtered blood. The virus is transmitted by the female fly to its offspring which become capable of causing infection after reaching maturity. The habits of the fly have been studied and plans devised for its control.[2]

Oriental Sore. — This is also variously called "Bagdad boil," "Biskra boil," "Aleppo button" and "Bouton d'Orient." It is also found in Panama and in Brazil, as well as in Asia and Africa. The parasite, *Leishmania tropica*, has been successfully cultivated. Inoculated into monkeys local lesion may result, but these animals seem not to be very susceptible. Although the parasites are not found in the blood it has been thought that certain biting insects may transmit the disease after becoming infected by feeding on the sores. Anopheles mosquitoes and the itch insect have been suggested. Wenyon[3] has made careful studies of this disease in Bagdad and has succeeded in getting a growth of the parasites in bedbugs and mosquitoes but not in ticks. As only the exposed parts of the body are

[1] Second Review of Recent Progress in Tropical Medicine, Khartoum, 1911, 371.

[2] Second Review of Recent Advances in Tropical Medicine, Khartoum, 1911, 248.

[3] Wenyon, Parasitology, 1911, IV, 273.

infected he thinks it improbable that bedbugs transmit the disease but suggests a sand fly, a species of *Phlebotamus*, or *Stegomyia fasciatus*. Wenyon also thinks that the virus may sometimes be carried mechanically by flies.

Typhus Fever. — According to Wilder,[1] Mexican physicians have long looked upon insects as carriers of "tarbadillo" or Mexican typhus. Recently Sambon suggested the louse as perhaps the transmitter of this disease, and in 1906 Hay[2] noted many epidemiological facts tending to implicate the flea. The first experimental work was done by Nicolle and his associates in Tunis, who succeeded in transmitting the typhus fever of that region from man to an ape. Ricketts and Wilder[3] and Anderson and Goldberger,[4] working with the Mexican type of the disease independently of Nicolle, demonstrated conclusively that the body louse, *Pediculus vestimenti*, can, under experimental conditions, easily transmit the disease from man to monkey and from monkey to monkey. They also showed that the virus is contained in the blood and is filterable and that one attack protects against another. Three of the investigators contracted typhus fever while engaged in this work and Ricketts died. One of the others, Dr. Goldberger, writes me that while experimenting on typhus fever he was bitten by a presumably infected louse. Five days later the symptoms of typhus fever developed.

Some experimental evidence was secured showing that in lice the infection is transmitted to offspring. Some work was done with bedbugs and fleas but no evidence was obtained except of a negative character. Wilder presents considerable epidemiological evidence to show that bedbugs and fleas are not likely to be the carriers of this disease.

[1] Wilder, J. Infect. Dis., Chicago, 1911, IX, 9.

[2] Pub. Health, Lond., 1906–7, XIX, 772.

[3] Ricketts and Wilder, J. Am. M. Ass., Chicago, 1911, LIV, 1304.

[4] Anderson and Goldberger, U. S. Pub. Health and Mar. Hosp. Serv., Pub. Health Rep., 1910, XXV, 177.

Epidemiological Evidence. — Typhus fever was formerly considered one of the most contagious diseases, and at the same time a typical filth disease. It was especially rife in camps and prisons and on shipboard. Physicians and nurses were frequently attacked. An impressive record of its contagiousness is a tablet in Bellevue Hospital, where I served as an interne, on which are inscribed the names of the medical men in the hospital who had died from it. In 1864 of 21 members of the staff 14 contracted the disease. Of late the contagiousness has apparently diminished. It is now a rare disease in western Europe and North America (except in certain parts of Mexico). Outbreaks are usually easily controlled and hospital infection is comparatively rare. Thus 600 cases were treated in the City Hospital, Liverpool, without a single case of hospital infection.[1] Wilder says that in the American Hospital in Mexico 144 cases were treated without transfer of the disease. Hay in Aberdeen, while noting instances of infection in the hospital during the outbreak of typhus in 1906, says that they were very few, as compared with former times, and confined to those who were brought in contact with the patients before or at entrance into the hospital. Those who handled the patients after they were cleansed escaped. In the typhus outbreak in New York in 1864, as stated above, 14 of 21 members of the hospital staff contracted the disease, while from 1881 to 1893, during which time there were 1897 cases, most of which went to the hospital, only one hospital physician was attacked, namely in 1884.

New Theory Explains the Facts. — The writer has always considered the decrease in typhus fever extremely puzzling. The old-time hygienists were in the habit of attributing it to improvements in "sanitation," meaning thereby better water supply and drainage, improved scavenging and better housing, but no one explained why all this had such a marked effect upon typhus and so little upon smallpox,

[1] Robinson and Potts, Brit. M. J., 1905, I, 1137.

scarlet fever and diphtheria. Again, if typhus is contagious by the same means as are the diseases just named, why should isolation "stamp out" typhus and do nothing of the kind for scarlet fever and diphtheria? Much light is thrown on the problem if, as now seems probable, the louse, or some similar insect, is the chief factor in the transmission of the disease. There is little doubt that there has been a vast improvement in the attitude of the public as regards these parasites, and the poverty and squalor which favor their presence has vastly decreased in the most progressive nations where the disease no longer prevails. In prisons, hospitals and similar institutions lice and bedbugs formerly abounded, but in all the better class of institutions a constant warfare is now waged against them. Thus a description of Bellevue Hospital in 1837, where typhus fever was then prevailing, reads "The patients were lying in their filthy blankets, destitute of sheets and pillow-cases and in some chronic cases they had not had a change in three months." Even when I was interne in 1879 the rooms of the staff were infested with bedbugs, pediculosis was quite common and the lodging house in the basement was outrageously filthy and full of vermin of all kinds. The contrast furnished by most modern hospitals is marvelous. If typhus fever is spread by lice no wonder that it has almost vanished from our institutions.

Seasonal Distribution. — Wilder calls attention to a number of points in which this mode of extension fits in with the epidemiology of the disease. Thus typhus is a disease of temperate climates, and lice are not as numerous in the tropics as in cooler regions, and on account of light and loose clothing their parasitism is not as close. In addition he found some evidence that warm weather shortened the persistence of the virus in the louse, also that the seasonal distribution of typhus in Mexico corresponds to the seasonal distribution of lice. In this connection it may be noted that Hamer found in London that the maximum seasonal prevalence of lice is in January and the minimum in April, May and June.[1] The seasonal distribution of typhus in London is not so marked as for most infectious diseases, but of 18,286 cases admitted to the London Fever Hospital the maximum number was in January and 30 per cent were admitted during the first three months of the year.[2]

The marked predilection of typhus for poverty and filth is well explained on this hypothesis. The only place in America where typhus prevails is on the Mexican plateau where Wilder says the masses are grossly lice infested. Even in the better quarters of the City of Mexico, the lousy lower classes, as servants and otherwise, are brought in such frequent contact with more cleanly people that pediculi and typhus are not rarely found among the latter. Hay called attention to a number of facts which he thought tended to implicate the flea. He found that in clean houses and among clean people the disease did not spread. The only hospital employees who contracted the disease were in contact with patients before the latter had been cleaned. Several were then attacked. No cases developed in the wards after the patients had been cleansed. He was perhaps led to suspect fleas because of the flea bites noted on the patients, but fleas and lice are often together, and Wilder and Anderson and Goldberger, judging from epidemiological as well as from experimental data, believe that the louse is the chief factor in the spread of the disease.

Such recent writers as McVail[3] and Ker[4] consider typhus above all things an air-borne disease, though they also state, as do others, that its "striking distance" is remarkably short. The short striking distance is easily explained if

[1] Hamer, Rep. Med. Off. Health to London Co. Council, 1909, Append. IV, 8.

[2] Blyth, A Manual of Public Health, Lond., 1890, 401.

[3] McVail, The Prevention of Infectious Diseases, Lond., 1907, 46.

[4] Ker, Infectious Diseases, Lond., 1909, 202.

lice are the carriers. So also it is easy to understand how clothing may at times transmit infection, as is said to be the fact. Thus Wilson[1] reports an instance in Belfast where the disease was probably carried in this manner in a shawl, yet according to the observations of Doty (page 216) such carriage is rare.

Identity of Typhus Strains. — There has always been some doubt as to the identity of Mexican typhus and the typhus of Europe, though very many think that they are one and the same disease. In his early experiments Nicolle, in Tunis, was not able to infect rhesus monkeys, but only the higher apes, while the experimenters in Mexico found the rhesus susceptible; but later Nicolle, by using larger doses, was able to cause infection just as could his American co-workers. No experimental difference was finally noted by the two groups of observers. Recently Brill[2] has reported cases of fever occurring in New York for many years which in many respects resembled typhus fever but which appeared to be much milder and less contagious. In New York it has been commonly called Brill's disease. Anderson and Goldberger,[3] by inoculation and immunizing tests with monkeys, now seem to have shown that Brill's disease, of New York, and Mexican tarbadillo are identical. If this is so the New York type has been greatly modified or else insect carriers are rare in New York, for the disease shows no tendency to spread in either the family or the hospital.

Dengue.

Transmitted by Mosquitoes. — The causation and mode of transmission of dengue are somewhat uncertain. Graham believes that he has demonstrated in the blood a protozoan

[1] Wilson, J. Hyg., Cambridge, 1910, X, 155.

[2] Brill, Am. J. M. Sc., Phil., 1911, CXLII, 196.

[3] Anderson and Goldberger, U. S. Pub. Health and Mar. Hosp. Serv., Pub. Health Rep., 1912, XXVII, 149.

which he considers the cause of the disease, but his findings have not been substantiated. Ashburn and Craig [1] demonstrated that it is possible to transfer the disease to healthy men by the inoculation of blood from the sick, and that the virus is contained in the filtered blood. They also proved that the disease can be transmitted by a mosquito, *Culex fatigans*, and they consider that this is probably the most common mode of transmission. Stitt also believes that the mosquito is the bearer of the disease. Carpenter and Sutton could not transfer the disease by mosquitoes, but they did not experiment with *C. fatigans*. Ross has shown that while dengue prevailed elsewhere in Egypt, there was none in Port Said and Ismailia, where the mosquitoes had been exterminated. Balfour,[2] from whose review this information is chiefly taken, states that in Khartoum, which was comparatively free from mosquitoes, especially *C. fatigans*, there was no dengue, though persons with the disease in all probability came there from Port Sudan and Halfa. It appears probable, therefore, that the contentions of Ashburn and Craig are correct.

Relapsing Fever.

Varieties. — According to Craig,[3] there are at least four forms of relapsing fever, each due to a particular kind of spirocheta, and each apparently limited in geographical distribution. It is still uncertain whether these spirochetæ are bacteria, as was formerly believed and as is strongly urged by Novy and Knapp, or protozoa, similar to the trypanosomes, as is maintained by Schaudinn, Prowazek, Leishman and others. Whatever they may be, there is no doubt that at least one form of the disease is carried from person to person by means of ticks.

[1] Ashburn and Craig, J. Infect. Dis., Chicago, 1907, IV, 440; also Philippine J. Sc. [B. Med.], II, 93.

[2] Supplement to the Third Rep., Wellcome Research Lab., Khartoum, 1908, 37.

[3] Craig, The Malarial Fevers, New York, 1909, 445.

Ticks. — The African form of relapsing or tick fever is caused by *S. duttoni*, which was discovered by Dutton and Todd, and also by Ross and Milne in 1904, the first named of whom, Dutton, lost his life while studying the disease. Dutton and Todd demonstrated beyond question that the disease may be carried from man to man by a tick, *Ornithodorus moubata*, and their observations were confirmed by Ross and Milne and by Breinl and Kinghorn. It was also shown that the disease is hereditary in ticks, according to Möllers,[1] even to the second generation. Unlike the malarial parasites and the trypanosomes, these spirochetæ soon disappear from the blood, and chronic latent infections do not seem to exist. Koch, however, suggests that the spirochetæ may ultimately be found in rats, and that these rodents may be the real source of this disease, as they are of plague. The tick, however, is said to be exclusively a human parasite. It is found in the floors and crevices of houses and native huts, where it hides during the day and feeds at night. The spirochetæ undergo a certain development and multiplication in the tick, but whether they pass through a definite cycle of development, like the protozoa, is not known. Ticks have been known to be infective for a year and a half.

Bedbugs. — Even before the discovery of the spirocheta it was suggested that the bedbug might be the carrier of the disease, but, according to Balfour,[2] Breinl and Kinghorn, and Todd have by experiment shown that this is probably not so.

Less is known about the other forms of relapsing fever. Tictin in 1897 believed that the recurrent fever of Europe is transmitted by the bedbug, and he claimed to have demonstrated its possible transmission in this way, but the experiments were not entirely satisfactory and have not been substantiated.

[1] Möllers, Ztschr. f. Hyg. u. Infectionskrankh., Leipz., 1908, LVIII, 277.

[2] Supplement to the Third Report, Wellcome Research Lab., Khartoum, 1908, 190.

The Indian form of the disease is caused by *S. carteri*, and has been much studied. Mackie could demonstrate the spirochetæ in bedbugs fed on relapsing-fever patients, up to the sixth day, but he found no evidence of their increase. Of fifty-three bugs found in a fever ward, only one contained spirochetæ. He also placed infected bedbugs in cages with six monkeys, and only one of the monkeys contracted the disease. Other sources could not be excluded.

Lice. — Recently the same author has found the spirochetæ in from two to fourteen per cent of body lice found in fever wards, and he showed that the parasites increased in number in the lice. Sergent and Foley, in Algeria, have made observations and experiments tending to implicate the clothes louse, *Pediculus vestimenti*.

Rocky Mountain Fever.

Transmitted by Ticks. — Rocky Mountain tick fever probably appeared in Idaho about 1885, and is now found in Idaho, Montana, Washington, Oregon, Wyoming and Utah. It is an acute fibrile disease with a high mortality, usually exhibits an eruption on the skin, and is followed by immunity. According to the investigations of Ricketts,[1] the disease is transmitted by means of ticks, probably from some of the small wild animals of the country. He showed that it is possible to transmit the disease to monkeys, guinea pigs, gophers, chipmunks, rock squirrels and other animals by allowing ticks (*Dermacenter andersoni*) to bite first an infected animal, and later a healthy animal, which soon becomes infected. There is evidence that the virus of the disease develops in the body of the tick and is transmitted to its offspring. Ricketts has shown by inoculation experiments that the virus is contained in the blood serum of infected animals, and he recently[2] reports the discovery of a bacillus which he believes to be the cause of the disease.

[1] Ricketts, Rep. St. Bd. Health, Montana, 1907–08, 88.
[2] Ricketts, J. Am. M. Ass., Chicago, 1909, LII, 379.

Biological Carriers Distinguished from Mechanical Carriers. —In most of the diseases thus far considered in this chapter the parasite which causes the disease passes through a definite cycle of its existence in the insect as well as in man. The insect is in most cases the true host of the parasite and has been called a "biological carrier" of disease. Most of the parasites transmitted in this way belong to the protozoa.

On the other hand, insects may be merely "mechanical carriers" of disease. The blood which contains the germs of the disease may be carried on the mouth parts of the insect and inoculated into the next person bitten, just as it might be carried on the point of a lancet.

Plague.

Discovery of Bacilli in Fleas. — According to Nuttall,[1] Ogata in 1897 found plague bacilli in fleas taken from the body of a rat dead of bubonic plague, and this observation was confirmed by the German Plague Commission the same year. In 1898 Simond noted that persons who handle dead rats not rarely die of the plague, but he found that infection never occurred if the rats had been dead over twenty-four hours. He also found that persons with plague occasionally presented on their skin what appeared to be flea bites, and he was able to demonstrate plague bacilli in these supposed bites. He was able also to demonstrate plague bacilli in fleas taken from rats dead of the plague.

Plague derived from Rodents. — Simond's observations led to much study and experiment and to still more controversy. It has been shown by large numbers of observations that plague is primarily a disease of the lower animals, particularly of rodents, many species of which easily become infected. It has been shown also that plague in man is generally derived from the same disease in rats, or more rarely mice, and recently in California from ground squirrels (*Citellus beecheyi*).

[1] Nuttall, Johns Hopkins Hosp. Rep., Balt., 1899, VIII, 1.

Epidemiological Evidence. — The very careful observations of Thompson[1] in Australia showed that outbreaks of human plague were preceded by outbreaks of rat plague, that human cases were connected in one way or another with foci of rat infection, and that the dispersal of human cases did not result in the dispersion of plague. He showed that while human plague had a local association with rat plague, the association was not a direct one, but was such as to render necessary the assumption of some such intermediary as the flea. It also seemed to him that the location of the buboes was in accord with the theory of flea infection.

Experimental Work. — Objection had been made by Nuttall and others to the flea theory on the ground that rat and human fleas are of different species, but Tidswell in Sydney[2] showed that rat fleas when hungry will bite man. This has been substantiated by many other observers, some of whom have also shown that *Pulex irritans*, the human parasite, will occasionally bite rats. It has also been shown that fleas speedily leave a dead animal, and then, impelled by hunger, they attack the nearest victim. As was shown by Nuttall, plague bacilli may live in fleas for several days. The English Plague Commission found as many as 5000 bacilli in the stomach of a single flea, and they believe that they increase in number for a while and sometimes live for fifteen days, but in starved fleas do not live over a week.[3] Verjbitski[4] has also confirmed these observations. He has shown, too, as did Nuttall, that bedbugs may become infected and harbor the germs for some days. According to Tidswell,[5] rats are frequently infested with bedbugs (*Cimex lectularius*), but there is no evidence as yet that these play any important part in

[1] Thompson, Reports of Plague in Sydney, 1902 to 1907.

[2] Tidswell, Rep. on Second Outbreak of Plague in Sydney, 1902, 73–75.

[3] J. Hyg., Cambridge, 1907, VII, 419.

[4] Verjbitski, J. Hyg., Cambridge, 1908, VIII, 162.

[5] Loc. cit.

the causation of the disease. Verjbitski showed that if the biting insect is crushed on the skin, either the bite or neighboring scratches are easily infected.

Demonstrations in India. — Finally, the very beautiful experiments of the English Plague Commission[1] showed conclusively that infection by fleas was practically the only way in which experimental animals could be infected under natural conditions. These experiments have been referred to on pages 246 and 312. In one experiment, a plague-infected village was cleared of its human inhabitants and guinea pigs placed in the houses, and it was demonstrated that infection took place only through the medium of fleas. The experimental and epidemiological evidence is that the bubonic form of human plague, which is by far the most common form, is caused by the transference of the bacilli from rodents to man by means of fleas.

Plague rarely spread except by Fleas. — While it is true that the flea is the chief agent in the transmission of plague, the disease may possibly be, and doubtless occasionally is, spread in other ways. In experimental animals it is possible to induce it by the ingestion of infected food, and the contact of the abraded or injured skin with any substance containing plague bacilli may result in infection. The pneumonic form of plague, when no precautions are taken, is highly contagious, for the sputum contains the bacilli. In some outbreaks of plague the pneumonic form prevails. In some localities the overcrowding, filth and habits of the people may cause contact infection or infection by food to assume some importance, but in Western Europe, Australia and America there can be little doubt that plague is chiefly a flea-borne disease.

Measures against Plague. — Measures against the plague ought, then, to involve the isolation of the sick, particularly those sick with the pneumonic form. In India evacuation

[1] J. Hyg., Cambridge, 1906, VI.
See also Summary of Work of Commission, 1908, Calcutta, Supt. of Gov. Printing.

of infected villages, that is, the removal of the population from the vicinage of the plague rat, is a measure of value. Disinfection, if it includes the killing of fleas and rats, is an important measure. Haffkine's serum has been found to prevent attacks for several months, and its general use is often of value in preventing the development of individual cases. But the chief anti-plague measures must be directed, not against the flea, but against rats and other rodents. The most obvious procedure is to attempt the destruction of the rats, but thus far this has proved to be a rather hopeless undertaking. Poisoning, trapping and destruction by infectious disease have proved only palliative or adjuvant measures. In Japan, in Australia and in California the most energetic rat destruction has not materially reduced their numbers. Thompson [1] says: "Prevention of epidemic plague consequently lies in maintaining a distance between the rat and man. The requisite separation between rat and man will be better secured by improving the construction of buildings than by attempts to exterminate the rat." In Sydney large sums are being spent in rebuilding wharves and warehouses so as to render them rat-proof. In San Franscisco [2] every effort has been made to prevent the growth of rats by cutting off their food supply, by improved scavenging, and by providing metal garbage pails and rat-proof receptacles for all kinds of food and grain likely to attract rats. But the chief effort was directed to rat-proofing, by the use of concrete construction, of stables, markets, provision and produce warehouses and wharves.

Anthrax.

Nuttall, in his valuable discussion and bibliography of the subject of insect carriers of disease,[3] cites a large number of

[1] Thompson, Internat. Cong. f. Hyg. u. Demog., Berl., 1907, III, 672.

[2] Eradicating Plague from San Francisco, Rep. of Citizens' Health Com., 1909.

[3] Nuttall, Johns Hopkins Hosp. Rep., Balt., 1899, VIII, 1; see also Rep. to Local Gov. Bd., Lond., on Pub. Health, 1909, n. s., 16.

authors who suggest that anthrax may at times be transmitted by any biting insects which pass from cattle to man. Numerous instances are given of persons who date the beginning of their pustule from the sharp sting of an insect, but, as was well said, it is probable that often the first noticeable sensations in the development of the pustule are wrongly considered as due to the bite of an insect. In a few cases a fly was felt to bite and was killed, and on the spot a malignant pustule developed. Most of the score or more of writers quoted urge this mode of infection on purely *a priori* grounds, and it is certainly highly probable that where anthrax is at all prevalent among animals, and biting insects pass from the lower animals to human beings, the disease is sometimes transmitted in this way; but, as has been suggested, if this happened often, the disease would be more common than it is. Certainly in England and the United States practically all human anthrax results from handling infected material.

Nuttall[1] allowed bedbugs to suck blood from mice infected with anthrax, and then caused them immediately to bite healthy mice. In all, 136 infected bugs were used, but in no instance did they transmit the disease. In six instances the bugs were crushed while biting, but these experiments were, like the others, without result. Nuttall also made a few similar experiments with fleas, with like negative results. He found that anthrax bacilli remained alive in bedbugs only for from two to four days, and died off even more quickly in fleas.

Nuttall carried on similar experiments with bedbugs and chicken cholera, but these were equally unsuccessful.

Septic Infection.

Nuttall cites Faure, Paltauf, Chrzaszczewski, Joseph and Berry as having noted instances of septic infection following the bites of insects, and others are occasionally noted in medi-

[1] Nuttall, loc. cit., 13.

cal literature. That this accident should sometimes happen seems very probable.

Typhoid Fever.

Dutton[1] caused bedbugs to bite a typhoid-fever patient and after twenty-four hours' fasting to bite two other healthy persons, both of whom developed typhoid fever in twelve and fourteen days respectively.

Insects carry Germs on Bodies. — The insects thus far considered inoculate disease by means of their bites, but it is evident that some diseases may be carried by them in other ways. If infective material exists in considerable quantity, and is accessible to insects, they are almost certain to get it on their legs and bodies, and may then carry the germs to other human beings. The chance of their doing this varies greatly with varying conditions. If the insects fly, the danger would seem to be much greater. If the infective material is large in amount and freely exposed, as typhoid excreta in privy vaults, the danger of fly infection is increased, and it is also greater if there is a possibility of infecting food which insects love to visit. Flies, particularly the common house fly, *Musca domestica*, have been most often accused of thus carrying infection, but othor insects have not escaped suspicion.

Cockroaches and Other Insects. — Engelmann[2] reports cockroaches extremely numerous in certain houses in Chicago where typhoid fever prevailed, and she attributed the spread of the disease to these insects. Weber[3] accuses various species of *Psocidæ* of carrying tubercle bacilli from cow to cow, and states that he demonstrated the germs in one of these insects found in a manger. In fact any "domestic" insect with power of active locomotion, and of filthy habits, may be considered as a possible carrier of disease germs.

[1] Dutton, J. Am. M. Ass., Chicago, 1909, LIII, 1248.
[2] Engelmann, Med. News, N. Y., 1903, LXXXII, 225.
[3] Weber, N. York M. J. [etc.], 1906, LXXXIV, 884.

But the house fly is undoubtedly the most numerous and ubiquitous and the most "domestic" in its habits, and it is rightly suspected of playing a larger part as the mere passive carrier of disease germs than is any other insect.

Mayer[1] states that some ants were seen to pass between cages containing mice, some of which were sick with mouse typhoid and some well. The well mice soon developed the disease, and agar plates, so placed that the ants ran over them, showed numerous colonies of the *B. murium typhi*.

Flies seen to carry Infective Material. — A large number of observers, noting the passage of flies from infected matter to human beings or to food, have become convinced that these insects are important carriers of disease. According to Nuttall, Budd as long ago as 1862 considered it proved that Egyptian ophthalmia is carried from child to child by the flies that can be observed in great numbers crawling over the face and eyes. Laveran noted the same conditions in Biskra, and he and many others believe that oriental sore is spread in the same way. Nuttall also cites several of the earlier writers as believing that anthrax, cholera and plague are transmitted by flies.

Experimental Work. — With the development of bacteriology, experiments began to supplement conjecture, and it was definitely determined that bacteria might be carried on the bodies of insects, which indeed is self-evident, and also that they might in a living state pass through the stomach and be voided in the feces. According to Nuttall, Raimbert, Davaine and Ballinger demonstrated living anthrax bacilli on flies of various kinds that had been feeding on infected material. Nuttall himself showed that house flies could carry for 48 hours living plague bacilli which they had derived from material they had fed on, and Hankin showed the same for ants. Nuttall, in the monograph previously cited, reviews the early literature, and many useful references as well as accounts of original work

[1] Mayer, München med. Wchnschr., 1905, LII, 226.

are to be found in Howard's[1] recent work and in the valuable reports to the Local Government Board.[2]

Cholera Spirilla on Flies. — In 1886 Tizzoni and Cattani caught flies in a cholera hospital in Bologna and found that cultures made from them showed cholera spirilla. Simmonds made similar observations in Hamburg in 1892. Macrae in India, in 1894, exposed boiled milk in different parts of a jail where cholera prevailed, and found that it became infected with cholera germs. Tsuzuki, in 1904, captured cholera-infected flies in a house in Tientsin where there were cases of the disease. Chantemesse and Gagnon have shown that flies may carry virulent germs for 17 and 24 hours respectively. Maus[3] says that cholera spirilla were found on several bluebottle flies caught in infected houses in the Philippines. Graham-Smith[4] in eight experiments could recover cholera spirilla from the legs and wings of flies only once later than 5 days after infection. Even in the crop and intestines the numbers rapidly diminished, all cultures after 48 hours yielding negative results.

Typhoid Bacilli on Flies. — The earlier observers were merely content to show that flies could transfer pathogenic germs, and made little attempt to show in what way and for how long they could be carried. Thus Manning[5] and Buchanan[6] caused flies to walk over typhoid feces and then over Petri plates with the result that somc of the plates became infected. Firth and Horrocks[7] showed that typhoid bacilli could be carried on the legs, wings, head and bodies of flies and that they could be found in their excreta after the insects had been fed on infected material, but they did

[1] The House Fly, Disease Carrier, N. York, 1911.

[2] Reports on Pub. Health and Med. Subjects, Nos. 5, 16, 40, 53.

[3] Maus, Abst. Med. News, N. Y., 1902, LXXI, 318.

[4] Rep. to Local Gov. Bd., Lond., 1910, No. 40.

[5] J. Am. M. Ass., Chicago, 1902, XXXVII, 1291.

[6] Lancet, Lond., 1907, II, 216.

[7] Brit. M. J. Lond., 1902, II, 936.

not consider that they had definitely proved that the germs passed through the intestinal tract. Faichnie[1] believes that typhoid bacilli are more often carried in the intestines of flies than on their legs. He bred flies in earth infected with typhoid feces. From the intestines and from the excrement of flies so bred he recovered typhoid bacilli up to the sixteenth day. Similar breeding experiments were carried on in earth impregnated with feces containing *B. paratyphosus A.* and bacilli were obtained from the flies up to the tenth day. Graham-Smith[2] fed flies on syrup containing typhoid bacilli and endeavored to determine the persistence of the germs on their feet, in their intestines and in the "specks" or excreta. Bacilli were not found on the feet or in the specks longer than 48 hours but were recovered from the intestines for at least 6 days. Similar experiments carried on with *B. enteritidis* (Gärtner) showed that while the bacilli could rarely be found on the legs they could be recovered from the "crop" and intestines up to 7 days and probably longer. Hewitt[3] allowed flies to walk over thin smears of typhoid feces and then kept them in cages for 24 hours and after that allowed them to walk over culture media. No typhoid colonies were found and only a few of *B. coli*. Similar experiments were made with *B. prodigiosus* with negative results, though the germs were recovered from the feet of the flies after 12 hours.[4]

Typhoid Bacilli on Flies from Infected Places. — Hamilton[5] in Chicago, and Fricker in Hamburg, in the same year, recovered typhoid bacilli from flies in houses where there were cases of the disease. Klein[6] also recovered typhoid bacilli from flies from houses where there was typhoid fever.

[1] J. Roy. Army M. Corps, Lond., 1909, XIII, 672.
[2] Rep. to Local Gov. Bd., Lond., 1910, No. 40.
[3] Hewitt, Quart. J. Micr. Sc., 1909, n. s., LIV, 394.
[4] Ibid., 403.
[5] Hamilton, J. Am. M. Ass., Chicago, 1903, XL, 576.
[6] Klein, Brit. M. J., Lond., 1908, II, 1150.

Faichnie, above cited, proved the presence of typhoid bacilli on flies caught in barracks at Ramptee, India, where there was an outbreak of the disease, and later he reported finding typhoid-infected flies on nine other occasions in various localities. Bartarelli,[1] in studying a house outbreak near Turin, found typhoid bacilli on 8 of 120 flies caught in the house and on 2 of 35 caught in the yard. On the other hand, as might be expected, some have failed to find the bacilli under similar circumstances, as Buchanan at Glasgow, Gorham at Providence and Gunn at Orange, N. J.

Tubercle Bacilli carried by Flies. — Spillmann and Haushalter found tubercle bacilli in the intestines and in the dejecta of flies that had fed on tuberculous sputum. Hoffmann found tubercle bacilli in 2 of 4 flies captured in a room occupied by a tuberculous patient, and also in the excreta of flies scraped from the walls and furniture of the room. Lord[2] found virulent bacilli in flyspecks, but could not induce the disease by causing guinea pigs to breathe air drawn over infected specks. Hayward[3] demonstrated living bacilli in flyspecks after the flies had been fed on sputum in such a way as to preclude the possibility of the infection of their feet or bodies. André[4] demonstrated tubercle bacilli in the excreta of flies by inoculation tests, and he found that they appeared in the feces about six hours after feeding and continued for five days. Flies may also become infected by eating tuberculous dust.

Graham-Smith[5] after feeding flies for several days on syrup infected with a culture of human tubercle bacilli determined that the bacilli may "be present in the crop for 3 days. In the intestines, however, they may be found for much longer periods, being present in considerable numbers

[1] Centralbl. f. Bakteriol. (etc.), I, Abt., Jena, 1910, LIII, 486.
[2] Lord, Boston M. & S. J., 1904, CLI, 651.
[3] Hayward, N. York M. J. [etc.], 1904, LXXX, 643.
[4] André, 6th Internat. Cong. on Tuberc., Wash., 1908, I, 162.
[5] Graham-Smith, Rep. to Local Gov. Bd., 1910, No. 40.

for at least 6 days. Subsequently their numbers diminish, but they may be discovered by careful search for 12 days or even longer. In the fæces they are numerous up to the fifth day, and occasional specimens may be found in fæcal material deposited between the sixth and fourteenth days after infection." Flies fed on sputum, only, contained the bacilli for 4 days, but flies cannot stand forced feeding with sputum as they do with infected syrup.

Anthrax Bacilli carried on Flies. — As has been stated, several early observers noted the ability of flies to transfer anthrax germs. Graham-Smith, however, has shown the period during which the flies may remain infective. He found that after flies have fed on the blood of an animal dead with anthrax the spore-free bacilli do not remain alive on the external parts of the fly for more than 24 hours. They may, however, persist in the intestine for 3 days and in the crop for 5 days. When flies are fed on anthrax spores the latter do not develop in the fly. They tend to disappear gradually from both the exterior of the body and from the intestine, and in one experiment none were obtained from legs or wings after the tenth day and from the crop only once after that, namely on the sixteenth day. In another experiment the spores persisted both outside and inside the fly up to the twentieth day, when the experiment terminated.

Other Disease Germs on Flies. Dysentery. — Auché[1] allowed flies to become contaminated with cultures of the dysentery bacillus, and found that they could carry the germs for hours, and that the flies would take up the bacilli from feces as well as from cultures.

Graham-Smith experimented by feeding flies on an emulsion of a diphtheria culture and showed that the bacilli seldom remain alive on the legs and wings for more than a few hours, but may live in the alimentary canal for 24 hours or even longer.

[1] Auché, Compt. rend., Soc. de biol., Par., 1906, LXI, 450.

He also made use of the Danysz rat virus: " A number of flies were allowed to feed for 1 hour on a broth culture of virus, recently recovered from the body of a rat, and were then transferred to a fresh cage. A piece of bread, soaked in milk, was put into the cage daily and the flies allowed to settle and feed on it. After 1 hour the bread was removed and given to a mouse.

" A mouse was also fed on bread soaked in milk containing an emulsion of fæces, passed about 48 hours after infection, scraped from the walls of the cage. The animal died in 2 days, and the organism was isolated from it.

" These experiments show that flies which have fed on virus are capable of infecting food on which they settle and feed to such an extent that mice fed on it become infected."

According to Nuttall and Jepson, Welander found that flies could carry living gonococci on their feet for 3 hours.

Nuttall showed that plague bacilli could be carried by flies, and Graham-Smith states that Yersin in Hong-Kong observed dead flies lying about where he made his autopsies on animals which had died of the plague and demonstrated that the flies contained virulent plague bacilli.

Although no specific germ of poliomyelitis has been discovered the infectivity of the fluids and other tissues can be tested on monkeys, and modes of infection can in this way be studied. Flexner and Clark[1] allowed flies to feed on the fresh spinal cord of a monkey which had the disease, and determined by inoculation that the virus would persist on or in the flies for at least 48 hours. Experiments after a longer interval were not tried.

Mechanism of Infection by Flies. — Graham-Smith has shown that flies often discharge the contents of their crops, especially when feeding on dry substances. The regurgitated material frequently contains pathogenic bacteria for some days after these have been taken up by the flies. Such bacteria are also discharged in the excrement. The germs

[1] J. Am. M. Ass., Chicago, 1911, LVI, 1717.

usually do not live more than a day or two, perhaps less, on the legs and wings but persist much longer in the alimentary tract. Flies allowed to walk over food material may infect it not only by means of the germs on their feet but also by the matter which they disgorge when they stop to feed and also by their excrement. There is less chance of infecting liquids, as then the flies do not need to disgorge to soften their food. Many of Graham-Smith's experiments were made with *B. prodigiosus* because of the ease with which it may be recognized. Yet in his experiments he could not once infect milk with this bacillus either by allowing infected flies to feed on it or to drown in it.

These experiments seem to show that while infection by flies is possible it is not as easy as might at first sight appear. Nevertheless, given much infected material and large numbers of flies, it is entirely conceivable that a large amount of disease may be caused by fly-borne infection. That food may, under natural conditions, become infected is shown by the observations of Macrae in regard to cholera. In 1899 the writer, with the assistance of Prof. F. P. Gorham, exposed agar plates and dishes of milk in the pantry of a house, and poured large amounts of a culture of *B. prodigiosus* into the near-by privy vault. Of nine tests, four showed infection with *prodigiosus*, while all of five plates exposed near the vault were so infected. Plates covered with wire netting were not infected. Flies were very numerous and were constantly walking over the plates.

Such a mode of infection is also indicated by the observations of Vaughan,[1] who reports that during the Spanish War flies covered with a white coating of lime were often seen crawling over the food, the lime showing that they had just come from the latrines where lime had been thrown over the fecal matter.

Wild Flies carry Fecal Bacteria. — Flies caught in the open have been shown to be at times loaded with fecal bac-

[1] Vaughan, J. Am. M. Ass., 1900, XXXIV, 1456.

teria, thus indicating at once their habits and the possibility of their carrying certain diseases. Jackson[1] found as many as 100,000 fecal bacteria on a single fly, and as a general thing the nearer the flies were to the sewer outlets the more numerous were this class of bacteria. Graham-Smith[2] found fecal bacteria on 23.6 per cent of 148 flies examined in Cambridge, England. For a part of them the surface of the body only was examined, and for a part the intestine only. Surface infection was about two and a half times as frequent as intestinal infection. The highest degree of infection was found among flies caught near decaying animal matter, and the next highest among those caught near manure. Nash[3] recovered *B. coli* from a fly caught in a hospital ward. Delépine[4] found bacilli of the colon type in four of thirty-five collections of flies caught in Manchester.

More Fecal Germs in July and August. — Recent observations by Torrey[5] indicate that flies may be more dangerous late in the summer. He found that fecal bacteria of the colon type were first encountered in abundance in the early part of July. The bacteria in the intestines of the flies were 8.6 times as numerous as on the surface of the insects. On the surface of the flies the colon-group of bacteria constituted 13.1 per cent of the total; and within the intestine 37.5 per cent of the total. Of the lactose fermenters, isolated and identified, 79.5 per cent belonged in the colon-aerogens group and 20.5 per cent in the acidi lactici group. Fifteen cultures of streptococci, isolated and identified, were distributed among the equinus, fecalis and salivarius groups. There were none of the pyogenes type. Most

[1] Jackson, Rep. to Com. on Pollution [etc.], of the Merchants' Ass. of N. York, 1907, 16.

[2] Graham-Smith, Further Preliminary Rep. on Flies [etc.], Rep. to Loc. Gov. Bd. on Health, n. s., 1909, 16.

[3] Nash, J. Hyg., Cambridge, 1909, IX, 141.

[4] Delépine, Rep. on Health of Manchester, 1906, 85.

[5] Torrey, J., Infect. Dis., Chicago, 1912, X, 166.

important was the isolation of three colonies of *B. paratyphosus, A.* Bacteria of the paracolon type causing a final intense alkaline reaction in litmus milk and fermenting only certain monosaccharids were frequently encountered during August.

Range of Flight. — As stated by Howard, probably the distance traversed by the house fly varies greatly under different circumstances, being greater if with the wind and if suitable food or breeding places are not at hand. Howard cites Forbes as observing a flight of half a mile from the tuberculosis hospital to the general hospital of Cook Co., Ill. He also cites Hine as finding marked flies at a distance of 40 rods on the third day but never as far as half a mile. Austen [1] after liberating marked flies found them at distances varying from 300 to 1700 yards. Under the direction of Delépine 300 flies were liberated in the administration building of a hospital, and within 5 days 4 were caught in wards distant from 30 to 190 yards. At the Worcester State Hospital Orton and Dodd [2] observed flies carry *B. prodigiosus* from the laundry to the kitchen and to all of the wards although the hospital was well screened.

Seasonal and Local Distribution of Flies. — There is a disposition in many quarters to rely upon a study of the relation of fly distribution to disease to throw light upon the causative relation of the insects to the disease under consideration. Such studies are not likely to prove very convincing and they are of little value unless extensive. Proper studies of the seasonal distribution of flies have been undertaken in only a few localities and for a few seasons. There have been still fewer observations on the local distribution of the insects in relation to the local distribution of disease. Even if a quite constant correlation of seasonal fly distribution and disease distribution is determined, the causative relation between the insects and the disease is

[1] Rep. to Local Gov. Bd., Lond., 1911, No. 53.
[2] Boston M. & S. J., 1910, CLXIII, 863.

far from established, as both phenomena might be dependent on some other cause.

Species of Flies. — Various species of flies are found in and about houses which may possibly serve as the mechanical carriers of disease. Of these by far the most common in dwellings is the house fly, *Musca domestica,* though other flies are not infrequently found. In New York Jackson found that 98 per cent of all flies captured were *M. domestica.* In London in 1908 Austen [1] found that next to the house fly the most common species were *Homalomyia canicularis, Calliphora erythrocephala* and *Muscina stabulans.* In Providence in 1909 Sykes [2] found all the above, and also considerable numbers of *Lucilia cæsar, Sarcophaga sarraceniæ* and *Stomoxys calcitrans,* and a few *Scenopinus fenestralis,* but 99 per cent of the flies caught indoors were *M. domestica.* The bluebottle fly, *Lucilia cæsar,* has been accused by Dutton[3] of transmitting typhoid fever. Maus in the Philippines blames bluebottles for the spread of cholera.

Transmission of Disease by Flies. — Of this we have very little actual knowledge. Because flies are seen to pass from sputum and feces to human lips and to food, and because it is shown that flies may carry disease germs on their bodies, it is assumed that these insects are the frequent carriers of disease. Again, because of a correspondence between the curves of fly distribution and disease prevalence, though this correspondence in some instances is found not to exist, it is assumed that flies are a prolific cause of sickness. There has been almost no experimental work under natural conditions. All that I have been able to find are the two negative experiments of Peters, to be referred to, in regard to summer diarrhea. To determine with any degree of certainty the part really played by flies in the transmission of disease, we need a large amount of

[1] Austen, Rep. to Local Gov. Bd. on Pub. Health, n. s., 1909, No. 5.

[2] Sykes, Rep. Supt. of Health, Providence, 1909, 13.

[3] Dutton, J. Am. M. Ass., Chicago, 1909, LIII, 1561.

epidemiological evidence such as would be afforded by changes in disease incidence following control of the fly nuisance. At present there is very little of such evidence and none at all until very recently. We may now consider what is said and known about the fly carriage of certain diseases.

Murrina.

Due to Flies. — Darling [1] has reported a disease occurring among horses and mules on the Isthmus of Panama. It is apparently caused by a trypanosome, *T. hippicum.* Darling has given careful attention to the cause of the disease and is satisfied that it is transmitted by a biting fly, *Stomoxys calcitrans.* He has never been able to demonstrate the growth of the trypanosome in the body of the fly, and he believes that the disease is carried mechanically. He does not think that it is introduced by the bite of the insect but only through abraded surfaces on the bodies of the animals. Only animals having superficial sores become infected.

Tuberculosis.

Due to Flies. — Cobb [2] watched flies passing from tuberculous sputum to food, and he attributes to these insects a large proportion of tuberculosis in man. Many health officials and anti-tuberculosis leagues have issued lurid bulletins illustrating the agency of flies in transmitting the germs of "the great white plague." While it is certainly possible for the disease to be transmitted in this way, there is absolutely no evidence that it is a factor of appreciable importance. The opportunities for infection with tubercle bacilli in other ways are so much greater and more numerous that we are not justified in considering infection by flies of much importance.

[1] Darling, J. Infect. Dis., Chicago, 1911, VIII, 467.
[2] Cobb, Am. Med., Phila., 1905, IX, 475.

Cholera.

Due to Flies. — Cholera has of late been considered to be to a considerable extent a fly-borne disease. This has been the view of Chantemesse and Borel,[1] as well as of many of our officials in the Philippines,[2] as Heiser,[3] Woodruff [4] and McLaughlin,[5] though all of the latter seem to consider contact infection a good deal more important than infection by means of flies. Nuttall cites Flügge, Macrae, Buchanan and Tsuzuki as considering flies of great importance in this disease. Heiser [6] says that cholera was spread in Bilibid prison in Manila by flies passing from the imperfectly disinfected latrines to the food. At mealtime they were seen to pass in swarms to where the food was served. After screening cholera ceased.

Dysentery.

Due to Flies. — In a recent outbreak of dysentery in an asylum at Danvers, Mass., involving 156 cases, and carefully studied by Ryder,[7] flies were believed to be the chief factor in the extension of the disease. In 1910 Orton and Dodd [8] reported an outbreak of 136 cases and 22 deaths, occurring in July and August, which they believed must be due to flies, as all frank cases were well isolated, screened and disinfected. They believed that contact infection from these cases was out of the question, but the possibility of infection from carriers does not seem to have been eliminated. The buildings were well screened, but many flies found their

[1] Chantemesse and Borel, Bull. Acad. de méd., Par., 1905, 3 s., LIV, 252.

[2] Maus, Abst., Med. News, N. Y., 1902, LXXXI, 318.

[3] Heiser, J. Am. M. Ass., Chicago, 1907, XLVIII, 856.

[4] Woodruff, J. Am. M. Ass., Chicago, 1905, XLV, 1160.

[5] McLaughlin, J. Am. M. Ass., Chicago, 1909, LII, 1153.

[6] Heiser, Bull. State Bd. Health, N. Y., Sept., 1911.

[7] Ryder, Boston M. & S. J., 1909, CLXI, 681.

[8] Orton and Dodd, Boston, M. & S. J., 1910, CLXIII, 863.

way in nevertheless. Dodd[1] reports much the same conditions, though with only 99 cases and 14 deaths, in 1911. Dick[2] states that dysentery, in which both Flexner and Shiga types of bacilli were present, was endemic for several years in an asylum at Dunning, Ill. Flies were thought to play an important part, and the disease disappeared from one of the wards after screening and the practice of strict medical asepsis. Hamer[3] refers to an outbreak of dysentery in an asylum near London in 1906 alleged to have been caused by flies.

Diarrhea.

Due to Flies. — Many of the English have been inclined to attribute considerable influence to the fly as a factor in the causation of the summer diarrheas of infants. Newsholme, who believes that diarrhea is due chiefly to infection of the milk in the house, says that opened cans of condensed milk are often seen to be black with flies, attracted by the sugar in the milk, and attributes to them no inconsiderable share in the causation of the disease. Sandilands,[4] like Newsholme, finds diarrhea especially prevalent among the users of condensed milk, and he thinks that the milk is probably infected by flies after the can is opened. Nuttall cites Copeman as seeing in flies the possible cause of an outbreak of diarrhea investigated by him. Nash[5] in 1903 stated his belief that the house fly played the chief part in the epidemiology of summer diarrhea. This also is the view of Sandwith.[6]

Seasonal Distribution of Diarrhea and Flies. — Observations made in widely different localities have shown a

[1] Dodd, Boston M. & S. J., 1912, CLXVI, 211.
[2] Dick, J. Infect. Dis., Chicago, 1911, VIII, 386.
[3] Rep. Med. Off. Health, Co. of Lond., 1907, Append. II.
[4] Sandilands, J. Hyg., Cambridge, 1906, VI, 77.
[5] Nash, J. San. Inst., Lond., 1903, XXVI, 495.
[6] Sandwith, Clin. J. Lond., 1911, XXXIX, 19.

certain relation between the seasonal distribution of flies and summer diarrhea. Stations are established at various places in a town and flies are caught in traps or by means of fly paper, and the number of flies is compared with the number of deaths from diarrhea. Niven[1] in Manchester, in 1903, found that the "fly curve" and the curve for diarrheal deaths corresponded very closely, and the same agreement was noted in 1905 and 1906.[2] The table given by him shows both the date of inception and the date of death of the fatal cases of diarrhea. In both years the maximum number of cases occurred at almost exactly the same time as the maximum number of flies, and the maximum number of deaths about a week later. In 1905 the maximum was about August 1, and in 1906 about September 5. Robertson in Birmingham[3] found a similar correspondence in that city. Jackson in New York[4] showed a similar close relation between flies and diarrhea, as has Ainsworth[5] for Poona in India. Nash,[6] showing the seasonal distribution of flies, states that in 1902, at Southend, there were few flies and little diarrhea in August, and that diarrhea increased in September as the flies increased. Both 1902 and 1903 had cool summers with few flies and little diarrhea, while 1904 and 1906 had plenty of flies and plenty of diarrhea. In 1904 there was a heavy local incidence near a large dump where flies abounded. Hamer[7] made a careful study of the seasonal distribution of flies in London, and he shows that while there is an apparent agreement between the fly curve and that of diarrheal deaths, the latter begins to fall before the former, which he thinks that it would not

[1] Niven, Rep. on Health of Manchester, 1903, 123.

[2] Rep. on Health of Manchester, 1906, 82.

[3] Robertson, Rep. Med. Off. Health, Birmingham, 1910, 111.

[4] Jackson, Rep. to Com. on Pollution [etc]., of the Merchants' Ass. of N. Y., 1907, 17.

[5] Ainsworth, J. Roy. Army Med. Corps, Lond., 1909, XII, 485.

[6] Nash, J. Hyg., Cambridge, 1909, IX, 141.

[7] Hamer, Rep. Med. Off. Health, Co. of Lond., 1907, Append. II.

be likely to do if flies were the chief cause of the disease. Hamer[1] in a later report shows that the relation between the fly curve and the diarrhea curve varies considerably in different years. He thinks that if flies have any part in the causation of diarrhea it is much obscured by other influences and that too great importance should not be attached to correspondence in any one year. He also says that the period of maximum infections (not dates of attacks) in typhoid fever in both England and America is some three weeks later than in diarrhea and that this is not reconcilable with the theory that the seasonal distribution of both diseases is determined solely by the distribution of the fly.

Maximum of Diarrhea before Maximum of Flies. — As regards this phenomenon Peters[2] has suggested that it is exactly what might be expected. If flies are the chief factor in the spread of diarrheal disease the diarrheal curve ought to lag a little behind the fly curve in the early part of the summer outbreak, for the increase in flies approaches an ordinary arithmetical progression while the diarrheal increase, he says, starting from an amount of infection relatively small, but proceeding more by geometrical progression, later on rises faster than the fly curve and reaches its maximum at about the same time. The fall of the diarrhea curve before the fly curve is due, he believes, to the exhaustion of infection, or of material to infect, and would doubtless occur even if the fly prevalence continued without a decline. A general agreement between the fly curve and the diarrhea curve, but with a certain definite lack of correlation, is, on theoretical grounds, to be expected, and Peters states that just this correlation exists in each of the eight seasonal charts of fly and diarrhea distribution prepared by Niven and Hamer before referred to.

Problem still Unsolved. — Peters in this paper gives the details of his exceptionally careful and valuable epidemio-

[1] Hamer, Rep. Med. Of. Health, Co. of Lond., 1909, Append. IV.
[2] Peters, J. Hyg., Cambridge, 1910, X, 602.

logical study of diarrheal disease in Mansfield. He found that many of the local conditions were well explained by the fly theory of transmission and that no facts were met with which were directly contradictory, yet he arrives at no more positive conclusion than "that the whole question merits the most thorough and laborious investigation." He suggests that a "positive experiment" in which "households duly protected against all other chance of infection, and in which flies from infected houses have been liberated, develop abundant diarrhea" would afford convincing evidence. Such an experiment he tried on two occasions without positive results. He also suggests "negative experiments" to determine whether screened houses in the midst of infection remain free.

Parallel Seasonal Distribution not Conclusive. — Although there is considerable evidence of a close parallelism between the seasonal distribution of flies and of diarrhea, this parallelism is no proof that the latter is dependent upon the former. Even as corroborative evidence it has little value. The return of the sun from the equator results in a great variety of phenomena, many of which, though closely related in time, have no causative relation one with another. The presence of flies seems to be closely correlated with the temperature, though it may be that the connection is far from direct. So also are a vast number of other events correlated with the temperature, though they have no causative connection with flies. A few years ago it was discovered that summer diarrhea developed only when the temperature of the soil had reached a certain point, and this was by many considered a demonstration that the germs of the disease developed in the soil. Now it is the fashion to say that diarrhea is due to flies because at times the increase in flies precedes by a little the increase in diarrhea. While it may be that flies have much to do with the causation of infantile summer diarrhea, as yet we have no proof of it.

Local Distribution of Flies and Diarrhea. — Jackson in his report has a map on which are located all the deaths from intestinal disease. This map shows that the great bulk of these are at no great distance from the water front, where the flies swarm about the sewer outlets. It is just there that the tenements crowded with poor children are situated, and to maintain his argument it would be necessary to show an excess over and above the excess of diarrhea always found in tenements, and to eliminate the other unfavorable factors associated with poverty.

A close relation between an excess of flies in a neighborhood and an excess of diarrhea has not been found by Davies in Woolwich, Dudfield in Kensington, Harris in Islington and Porter in Finsbury.[1] Hamer also calls attention to the fact that among English towns many which have a very high typhoid death rate have a low diarrheal death rate and vice versa. If both diseases are largely dependent on flies this needs explanation. In our own country Fall River, which, for the five years 1904–1908, had a death rate from typhoid fever of 13.2 (less than half the average of the registration cities), had a diarrheal death rate of 380 (over three times the average of the registration cities and the highest of all of them).

Typhoid Fever.

Flies in Spanish War. — More attention has, however, been bestowed on the relation of the fly to typhoid fever than to any other disease. Sedgwick [2] was the first that I know of to call attention to the importance of flies as a means of spreading typhoid fever, but the excessive typhoid death rate in the home camps of our soldiers during the Spanish-American War did more than anything else to call attention to the possible importance of the fly as a distributer of the germs of this disease. Surgeon General Stern-

[1] Rep. Med. Of., Co. of Lond., 1909, Append. IV, 7.
[2] Sedgwick, Rep. Bd. Health [etc.], Mass., 1892, 736.

berg had issued orders to guard against flies, but they had little effect. Veeder [1] clearly set forth the possibility of the transfer of fecal matter to food by means of flies, and he declared that flies were the principal cause of the prevalence of the disease in the camps. The report of the commission to investigate the cause of the fever, although laying chief stress on contact infection, forcibly emphasized the part played by flies in the spread of the disease.[2] Vaughan, a member of the commission, personally urged the importance of flies in the spread of this disease.[3] Ever since, great popular and scientific attention has been bestowed upon the fly in the United States and also in other countries.

Other Reports of Typhoid Fever due to Flies. — Nuttall cites Quill, Tooth and Calverly, Smith, Austen, Straton and Jones as attributing much of the army typhoid in South Africa and India to the presence of flies. Numerous writers on typhoid fever in civil life have referred to the fly as a most active agent in the transmission of this disease. In "The House Fly at the Bar," published by the Merchants' Association of New York in 1909, are printed opinions of seventy or more health officials and others, all but nine or ten of whom are emphatic in their statements that flies are very important carriers of disease germs. Some few, however, consider that the case against the fly has not been proved, though some circumstances are suspicious. Several give instances of fly infection that have come to their notice. Hurty writes of an outbreak in an asylum following the brief use of the privy by a walking case of typhoid fever. Flies abounded and there was no chance for contact. Taylor, of Denver, reported typhoid fever at a dairy. The milk became infected, he thinks by flies, for the privy was near the milk house, and gelatine cultures exposed near the privy

[1] Veeder, Med. Rec., N. Y., 1898, LIV, 429.

[2] Abst. of Rep. on the Origin and Spread of Typhoid Fever in U. S. Military Camps during the Spanish War, 1898, 183.

[3] Vaughan, J. Am. M. Ass., Chicago, 1900, XXXIV, 1451, 1496.

and in the milk house showed colonies of typhoid bacilli, presumably deposited by flies! Dr. H. W. Hill, the exceedingly cautious epidemiologist of the Minnesota State Board of Health, writes me that from his observations in that state he "firmly believes that flies are an important factor in the spread of typhoid in such places as mining and lumber camps, and that the small country village with its exposed outdoor closets parallels the camp conditions exactly." He further states that Wald noted that in a certain camp the Italians did not contract the disease because, as he thought, they did not eat between meals, while the Finns suffered severely because they kept their food laid out on the table all the time, where it was exposed to innumerable flies, and helped themselves during the day at random.

Pease[1] refers to an outbreak of 50 cases at Castleton from June to September all in the vicinity of a yard where typhoid excreta were thrown and where flies abounded. Dutton[2] accused bluebottle flies of carrying infection from the feces of a carrier to 4 other members of the family. In 1906 an outbreak of typhoid fever near London was thought by Ransome and Young to be due to swarms of flies which bred in a manure dump near by.[3] In none of these alleged instances of fly-borne infection are other modes excluded, and often it is quite as probable that the cases were due to contact, and in scarcely any of them is there more than a possibility that the disease was caused in the manner alleged.

Numerous bulletins and circulars have been issued by state and municipal health officials, some of which depict, in exaggerated language and with extravagant illustration, the danger to be feared from this household pest, and a distinguished entomologist has urged that the familiar name of *M. domestica* be changed from house fly to typhoid fly.

[1] Long Island M. J., Brooklyn, 1910, IV.

[2] Dutton, J. Am. M. Ass., Chicago, 1909, LIII, 1561.

[3] Rep. Med. Off. to Lond. Co., Council, 1907, Append. III.

Flies suspected from their Habits. — The chief reason why the fly is believed to be the carrier of diarrhea, cholera and typhoid fever are that flies are seen to pass from feces to food; that they have been shown to carry fecal bacteria, and in several instances the specific bacteria of cholera and typhoid fever; and that they often swarm in unusual numbers at times and in places where there is an exceptional prevalence of disease. The very definite observations of Hamilton, Fricker, Klein, Simmonds, Bartarelli Faichnie, Mann and Tsuzuki as to the finding of infected flies in infected houses, and the accounts given by Veeder, Vaughan, Tooth, Smith, Hill and others, of the contamination of food by flies in camps, military and civil, certainly render it probable that these insects do at times cause sickness, and may under certain conditions, such as prevail in camps, be an important factor in outbreaks. But these observations are far from a demonstration of what is now generally claimed, that flies are the chief factor in the spread of typhoid fever, and perhaps of summer diarrhea, in well-ordered civil communities.

Dr. Howard's Views. — Howard in his admirable work on the house fly, before cited, devotes 174 pages to the "Carriage of Disease," a large part of which is taken up by a consideration of typhoid fever; he quotes many of the writers referred to in the last few pages of this book and also some others as Wanhill in Bermuda, and Washburn in Minnesota, who, noting the filthy habits of flies and their seasonal distribution in relation to typhoid fever, are convinced that flies are an important factor in the causation of this disease. Very little convincing epidemiological evidence is offered. Howard apparently bases his own view on this matter upon the habits of the fly, for he says that "the correlation or non-correlation of the curve of house fly abundance and the abundance of typhoid has practically no effect upon our conclusions as regards the possible transfer of the disease by flies." Howard cites as significant the experience of Palmer in Georgia who offered to care for, without charge, any typhoid patient living in a fly-proof house, but none applied. He also found no secondary cases in families which controlled flies as directed. This does not appear to throw much light on the subject, for, if there were no secondary cases, his families must have been wonderfully well trained in avoiding contact infection; and this is doubtless the complete explanation.

Seasonal Distribution of Flies and Typhoid Fever. — As the seasonal distribution of flies has been studied with reference to diarrhea, so has it been studied with reference to typhoid fever. Jackson, in his report to the Merchants' Association in New York before referred to, gives a chart showing the seasonal distribution of flies in New York and of deaths from typhoid fever, the latter being set back two months to allow for the assumed time between the date of infection and the date of death. Hamer thinks two months is too long a time. He thinks that it is nearer five weeks. The apex of the typhoid curve corresponds fairly well with the apex of the fly curve, but there is a rise in the typhoid curve in February, two-thirds as high as that of August, which certainly cannot be attributed to flies. Ainsworth in India [1] states that at Poona the maximum admissions of typhoid fever to the hospital occur about one month after the maximum fly catch. Judging from Ainsworth's paper, there appears to be great seasonal variation in the number of flies in Poona, correlated closely with the temperature, as with us.

In Jacksonville [2] it is said that the fly curve and the typhoid-fever curve correspond closely, though Dr. Terry gives no figures or diagrams. According to Howard a similar correlation has been worked out by Purdy in New Zealand (1910) and Osmond in Cincinnati (1909).

[1] Ainsworth, J. Roy. Army Med. Corps, Lond., 1909, XII, 485.

[2] Am. J. Pub. Health, 1912, II, 14.

Evidence against Theory. — Niven [1] found that, while in Manchester in 1903 the maximum number of flies was caught about August 29, the maximum number of cases of typhoid was not reached until November, during the whole of which month the morbidity remained high. In 1906 [2] there was, as usual, a well-marked maximum of flies about September 1, and while the typhoid morbidity was high in September, being 65, it was somewhat higher in October, and there were 46 cases in November and 50 in January and only 21 in July and 23 in August. In Washington,[3] in 1908, the maximum fly catch was for the week ending June 24, after which it steadily and rapidly decreased. The maximum of typhoid cases, according to date of attack, was in the week ending July 22, but instead of falling rapidly, as did the fly catch, it continued high until the middle of September. There certainly is little parallelism between the two curves. The commissioners appointed to study the disease, and who make the report, say that the evidence is quite strong that flies play a relatively small part in the spread of typhoid fever in Washington.

In Providence the seasonal distribution of typhoid fever cases, according to date of first symptoms, for the six years 1904–1909, was as follows. All cases due to milk and all certainly contracted out of the city are excluded.

Jan.	Feb.	Mar.	Apr.	May	June
45	36	26	48	49	56
July	Aug.	Sept.	Oct.	Nov.	Dec.
80	161	133	117	96	59

According to observations of Sykes, the maximum fly catch out of doors was about the last of July, when it began to fall

[1] Niven, Rep. on Health of Manchester, 1903, 123.
[2] Rep. on Health of Manchester, 1906, 63, 84.
[3] U. S. Pub. Health & Mar. Hos. Serv., Hyg. Lab. Bull., No. 52, 30.

off quite rapidly. The observations as to the indoor catch were not very numerous, but it seems probable that the flies go indoors in greater numbers as the weather grows cooler in September. There is certainly not a very close agreement between the number of flies and the prevalence of typhoid fever. It is scarcely possible that the typhoid fever developing in November is due to flies, and yet there were 96 cases in November, and the November rate is higher than that of any other month except August, September and October. If we cannot attribute the excess in November to flies, why should it be thought necessary to attribute the excess of the preceding three months to flies? I can see nothing in the seasonal distribution of typhoid fever in Providence to warrant the assumption that flies are an important factor in its causation.

In London,[1] while the typhoid curve and the fly curve corresponded fairly well in 1907, in 1908 the greatest prevalence of flies was in the second week in August, while the maximum of typhoid fever notifications was in the second week in November. In 1909 there was only a slight autumnal rise of typhoid fever, the maximum being in January, while the maximum fly prevalence was in August.

Correlation of Typhoid Fever and High Temperature. — I have been able to find only the very few observations noted above as to the correlation of fly distribution and typhoid fever, and these few do not indicate that there is any reason to assume that the flies stand in causative relation to the fever. The very careful work of Sedgwick and Winslow[2] shows that throughout the world, and in both hemispheres, there is a distinct relation between this disease and the seasonal rise in temperature. These authors, though they recognized a certain amount of infection by flies, explained the autumnal increase in typhoid fever as due to the direct

[1] Rep. Med. Off. Health, Co. of Lond., 1907, 1908, 1909.

[2] Sedgwick and Winslow, Mem. Am. Acad. Arts & Sc., 1902, XII, No. 5.

and favorable action of high temperature on the life of the bacillus outside the body. This view hardly seems tenable from what has since been learned of the life habits of the bacillus, and I think is now no longer held by the authors. It is the custom now for most writers to attribute to flies the chief rôle in the autumnal excess of typhoid fever, but from the evidence at hand it seems wiser, while admitting the fact of seasonal distribution, as determined by Sedgwick and Winslow, to await further study before attributing this definitely to any one cause or group of causes.

Epidemiological Evidence, Minnesota. — More direct evidence of fly carriage is offered by Hill.[1] He reports three large insane hospitals, with 1400 to 1800 patients each, having outbreaks of typhoid fever at about the same time in the summer. In one, the wards of the institution, though screened, were full of flies, which followed the food from the kitchen, which was unscreened and swarming with the insects. In a second hospital the disease was confined almost exclusively to the men, whose dining rooms, and wards too, were swarming with flies, while the women's side was comparatively free. In both these institutions the outbreak continued until cold weather. In another hospital the flies were so numerous that when they settled on the slender wire supporting the electric lamps they gave it the appearance of an inch rod! The management determined to exterminate the flies, which they did, and though it was two months before cold weather, no more cases developed after the period of incubation had passed. Such a bit of evidence is not conclusive, but, if observed often enough, would be cumulative and would indicate a real causative relation between typhoid fever and flies as can no amount of watching the habits of flies or comparing fly curves and typhoid curves.

Evidence from Jacksonville, Richmond and Asheville. — The health officers of the two cities first named have very

[1] Hill, Rep. State Bd. Health, Minn., 1911, 206.

forcibly called attention to the much greater liability of infection by flies in the comparatively more "unsanitary" cities of the south and have criticized the present writer for an apparent disregard of this, and it is true it must be admitted that a large part of what is here written about the comparative unimportance of nuisances in general and the fly nuisance in particular is based upon conditions studied in the cities in the northern states and in England. According to Terry,[1] Jacksonville, with its large numbers of poorly made privies and enormous swarms of flies, has in the past been no better than an old-time army camp as regards conditions favoring the spread of typhoid fever. Late in 1910 a most energetic campaign was begun against the fly and for the construction of fly-proof privies. In 1911 there were reported only 142 cases of typhoid fever as against 321 for the same period of 1910. Formerly 60 per cent of the cases had been in the privy section and 40 per cent in the sewered section, though the distribution of the population was the reverse of these figures. After the fly campaign there was little difference in the incidence of the disease in the sewered and unsewered portions. The high typhoid rate of several Georgia cities showed no falling off in 1911. It would have been well if Terry had given the typhoid fever figures for a number of years and had also shown the seasonal distribution so that it might be seen whether the decrease was confined chiefly to the fly season. Still the figures as they stand are striking and call for continued effort along the same lines. Just as this is going to press the Report of the Board of Health of Jacksonville for 1911 has come to hand and on page 16 is a diagram which shows that reduction in typhoid fever incidence in 1911 was confined to the May–August period, the time of fly prevalence.

In Richmond, Levy[2] has been carrying on an energetic and well-directed campaign against typhoid fever since

[1] Terry, Am. J. Pub. Health, 1912, II, 14.

[2] Levy, Rep. Health Dept., Richmond, 1910.

1907, with the result that the death rate per 100,000 fell from nearly 50 in the preceding five years to 24.1 in 1909, 21.9 in 1910 and 17.8 in 1911. In 1910 strong effort was made to prevent fly infection by screening privies and patients, and by reducing the number of flies. In a letter Dr. Levy states that the number of flies is still large but that the screening has been very effective. I judge that he attributes a good deal of the typhoid reduction to this, but it is difficult to disentangle this factor from supervision of cases, instruction of attendants, disinfection of excreta and better notification. It is worth noting that the decrease does not seem to be greater for the summer months than for the winter when flies can scarcely be a factor.

In Asheville, N. C., so Dr. McBrayer writes me, there was a reduction in typhoid fever cases from 119 in 1910 to 60 in 1911, due chiefly, he believes, to strict control of privies which are now required to be made fly-proof.

Privies, Flies and Typhoid Fever. — That an excess of typhoid fever is found in cities or sections of cities where there are many open privies has often been noted. Of late some have attributed this to the transference of infected matter by flies. There is little warrant for this assumption, though Terry says that in Jacksonville after the screening of the privies there was no excess of typhoid fever in the unsewered parts of the city. But meanwhile an active campaign against typhoid fever was being waged, and more cleanly privies and better care of cases would do much to prevent contact infection. That the excess of typhoid fever in privy districts is doubtless largely due to contact is shown by the fact that, as has recently been noted in Providence, localized outbreaks among careless people using privies have occurred out of fly time. In Washington [1] investigation has shown that in the fly season the users of privies furnish a higher percentage of typhoid fever as com-

[1] U. S. Pub. Health and Mar. Hosp. Serv. Lab., Bull. 78, 1911, 66, 160.

pared with the users of water-closets than they do in the winter time. The percentage of cases furnished by the users of privies in fly time was 13.3, in the winter 7.7, but the figures were not large. It was also found in Washington that during 1908 and 1909 the 32 per cent of the population living in unscreened houses furnished about 59 per cent of the cases occurring in the summer and fall. But, as the report suggests, people living in unscreened houses are more likely to have other unsanitary surroundings and to be of careless habits.

Sykes' investigations in Providence showed that flies are 25 to 30 times more numerous in the uncleanly parts of the city than they are in the clean parts, and the differences in the indoor catch is even greater. Though, as shown above, there appears to be some excess of typhoid fever in the fly-infected and privy-using parts of cities, the difference bears no comparison to the difference in fly distribution.

Unwise to Claim Too Much. — While the fly is a nuisance and it is highly desirable to get rid of it, and while it seems likely that it is to some extent a means of spreading disease, it is extremely unwise to make definite statements that it is the chief source of diarrhea, of cholera or of typhoid fever, unless we have very exact proof, and it is unwise, unless such proof is at hand, to urge large expenditures to get rid of flies, promising thereby the eradication of typhoid fever and other diseases. If it should chance that a mistake has been made, and that the fly is not the chief disseminator of typhoid fever, and the disease still persists after the fly has disappeared, we need not be surprised if the public fail to take us seriously when we advise, on knowledge that is well established, that mosquitoes are the sole carriers of malaria and yellow fever; that escape from the tsetse fly means escape from sleeping sickness; and that a rat-proof city will be a plague-proof city.

Control of Flies. — As flies are a great nuisance and a possible source of danger it is very desirable that they should be eliminated as far as possible, but too much money should not be expended in the experiment and too large results should not be promised. Each individual family can very effectually control these pests by good screening and the use of fly paper. It is desirable that people should be educated to dislike flies. Chantemesse says that the housewife should think it as much of a discredit to have flies in her house as bugs in her bed. Circulars of information may be distributed, but care should be taken to avoid exaggeration and not to promise too much either as to the effectiveness of remedies or the resulting decrease in disease. We know even now far too little about the habits of flies and the best ways of attacking them. Packard and Howard gave us our first definite knowledge, but this has been much extended by Newstead,[1] who showed that the fly is far less exclusive in its choice of breeding places than was supposed.

Howard in his "The House Fly — Disease Carrier" gives a summary of our present knowledge which contains much information. The recent papers by Terry and by Dodd previously cited recite interesting and suggestive experiences. It appears that effective scavenging is the most important means of getting rid of flies. If yards, streets and vacant lots were kept clean, market refuse removed promptly, and all garbage kept covered, there would be an enormous reduction in the number of flies about dwellings. The most practicable way to prevent the breeding of flies in stable manure is to compel its removal once a week. Wherever it is possible the privy vault should be abolished. When this is impossible, the fly-proof privy has been urged and the Federal Government has issued a detailed account of how one may be economically constructed.[2] This

[1] Newstead, Rep. on the Habits, etc., of the House Fly, to the Health Committee, Liverpool, 1907.

[2] Stiles and Lumsden, U. S. Dept. Agriculture, Farmers Bull. 463, 1911.

has seemed somewhat visionary, but the energetic work done by the health officers of Richmond, Jacksonville and Asheville show that by means of constant supervision it is possible to make such privies effective. The question of covering food in markets and shops to protect it from flies as well as from dust has been much discussed. Slack [1] in an excellent paper concludes that the danger from this source in a well-ordered city is not very great, but that for æsthetic reasons the public might well demand, through ordinances or otherwise, that food be so protected. In this opinion the writer heartily concurs.

Summary. — After this brief examination of the evidence in regard to the rôle of insects in the transmission of disease we are justified in the following conclusions:

First. It is certain that yellow fever and malaria are transmitted solely by certain mosquitoes, and that by controlling the mosquitoes it is possible, even under very unfavorable conditions, to eradicate or reduce to a minimum these two diseases.

Second. It is highly probable that the relapsing fevers are transmitted solely by certain ticks, sleeping sickness by the tsetse fly, filariasis by the mosquito, pappataci fever by a fly and typhus fever by lice.

Third. The bubonic type of plague in human beings is usually transmitted from rat to man by the flea.

Fourth. It is probable that under certain conditions, as in military and civil camps and in filthy communities without sewerage, insects, especially flies, may be an important factor in the spread of the fecal-borne diseases, but there is no evidence that in a well-sewered city with few privies the house fly is a factor of great moment in the dissemination of disease.

[1] Slack, Am. J. Pub. Hyg., 1909, V, 159.

INDEX

PAGE

Actinomycosis . . . 366
African cattle fever . . . 122
Air, see Sewer air.
  bacillus influenzæ not carried by . . . 99–100
    tuberculosis in . . . 298–299
  bacteria found in . . . 282, 298–301
  danger of infection by . . . 300
  expired, free from germs . . . 287
  infection by, thought important . . . 137
    conclusions . . . 313–315
    experiments with anthrax . . . 312
      Mediterranean fever . . . 311–312
      plague . . . 281, 312–313
    not impossible . . . 281
    of wounds by . . . 300–301
  pneumococcus in . . . 300
  pus-forming bacteria in . . . 299–300
  swine plague bacilli in . . . 300
Air-borne anthrax . . . 285–286
  chicken pox . . . 270, 280
  disease in hospitals . . . 270–271, 279–280
    slight evidence of . . . 286
  infection indoors . . . 282
    in surgery . . . 283–284
    reasons for belief in . . . 259–260, 283
  influenza is not . . . 277
  malaria is not . . . 384
  measles . . . 272–280
  rubella . . . 280
  scarlet fever . . . 270–273, 280
    out of doors . . . 272–273
  small-pox, cases traced to other sources . . . 268–269
    conclusions . . . 269–270
    evidence against . . . 266–269
      of, in United States . . . 264–265
    from hospitals . . . 260–270
    infection of, denied . . . 263–270
    objections to theory . . . 265–266
  tuberculosis . . . 194, 202–203
  typhus fever . . . 281
  whooping cough . . . 280
Amebæ dysenteriæ, carriers of . . . 118
    grown on culture media . . . 24
    in soil . . . 24
    in well persons . . . 118
    on vegetables . . . 24

PAGE

Amebæ, intestinal parasites ... 112
species of ... 24
Amebic dysentery ... 24, 118
American hospitals ... 142–145, 279
Anchylostoma, see Uncinaria, Hookworms.
duodenalis ... 186
Anchylostomiasis, due chiefly to contact ... 186–187
Animals, diseases of, affecting man ... 371–373
spread tuberculosis by licking one another ... 204
Anopheles mosquitoes carry malaria ... 382–383
species and habits ... 385–386
Anthracosis ... 306–307
Anthrax, a dust-borne disease ... 285–286
an air-borne disease ... 285–286
and fomites ... 226–227
insects ... 416–417, 423
bacillus, see Bacillus anthracis.
due to food infection ... 2, 365
experiments in infection by air ... 312
from hair, hides ... 227
morocco factories ... 3
wool ... 227
wool refuse ... 3
perpetuated by direct contact ... 2
soil in relation to ... 2
spores in dust, hair, hides, wool ... 226–227
spread by unrecognized or concealed cases ... 2
Antisepsie médicale in French hospitals ... 198, 278–279
Antitoxin may favor spread of disease ... 386–387
Ants carry bacillus murium typhi ... 419
plague bacilli ... 419, 424
Aspergillus destroys mosquitoes ... 390
Asylums, bacillary dysentery in ... 183–184, 430–431
percentage of bacillus diphtheriæ carriers in ... 90
typhoid fever in ... 51–52, 442
Atoxyl to prevent sleeping sickness ... 402
Atypical cases, laboratory evidence of ... 123
not easily distinguished from carriers ... 130–131

Babies' Hospital, gonorrhea in ... 165–166
Bacillary dysentery, carriers of ... 67–69
caused by contact ... 183–184
culture of bacillus in eye ... 183–184
in camps ... 183
in institutions ... 183–184
mild cases of ... 68–69
Bacillus anthracis, see Anthrax spores.
carried by flies ... 419, 423
growth in ponds ... 3
relation to the soil ... 2, 4
saprophytic existence of ... 2
Bacillus coli communis cause of diarrhea ... 367
in dust of schoolrooms ... 294
on the hands ... 179, 192
on roller towel ... 192

PAGE

Bacillus diphtheriæ carried by flies........ 423
carriers in family........ 89–90
insane asylum........ 90
schools........ 90–94
investigation of, in Massachusetts... 83
of........ 82–99
found intermittently........ 98
in bread........ 26
carriers, varieties of........ 83
virulence of........ 82, 84–86, 91–92
clay........ 233
convalescents........ 82, 84–85, 98–99
dust........ 290, 294
holy water, on cups, pencils, drinking glass. 192
membrane........ 240
milk........ 25, 26
otitis........ 94–95
pupils cause disease in teacher........ 98
rhinitis........ 94–95
rooms........ 233, 241
scarlet fever........ 86–88, 91, 96
school children........ 82–86, 88, 90–94
soil........ 26
sore throat........ 93–94, 98–99
well persons........ 82–83
life of, in butter........ 251
may be air-borne........ 289
not in normal throats........ 84–85
on coat........ 227
drinking glass........ 192
fomites........ 192–193, 227, 240–241
virulence of........ 240
pencils........ 193, 233
resistance to drying........ 233, 290
saprophytic existence of........ 25

Bacillus dysenteriæ, carried by flies........ 423
cause of diarrhea........ 367
in carriers........ 67–69
feces........ 24
milk........ 15
soil........ 23
resistance to drying........ 234
saprophytic existence of........ 23

Bacillus enteritidis, cause of diarrhea........ 367
(Gaertner) in ice cream........ 250
in food poisoning........ 58, 371
sporogenes, cause of diarrhea........ 367

Bacillus influenzæ in droplets........ 298
not carried by air........ 99–100
saprophytic........ 26
persistence of........ 100
resistance to drying........ 238
widely distributed........ 100–101

Bacillus lepræ in droplets........ 297

PAGE
Bacillus morbificans in food poisoning 371
Bacillus paratyphi, cause of diarrhea 367
in feces 16
food poisoning 371
not found in healthy persons 59–61
Bacillus paratyphi A in carriers 58
Bacillus paratyphi B in carriers 59
Bacillus pestis carried by ants 419–424
in bodies of fleas 236
convalescent animals 69–70
convalescents 70
cow dung 23
dust 290–291
sputum 71
infection of soil by 22
not found on floors 235
on cotton goods 228
resistance to drying 235–236, 290–291
saprophytic existence of 22
Bacillus prodigiosus on flies 425
in droplets 295–297
sewer air 284
Bacillus pullorum, carriers of 71
Bacillus tetani in blank cartridges 6, 226
dirt of floors 239
gelatine 6, 284
intestines of animals 5
soil 6, 239
latency of 106
on lamp wick 6, 226
resistance of 6, 225–226
saprophytic existence of 6
Bacillus tuberculosis, carriers of 103–105
in air 298–299
butter 364–365
communion cups 195
droplets 295–296
dust 292–293
flies, and fly specks 422–423
lymphatic glands 203
milk 355–356
nose and mouth 103–104, 193, 203
railway carriages 292
room 235, 292
tonsils 203–204
tramcars 292
latency of 104–105
may be dust-borne 289–290
pass from stomach to lungs 305–308
not found in street dust 292
in expired air 287
on spirometer 195
saprophytic 26
so resistant as believed 234–235

PAGE
Bacillus tuberculosis, on a glass........ 195
dishes........ 195
fomites........194–195, 241–242, 292, 293
hands........193–194
napkin rings........ 195
sidewalks........ 194
telephones........ 195
tongue........ 203
perishes in light........234–235
proportion of human and bovine types...360–361
resistance to drying........234–235, 241–242, 291
swept from sidewalk by dresses........ 194
Bacillus typhi carried on fingers........169–170
flies and........420–422
in blood........34–35
bones........ 35
butter........ 16
cerebro-spinal fluid........ 35
dead animals........ 8
dust........ 290
feces........9, 34–36
gall bladder........35, 42
ice........13, 319, 340–341
kidneys........ 35
milk........ 15
ovaries........ 35
oysters........ 13
privy vaults........ 9–10
prostatic fluid........ 37
seltzer water........ 13
seminal vesicles........ 37
septic tank effluent........ 10
sewer air........ 284
soft drinks........ 13
soil........ 7, 10
epidemiological evidence of growth........ 16
spleen........ 35
sputum........37–38
tidal mud........ 8
tonsils........ 34
urine........ 37
persistence of........ 10
water........10–13
epidemiological evidence of growth........ 17
modes of contamination........ 320
recovered from........ 319
increase in milk........ 17
intermittent excretion of........46–47
moisture necessary to growth of........ 16
on blankets........ 227
vegetables........ 8
path of entrance........34, 178
resistance to drying........232–233, 290
saprophytic existence of........ 7, 16

PAGE

Bacteria and sewer air....284–285, 288–289
cultured less resistant than uncultured.... 11
effect of drying upon....231–232
found in air....298–301
inhalation of....304–305
not found in expired air.... 287
given off from moist surfaces....287, 288
of suppuration, see Pus bacteria.
on cups....192–193
fomites....239–242
hands....192–194
money....223–224
pencils....192–193
Bagging, yellow fever from.... 213
Balantidium.... 112
Ballast, yellow fever from.... 213
Bathing, typhoid fever from....324–325
Baths, public, encourage cleanliness.... 211
Bed clothing, bacillus diphtheriæ on.... 240
Bed, smallpox from.... 214
Bedbugs and anthrax.... 417
kala-azar.... 402
plague.... 414
relapsing fever....411–412
typhoid fever.... 418
Bedpan carries dysentery amebæ.... 183
Betel nut, cholera spread by.... 185
Biological carriers distinguished from mechanical carriers.... 413
Black-leg.... 4
Blank cartridges, bacillus tetani in.... 6
Blankets, bacillus typhi on.... 227
Blood, bacillus typhi in....34–35
infection of, cause of typhoid fever....34–35
meningococcus in.... 73
yellow fever virus in....393–394
Boer War, typhoid fever from dust in....275–276
flies in.... 436
Books, bacillus tuberculosis on.... 241
scarlet fever from.... 215
Boophilus annulatus and cattle fever.... 112
Botryomycosis.... 366
Bovine tuberculosis bacillus may infect man....353–354
Bread, bacillus diphtheriæ in.... 26
Brill's disease.... 409
Broad Street well....316–317, 325
Brush, bacillus diphtheriæ on.... 240
Bubonic plague, see Plague.
Butter, a source of diphtheria.... 350
bacillus tuberculosis in....364–365
typhi in.... 16
life of bacillus diphtheriæ in.... 251

Calliphora erythrocephala.... 428
Camps, bacillary dysentery in.... 183

PAGE
Camps, filthy condition of 180
typhoid fever in 170–171, 435–437
Caps and gowns to prevent infection 218
Carbolic acid in well water 324
Carriers a recent discovery 33, 38
source of protozoan disease 126
and mild cases, number of 124–125, 133–135
cause cattle fever 112
cerebro-spinal meningitis 74–81
cholera 65–67, 185
diphtheria 94–99
glanders 99
malaria 114–115
nagana 113
typhoid fever 47–54
definition of and classification of 38–39
during incubation 39
evidence against 55
of infectivity 127–131
explain spread of cerebro-spinal meningitis 78–81
in bacterial diseases 127
in institutions 50–52, 65, 67
infect food 47–51, 60, 65
milk 52–54
intermittent excretion in 46, 62
laboratory evidence of 123
less infective than the sick 155
more dangerous than things 225
not always dangerous 129
of amebic dysentery 118, 183
bacillary dysentery 67–69
bacillus pullorum 71
cattle fever 112
cerebro-spinal meningitis 72–81
cholera 61–67
diphtheria, importance of 149–152
dourine 113
glanders 99
gonorrhea 102
influenza 99
lepra bacilli 105
malaria 114–115
measles 111
Mediterranean fever 72
nagana 113
paratyphoid fever 58–61
plague 69–71
pneumococcus 101–102
poliomyelitis 118–121
pus organisms 105–106
scarlet fever 109
sleeping sickness 115–116
smallpox 109–110
tetanus bacilli 106

PAGE

Carriers of tubercle bacilli ... 103–105
 typhoid fever ... 38–55
 among different classes ... 39–44
 cannot be isolated ... 152
 duration of infection ... 45
 Vincent's angina ... 117
 relation to infectivity ... 125
 shade into missed cases and atypical cases ... 130–131
 virulence of germs in ... 126
Cartridges, bacillus tetani in ... 226
Cattle fever ... 112, 122
Celery, typhoid fever caused by ... 379
Cerebro-spinal meningitis an accident of infection ... 81
 carriers of ... 73–81
 explain spread of ... 78–81
 contagiousness of ... 79–80
 due to pneumococcus ... 81
 infection by carriers ... 74–81
 isolation a failure in ... 81, 146
 path of infection ... 73
 prompt isolation in, a success ... 146
 secondary cases ... 79–80
Charbon symptomatique ... 4
Charts, bacillus tuberculosis on ... 241–242
Chicken pox air-borne ... 270, 280
Chicks, white diarrhea of ... 71
Children not cleanly ... 190
Cholera and contact ... 184–185
 flies ... 420, 430
 fomites ... 215
 atypical cases ... 65
 caused by washing soiled linen in running streams ... 325
 from betel nut ... 185
 carriers ... 65–67, 185
 clothing ... 215
 handling food ... 185
 rags ... 222
 shellfish ... 374
 soil ... 29
 unrecognized cases ... 20, 65
 water ... 325–326
 wells ... 325–326
 infection of nurses ... 185
 not dust-borne ... 289–290
 on shipboard due to infected water ... 326
 outbreaks in various places ... 20
 spirillum, see Spirillum choleræ.
Christmas presents, diphtheria from ... 215
Cimex lectularius, see Bedbug.
Citellus beecheyi ... 413
Clams, typhoid fever from ... 375
Clay, bacillus diphtheriæ in ... 233
Cleanliness, education in, needed ... 208–209
 municipality should encourage ... 210–211

PAGE

Cleanliness, neglected 206–208
  rare 178–180
    in children 190
  teaching of, in school 209–210
  versus disinfection 257
Cloth, yellow fever from 213
Clothing as fomites 216
  bacillus tuberculosis on 242
  cholera from 215
  infection by, rare 217–219
  leprosy in 216
  scarlet fever not from 217
  typhoid fever from 219
  typhus fever not from 216–217
Coat, bacillus diphtheriæ on 227
  scarlet fever from 215
Cockles, typhoid fever from 375–376
Cockroaches and disease 418
Colon bacillus, see Bacillus coli communis.
Communion cups, bacillus tuberculosis in 195
  individual, adopted 210
Conductors not infected by money 224
Connorrhinus 403, 404
Contact by drinking cups 189–190, 192–193
  chief mode of infection 195–206
  indirect, vehicles for 188–190
  infection and fingers 188–189
    disregard of 207–208
    importance of 206
    in amebic dysentery 183
      bacillary dysentery 183–184
      cerebro-spinal meningitis 73–74, 76–77, 80
      cholera 184–185
      diarrhea 185
      diphtheria 196–202
      gonorrhea 165–167
      influenza 277
      measles 199
      Mediterranean fever 312
      scarlet fever 196–202
      syphilis 164, 167–169
      tuberculosis 204–205
      typhoid fever 17, 47–50, 169–183
        amount of 177–178
        evidences of 177
        in civil life 171–173
        in hospitals 198–202
        opportunities for 179–180
        rôle of privies 180–182
        Spanish war 170
        why disregarded 179–181
      uncinariasis 186
    less easy in some diseases than in others 187–188
    most obvious 164

PAGE
Contact infection, opportunities for......190–192
mode of infection between families......196–198
with missed cases, importance of......190–192
well carriers, importance of...... 191
Contacts, diphtheria carriers among...... 89
typhoid carriers among...... 43
Contagiousness, factors involved......153–155
less outside family......154–155
than believed......153–155
of carriers less than that of sick...... 155
Convalescents, cholera spirilla in......61–65
diphtheria bacilli in......84, 85
dysentery amebæ in...... 118
bacilli in......68–69
malarial parasites in......114–115
meningococci in......74–77
plague bacilli in......70–71
pneumococci in...... 101
typhoid bacilli in......40–41
Cornet, diphtheria from...... 215
Cotton goods, bacillus pestis on...... 228
smallpox from...... 214
Cow dung, bacillus pestis in...... 23
Cows, diphtheria in...... 347
scarlet fever said to occur in......346–347
Crawfish and typhoid fever...... 378
Cream, typhoid fever from...... 349
Cubicles for isolation in French hospitals......198–200
Culex, experiments with...... 383
fasciatus and yellow fever...... 392
fatigans and dengue...... 410
filariasis...... 399
Culicides......388–389
mosquito destruction by......390, 397
Culture method of diagnosis, introduction of......137–138
Cups, bacteria on......192–193

Danysz rat virus carried by flies...... 424
Dead animals, bacillus typhi in...... 8
bodies, spirillum choleræ in...... 19
Dengue transmitted by mosquitoes...... 409
Dermacenter andersoni...... 412
Diarrhea, bacteria which cause...... 367
due to condensed milk......368–369
contact......185, 367
dust......276–277
flies......431–435
milk......366–369
not always...... 185
water......327–329, 331, 334
explosive outbreaks...... 369
nature of......366–367
prevention of......369–370

PAGE

Diarrhea, relation of feeding to 367–369
white, of chicks 71
Diphtheria, atypical 92–94, 133
bacillus, see Bacillus diphtheriæ.
carried to homes by discharged scarlet fever cases 98
carriers, importance of 149–152
isolation of, often impossible 150–152
chronic 99
cultures introduced 137–138
value of findings 84–85
disinfection unnecessary after 247–250
extension in dwellings 197–198
family infection 89–90
from butter 350
carriers 95–99
Christmas presents 215
cornet 215
drinking glass 192–193
fomites 215–227
milk 96–97, 346–347
pitcher 97
sewer air 273
teacher 97
tools 215
in cows 347
Owatonna, Minn 144
Providence 136, 138
Willard State Hospital 144
isolation, duration in Providence 143
in institutions, failure of 143–145
principles of 149–152
mild cases found by cultures 138
not air-borne in hospitals 273–274
dust-borne 290
from soil 28
of extra-corporal origin 29
similarity to scarlet fever 106–107
warning sign in 151
with recurrent ear discharge causes infection 98
Disease rarely carried by physicians 217
Dishes, bacillus tuberculosis from 195
Disinfection, American views on 256
desirable at times 256–257
English views on 255–256
French views on 255
in Providence 137
abandoned 247–252
schools 254
objections to 257
of little value 247–256
unnecessary after diphtheria 247–250
in other diseases 252–254
scarlet fever 250–252
versus cleanliness 257

PAGE

Dog drinks from the drinking glass on train 190
Dourine, carriers of 113
Drainage, mosquito destruction by 390
Dresses, bacillus tuberculosis on 194
Drinking cups, contact infection by 189–190
 glass, bacillus diphtheriæ on 192
 common, abolished 210
Droplet infection 295–298
Droplets, bacillus influenzæ in 298
 lepræ in 297
 prodigiosus in 295–297
 tuberculosis in 295–296
 pneumococcus in 298
 streptococcus salivarius in 297
 versus dust 303–305
Drying, effect upon bacteria 231–232, 288–289
 resistance of bacillus diphtheriæ to 233, 290
 dysenteriæ to 234
 influenzæ to 238
 pestis to 235–236, 290–291
 tuberculosis to 234–235, 241–242, 291
 typhi to 232–233, 290
 gonococcus to 239
 meningococcus to 238–239
 micrococcus of Mediterranean fever to 233
 pneumococcus to 238
 protozoa to 242
 pus-forming bacteria to 236–237
 smallpox virus to 244
 spirillum choleræ to 237–238, 242, 291–292
 spirochete of syphilis to 239
 spores to 232
 vaccine virus to 242–244
Dust, anthrax spores in 227
 bacillus coli communis in 294
 diphtheriæ in 290, 294
 pestis in 290–293
 tuberculosis in 292–293
 typhi in 290
 danger from slight 294–295
 infection 288
 meningococcus in 289–290, 293
 micrococcus melitensis in 21, 300
 pneumococcus in 293–294
 pus organisms in 294
 streptococcus in 282
 versus droplets 303–305
Dust-borne disease 288–290
 anthrax 285–286
 diarrhea 276–277
 influenza 277
 Mediterranean fever 312
 poliomyelitis 278
 tuberculosis 288, 291–293, 301–311

PAGE

Dust-borne disease, typhoid fever 275–276
Dwellings, extension of diphtheria in 197–198
scarlet fever extension in 196–197
Dysentery, see Bacillary dysentery.
amebic 118, 183
due to chronic carriers 183
infection from bedpan 183
produced in men by amebæ grown in culture . 24
monkeys by amebæ 24
transmitted by contact 183
bacillus, see Bacillus dysenteriæ.
due to flies 430–431
infection by water 326–329, 331

Ear discharge causes diphtheria 98
Elephantiasis 399
Endemic diseases 29–30
English hospitals 139–142
isolation in 200–202
Entameba coli and entameba histolytica, distinction between ... 24, 118
Erysipelas from rags 222

Family, carriers in, cerebro-spinal meningitis 75
diphtheria 89
infection of, in house 28, 196–198
isolation in 160–161
typhoid fever by contact in 176
Feces, bacillus dysenteriæ in 24
paratyphi in 16
typhi in 9, 35–36
persistence of 10
intermittency of 46–47
hookworms in 187
spirillum choleræ in 19
Filaria bancrofti 398
Filariasis and mosquitoes 398–399
Filth theory of disease 27
Filtration of water 338
reduces typhoid fever 321
Fingers and contact infection 188–189
Fish, infection by fried 278
Fishermen, influenza among 277
Fleas and anthrax 417
plague 23, 312–313, 413–416
bacillus pestis in 236, 414–415
Flies a nuisance 445–446
and anthrax 419
cholera 430
diarrhea 431–435
dysentery 430
Egyptian ophthalmia 419
murrina 429
plague 419, 424
tuberculosis 429

PAGE
Flies and typhoid fever.....169–171, 182–183, 435–445
epidemiological evidence.....442–445
evidence against theory.....440–441
reports of outbreaks.....435–439
statistical evidence.....439–445
bacillus tuberculosis in.....422–423
carry bacillus anthracis.....419, 423
diphtheriæ..... 423
dysenteriæ..... 423
prodigiosus..... 425
typhi.....420–422
Danysz rat virus..... 424
fecal bacteria.....425–427
germs.....419–437
gonococci..... 424
lime from privies..... 425
poliomyelitis..... 427
spirillum choleræ..... 420
control of.....445–447
difficult to infect by..... 425
habits bring them in contact with excrement..... 438
infected, in typhoid houses.....421–422
local variation in distribution.....435, 445
mechanism of infection..... 424
range of flight..... 427
reduction of and decrease of typhoid fever.....442–444
seasonal and local distribution..... 427
species in houses..... 428
tuberculosis due to..... 429
Flock cough from rags..... 222
Floors, bacillus pestis not on..... 235
tetani in dirt of..... 239
Fly specks, bacillus tuberculosis in.....422–423
Fomites: Bagging..... 213
Ballast..... 213
Barbers' utensils..... 168
Barracks.....76, 216
Bedding.....168, 214
Blankets..... 227
Books.....215, 241
Brush..... 240
Cartridges.....6, 226
Charts.....241, 242
Christmas presents..... 215
Clay..... 233
Cloth..... 213
Clothing.....169, 215–216, 219, 242
Coat.....215, 227
Communion cups..... 195
Cornet..... 215
Cotton..... 214
Cotton goods..... 228
Cups.....192–193
Dentists' tools..... 168

PAGE

Fomites: Drinking glass........168, 189–190, 192–193, 195, 240
Floors........235, 239
Furniture........241
Gelatine........6, 226
Glass blowers' tubes........168
Grain........213
Hair........215, 226, 227
Handkerchief........168, 234, 240, 293
Hides........226, 227
House, see Room.
Lamp wick........6, 226
Letters........215
Linen, soiled........175, 214, 240
Lumber........214
Mattress........213
Merchandise........213
Mirror........240
Money........168, 223, 224
Napkin rings........195
Nursing bottles........168
Oyster buckets........213
Pencils........168, 193, 233
Pins........168
Pitcher........97
Rags........169, 222
Railway carriages........292
Roller towel........210
Room........214, 216, 219–222, 233, 235, 241, 292, 294
Rugs........223
Shawl........409
Shoes........218, 240
Spirometer........241
Spoons, etc........168
String........168
Surgeons' instruments........168
Telephones........195, 241
Thermometer........174
Tools........215
Toys........240
Tramcars........292
Wind instruments........168
Wool........226, 227

Fomites and anthrax........226–227
cholera........215
diphtheria........215, 227
plague, experiments in India........246–247
observations in Sydney........245–246
scarlet fever........214–215
smallpox........214
tetanus........225–226
tuberculosis, lack of experiments........247
typhoid fever........227
typhus fever........216–217, 409
yellow fever........213–214, 394

PAGE

Fomites and yellow fever experiments in Havana . . . 245
bacillus diphtheriæ on . . . 240–241
tuberculosis on . . . 241–242
bacteria of suppuration on . . . 25
on . . . 239–240
clothing as . . . 216
conclusions concerning . . . 258
definition of term . . . 212–213
evidence of infection by, unsatisfactory . . . 224–225
infection, bacteriological evidence . . . 230–231
evidence against . . . 229–230
few instances of . . . 228
reasons for belief in . . . 228–229
thought important . . . 137
Food, carriers infect . . . 47–51, 60, 65
handling by contacts . . . 162–163
infection and cholera . . . 185
tuberculosis . . . 364, 372–373
typhoid fever . . . 169–170, 364, 374–379
poisonings . . . 38, 60, 371–372
spirillum choleræ in . . . 20
Foot-and-mouth disease and milk . . . 366
French hospitals . . . 198–200
"Antisepsie médicale" in . . . 198
cubicles for isolation in . . . 198–200
screens for isolation in . . . 198–200
Furniture, bacillus diphtheriæ on . . . 241

Gall stones and typhoid fever . . . 36, 42
Gelatine, bacillus tetani in . . . 6, 226
Glanders, carriers of . . . 99
Glands, bacteria of suppuration in . . . 25
cervical and mesenteric, bacillus tuberculosis in . . . 203
Glass, bacillus diphtheriæ on . . . 192, 240
tuberculosis on . . . 195
contact infection by drinking from . . . 189–190
Glossina morsitans . . . 113
palpalis . . . 115, 399–401
Goats and Mediterranean fever . . . 21, 72, 365
Gonococci carried by flies . . . 424
Gonococcus, not saprophytic . . . 26
resistance to drying . . . 239
Gonorrhea, air-borne infection not possible . . . 166–167
believed to be spread by contact . . . 164–167
carried by nurses . . . 166–167
in Babies' Hospital . . . 165–166
infection by fomites impossible . . . 166–167
latency of . . . 102–103
not dust-borne . . . 289
persistence of . . . 102–103
Gown and cap for physicians and nurses in contagious cases . . . 218
Grain, yellow fever from . . . 213
Ground squirrels and plague . . . 413
Guinea pigs, bacillus pestis in . . . 69–70

PAGE

Hair, anthrax spores in 226–227
 scarlet fever from 215
Handkerchief, bacillus diphtheriæ on 240
 tuberculosis on 234, 293
Hands, bacillus coli communis on 179, 192
 tuberculosis on 193–194
 pus bacteria on 192–194
 should be washed 179–180
Hazens theorem 329
Hides, anthrax spores in 226–227
Holy water, bacillus diphtheriæ in 192
Homalomyia canicularis 428
Home isolation effective 160
Hookworms, see Uncinaria, Anchylostoma 186–187
 enter through skin 187
 grow in soil 186
 in feces 187
Hospital isolation, failure of 139–142
 in 161
Hospitals, air-borne disease in 270–271, 279–280
 bacillary dysentery in 183–184
 contact infection in 198–202
 diphtheria not air-borne in 273–274
 in America 142–145
 England 139–142
 France 198–200
 scarlet fever, not air-borne from 272–273
 smallpox, air-borne infection from 260–270
 typhoid fever by contact in 173–174
 value of 160
House, infection from family to family 28
 of, cause of scarlet fever 214–215
 tuberculosis infection in 205, 220–222
Houses, species of flies in 428

Ice, bacillus typhi in 13, 319, 341–342
 infection by 339–342
Ice cream, a source of disease 349–350
 control of 350
Incubation stage infective 39–40
Infection, former theories of 1
 not so easy as believed 84, 153, 191–192
Influenza among fishermen 277
 lighthouse keepers 277
 atypical cases 99
 bacillus, see Bacillus influenzæ.
 from rags 222
 not air-borne 277
 carried across Atlantic 277
 dust-borne 277, 289
 spread only by contact 277
Inhalation of bacteria 304–305
Insect-borne disease usually due to protozoa 380–381
Insects as biological and mechanical carriers 380–382

PAGE
Insects carry germs on bodies.... 418
first proof of transmission of disease by.... 381–382
infection by, importance of subject.... 380
Texas cattle fever first disease proved to be carried by.. 381–382
Institutions, carriers in.... 50–52, 65, 67
Intermittent excretion in carriers.... 46, 62, 68, 76, 98
Isolation a failure in cerebro-spinal meningitis.... 146
measles.... 145–146
smallpox.... 147
causes of failure.... 147–149
duration of.... 160–162
effective if prompt.... 146, 157–158
in Michigan.... 156–158
rare diseases.... 158–159
hospitals, failure of.... 139–142
in American cities.... 142–145
English hospitals.... 200–202
family.... 160–161
effective.... 160
hospital.... 161
Monsall Hospital.... 200–202
Providence.... 136, 160
villages.... 155–158
not effective in extensive outbreaks.... 158
to be too strict.... 151–152
of cerebro-spinal meningitis.... 146
diphtheria.... 136, 137–139, 143, 149, 156
duration in Providence.... 143
malaria.... 388
measles.... 145, 156
plague.... 415
rare diseases.... 158
scarlet fever.... 136, 139, 156
school children.... 162
sleeping sickness.... 401
smallpox.... 139, 147, 156
typhoid fever.... 152, 156
wage earners.... 152, 162–163
yellow fever.... 393
should vary.... 155
too rigorous.... 152–153
useless if many carriers.... 159
value of.... 151–152

Jews do not eat shellfish.... 376

Kala-azar and insects.... 402
Kissing means of spread of tuberculosis.... 202–203
spreading syphilis.... 168

Laboratory infection, bacillary dysentery.... 183–184
typhoid fever.... 175
tuberculosis infection in.... 308–309
Lamblia.... 112

PAGE
Lampwick, bacillus tetani on....6, 226
Latency of infection common....106, 122
Laundress contracts smallpox.... 214
typhoid fever.... 175
Laundries and disease....218–219
tuberculosis.... 219
Leishmania donovani.... 402
tropica.... 404
Leprosy, bacilli remain latent.... 105
in clothing.... 216
isolation of.... 156
Letters, scarlet fever from.... 215
Lettuce, bacillus typhi on.... 8
Lice and relapsing fever.... 412
typhus fever and....405–409
Light, bacillus tuberculosis perishes in....234–235
Lighthouse keepers, influenza among.... 277
Linen, soiled, smallpox from.... 214
typhoid fever from....175, 219
Lockjaw, see Tetanus.
Lucilia cæsar or "blue-bottles"....428, 437
Lumber, smallpox from.... 214
"Lung Blocks" in New York....220–222
Lupus due to inoculation with saliva.... 203

Malaria, an endemic disease....29–30
and insects....382–392
water.... 384
anointing the skin in.... 389
clearing of space about dwellings.... 389
discovery of insect transmission....382–383
experiments on infection of human beings.... 383
isolation sometimes necessary.... 388
killing of mosquitoes in houses.... 388
latency of....113–115
explanation....114–115
in children....114–115
percentage of....114–115
mosquito sole carrier of....383–385
not air-borne.... 384
due to soil infection.... 30
from water....335–336
on ship *Argo*.... 335
screening of patients.... 388
success of mosquito destruction....390–391
ways of prevention....386–390
Malta, Mediterranean fever exterminated at.... 72
Malta fever, see Mediterranean fever.
Mattress, yellow fever from.... 213
Measles an air-borne disease....278–280
carriers of.... 111
disinfection after.... 253
isolation in, a failure....145–146
not from soil.... 28

PAGE
Measles, number attacked . . . 111
per cent of children attacked . . . 145
Meat and tuberculosis . . . 372–373
infection by . . . 371–374
inspection, federal control of . . . 373–374
Mechanical carriers distinguished from biological carriers . . . 413
Mediterranean fever an endemic disease . . . 21
and contact infection . . . 312
dust . . . 312
goats . . . 21, 72, 365
caused by milk from infected goats . . . 21, 365
experiments in infection by air . . . 311–312
exterminated at Malta . . . 72
goats carriers of . . . 72
human carriers of . . . 72
in United States . . . 365
micrococcus of, resistance to drying . . . 233
on a steamship . . . 72
spread by urine . . . 22
Membrane, bacillus diphtheriæ in . . . 240
Meningitis, cerebro-spinal, see Cerebro-spinal meningitis.
Meningococcus causes rhinitis . . . 73
found intermittently . . . 76
only near sick . . . 77
in air . . . 77
contacts . . . 73–74, 76–77, 80
dust . . . 289–290, 293
families . . . 75–80
normal nose . . . 73
nose in sickness . . . 72
infection in barracks . . . 76
not saprophytic . . . 26
persistence of infection . . . 74–75
resistance to drying . . . 238–239
Merchandise, yellow fever from . . . 213
Michigan, isolation effective in . . . 156–158
Micrococcus albus . . . 24
aureus . . . 24
citreus . . . 24
melitensis, discovery and study of . . . 21
in dust . . . 21, 300
resistance to drying . . . 233
saprophytic existence of . . . 21
meningitidis, see Memingococcus.
pneumoniæ, see Pneumococcus.
Mild cases of infectious disease not recognized . . . 134–135
Milk and disease . . . 342–370
bacillus diphtheriæ in . . . 25–26
dysenteriæ in . . . 15
tuberculosis in . . . 355–356
typhi in . . . 15–17
carriers infect . . . 52–54
classification of . . . 363
condensed and diarrhea . . . 368–369

PAGE

Milk, diarrhea from 366–369
diphtheria from....96–97, 345–346
foot-and-mouth disease from.... 366
handling by contacts....162–163
increase of bacillus typhi in.... 17
infection by water.... 323
from human sources....347–348
Mediterranean fever from.... 365
mode of infection of....347–348
outbreaks, characteristics....342–343
few in large cities....344–345
frequency of....343–344
source of infection....346–347
pasteurization of....348–349
protection against tuberculosis from....362–363
of....348–349
rabies from.... 366
scarlet fever from....346–349
spirillum choleræ in.... 19
sterilization of vessels.... 348
streptococcus in.... 352
tonsillitis from....351–352
tuberculosis from....354–362
amount of 356–362
epidemiological evidence 361–362
instances of 360
tuberculous, consumed by children....357–360
typhoid fever from 51–54, 343–345
Mills-Reincke phenomenon 329–335
Miners, typhoid fever among.... 182
Minnesota, smallpox isolation abandoned in.... 147
Mirror, bacillus diphtheriæ on.... 240
Missed cases a recent discovery.... 33
Moist surfaces, bacteria not given off from....287–288
Money and disease....223–224
bacteria on 223–224
Monkeys, dysentery in.... 24
Monsall Hospital, isolation in....200–202
Montana, smallpox isolation abandoned in.... 147
Mosquito destruction by culicides....390, 397
drainage.... 390
oiling.... 390
prevention....389–391
Mosquitoes and dengue....409–410
filariasis....398–399
malaria....382–383
conditions for carrying....385–386
yellow fever....392–398
destruction of.... 397
habits 395
destruction of, in malarious houses.... 388
habits of.... 385
species which carry malaria....382–383, 385
success of measures for extermination....390–391

PAGE
Mosquitoes, transportation of ... 395
Mouth, bacillus tuberculosis in ... 103–104, 193
pneumococcus in ... 101–102
Mucous surfaces, bacteria of suppuration on ... 24
Mud dumped near intake cause of typhoid fever ... 320
Municipal versus personal prevention ... 208
Murium typhi, bacilli of, carried by ants ... 419
Murrina, flies and ... 429
Musca domestica (see Flies) ... 418, 428, 437
Muscina stabulans ... 428
Mussels, infection by ... 375–377
Myzomyia ludlowii ... 385

Nagana ... 113
Night soil as a fertilizer ... 9
North Boston well ... 317
Nose, bacillus tuberculosis in ... 103–104, 193, 299
meningococcus in, in sickness ... 72–73
in normal ... 73
tuberculosis of ... 204
Nurses, gown and cap for, in contagious cases ... 218
infect patients with typhoid fever ... 174
typhoid fever among ... 173–174

Oiling, mosquito destruction by ... 390
Ophthalmia, Egyptian, carried by flies ... 419
Opilacao due to connorrhinus ... 403
Opsonic index in typhoid carriers ... 42
Oriental sore and insects ... 404
Ornithodorus moubata ... 411
Otitis, bacillus diphtheriæ in ... 94–95
Owatonna, Minn., diphtheria in ... 144
Oyster buckets, yellow fever from ... 213
Oysters, bacillus typhi in ... 14
"fattening" of ... 377
infection by ... 374–378

Pail-closets cause typhoid fever ... 181–182
Pappataci fever and insects ... 404
Paratyphoid bacilli, see Bacillus paratyphi.
fever ... 58–61
Pediculis vestamenti and typhus fever ... 405–409
Pellagra and insects ... 403
Pencils, bacillus diphtheriæ on ... 193, 233
bacteria on ... 192–193
Personal versus municipal prevention ... 208
Persons, not things, are dangerous ... 225
Phlebotamus ... 404, 405
Physicians, gown and cap for, in contagious cases ... 218
rarely carry disease ... 217
Pigment to lungs from stomach ... 306
Piroplasma bigeminum ... 112, 381–382
Placards for contagious diseases ... 151

PAGE

Plague, air-borne ... 281
and bedbugs ... 414
fleas ... 23, 312–313, 413–416
epidemiological evidence ... 414–415
experimental work ... 414–415
flies ... 419, 425
fomites, experiments in India ... 246–247
observations in Sydney ... 245–246
ground squirrels ... 413
other rodents ... 413–416
rats ... 23, 69–70, 413–416
rugs ... 223
atypical and chronic in animals ... 69–70
human ... 70
bacillus, see Bacillus pestis.
experiments in infection by air ... 312–313
isolation of ... 415–416
not dust-borne ... 289–290
Plasmodium ... 113, 384–385
Pneumococcus cause of meningitis ... 81
in air ... 300
convalescents ... 101
droplets ... 298
dust ... 293–294
normal mouths ... 101–102
may be air-borne ... 289
not dust-borne ... 290
saprophytic ... 26
persistence of ... 101
resistance to drying ... 238
virulence of, in carriers ... 101–102
Pneumonia and water ... 333
Poisoning by food ... 371–372
Poliomyelitis a dust-borne disease ... 278
atypical cases ... 121–122
carried by flies ... 427
carriers of ... 118–121
Privies and water-closets usually filthy ... 179–180
encourage uncleanliness ... 182, 211
infect water supplies ... 320
removal of, causes decrease of typhoid fever ... 181–183
typhoid fever from ... 169–170, 179–183
Privy vaults, bacillus typhi in ... 9–10
Prosodemic infection, typhoid fever by ... 172
Prostatic fluid, bacillus typhi in ... 37
Proteosoma in birds ... 383
Protozoa, difficult to cultivate ... 27
not saprophytic ... 26
resistance to drying ... 242
Protozoan disease, carriers a source of ... 126
latency in ... 111–112
Psocidæ and disease ... 418
Pulex irritans ... 414
Purification of water ... 338–339

PAGE
Pus bacteria 24
distribution of 240
in air 299–300
dust 294
glands 25
schoolrooms 294
skin and mucous surfaces 24
tonsils 24
water 25
may be dust-borne 289–290
on fomites 25
resistance to drying 236–237
saprophytic existence of 24–25

Quarantine and sleeping sickness 401
yellow fever 396
Quinia prevents malaria 386–388

Rabies from milk 366
Radishes, bacillus typhi on 8
Rags and disease 222–223
cholera from 222
erysipelas from 222
flock cough from 222
influenza from 222
scarlet fever from 222
septicemia from 222
smallpox from 222–223
typhoid fever from 222
Railway carriages, bacillus tuberculosis in 292
Rat-proofing of buildings 416
Rats and plague 23, 69–70, 413–416
carriers of plague 70
chronic plague in 69
destruction of 416
Relapsing fever and bedbugs 411–412
lice 412
ticks 410–411
infectious during afebrile period 116
types and parasites 116
Resistance of bacteria less in cultures 11
Rhinitis, bacillus diphtheriæ in 94–95
caused by meningococcus 73
Rhode Island, death rate from typhoid fever 18
Rice, spirillum choleræ in 20
Rocky Mountain fever and ticks 412
Rodents, plague derived from 413–416
Roller towel, bacillus coli communis on 192
should be abolished 210
use of, forbidden 211
Room, bacillus diphtheriæ in 233, 241
tuberculosis in 235
infection cause of typhoid fever in barracks 216
Rooms, infection of 205, 214–215, 219–222

PAGE
Rubella, air-borne 280
Rugs and plague 223

Saliva, inoculation with, cause of lupus 203
  transfer of 189
  vehicle of infection 188–190
Sarcophaga 428
Scarlet fever, air-borne 270–273
    out of doors 272–273
  and books 215
    clothing 217
    coat 215
    fomites 214–215
    house infection 214–215
    letters 215
    milk 346–347
    rags 222
  atypical 107–109
  disinfection unnecessary after 250–252
  due to ice cream 350
  extension in dwellings 196–197
  hospital temporarily closed in Leicester 141
  hospitals in England 139–142
  in cows 346–347
  in Providence 136
  like diphtheria 106–107
  not air-borne from hospitals 272–273
    from soil 28
  virulence varies in 140
Scenopinus fenestralis 428
Schizotrypanum cruzi 404
School children, isolation of 162
  disinfection 254
  teaching cleanliness in 209–210
Schoolrooms, bacillus coli communis in 294
  pus organisms in 294
Screening for protection against malaria 388
  of cases of malaria 388
    yellow fever 396–397
Screens for isolation in French hospitals 198–200
Sedgwick, typhoid fever outbreak in Bondville, Mass. 169
Seltzer water, bacillus typhi in 13
Seminal vesicles, bacillus typhi in 37
Septic infection and insects 417–418
  tank effluent, bacillus typhi in 10
Septicemia from rags 222
Sewer air and bacteria 284–285
    diphtheria 273
    typhoid fever 274–275
  bacillus prodigiosus in 284
    typhi in 284
  infection by 297, 299
Sex of smallpox cases 267
Sheet hung before door to prevent infection 282

PAGE

Shellfish, infection by 374–378
Shipboard, influenza on 277
  malaria on 335
  typhoid fever by contact on 176
Ships for smallpox hospitals 262–263
Shoes as carriers of infection 218
  bacillus diphtheriæ on 240
Shuttle, infection from 192
Sidewalks, virulent bacilli tuberculosis on 194
Simulium 403
Skin, bacteria of suppuration in 24
  hookworms enter through 187
Sleeping sickness, an endemic disease 30
  and tsetse flies 399–401
  atoxyl to prevent 402
  discovery of trypanosome 399–400
  in lower animals 400
  is it carried mechanically? 400–401
  modes of transmission 399–401
  not due to soil infection 30
  per cent of carriers 115–116
  persistence of infection 115–116
  prevention of 401–402
  quarantine 401
Smallpox, air-borne, conclusions 269–270
  evidence against 266–269
  infection of, denied 263–270
    in United States 264–265
  objections to theory 265–266
  sex of cases 267
  and fomites 214
    rags 222–223
  atypical cases 109–110, 133
  carriers 109–110
  hospital ships 262–263
  isolation in, often a failure 147
  mild cases of 109–110
  not from soil 28
  virus, resistance to drying 244
Soft drinks, bacillus typhi in 13
Soil, amebæ dysenteriæ in 24
  bacillus diphtheriæ in 26, 28
    dysenteriæ in 23
    pestis in 22
    tetani in 239
    typhi in 7, 10
  hookworms grow in 186
  infection, cholera from 29
    in common diseases 28
    typhoid fever from 29
  melitensis micrococcus in 21
  not infected with cattle fever 30
    malaria 30
    measles 28

PAGE

Soil, not infected with scarlet fever........ 28
sleeping sickness........ 30
smallpox........ 28
Texas cattle fever........ 30
yellow fever........ 30
spirillum choleræ in........ 19–20
Sore throat and milk........ 351–352
Spanish-American War, typhoid fever in........ 17, 56, 435
from dust in........ 275–276
flies........ 435–436
Spirillum choleræ carried by flies........ 420
found in water........ 326
grow only in human body........ 20
in convalescents........ 61–62
cooked food........ 20
dead bodies........ 19
feces........ 19
gall bladder........ 62
healthy persons........ 62–65
milk........ 19
soil........ 19, 20
water........ 19
intermittent excretion........ 62
resistance to drying........ 237–238, 242, 291–292
saprophytic existence of........ 19
Spirocheta carteri........ 116, 412
duttoni........ 116, 411
Spirochete of syphilis, latency of........ 116
not saprophytic........ 26
resistance to drying........ 239
Spirometer, bacillus diphtheriæ not on........ 241
tuberculosis not on........ 195
Spitting should be forbidden........ 211
Spores may be dust-borne........ 290
resistance to drying........ 232
Springs as sources of infection........ 324
Sputum, bacillus pestis in........ 71
typhi in........ 37–38
Squirrels, see Ground squirrels (Citellus beecheyi).
Stamp out disease, failure to........ 135–136
Stegomyia calopus........ 392, 395, 405
Sterilization of municipal water supplies........ 339
Stomach, bacillus tuberculosis may pass to lungs from........ 305–308
Stomoxys calcitrans........ 428
Storage of water........ 338
Street dust, bacilli tuberculosis not found in........ 292
Streptococcus enteritidis, cause of diarrhea........ 367
in dust........ 282
milk........ 352
may be air-borne........ 289
pyogenes........ 24
salivarius in droplets........ 297
Suppuration, bacteria of, in healthy organs........ 105–106
latency of bacteria of........ 105–106

PAGE

Suppuration, result of infection by bacteria ... 24
Surgery, air-borne infection in ... 283–284
Swine infected by bacillus tuberculosis through the tonsils ... 203–204
  plague bacilli in air ... 300
Syphilis, air-borne infection not possible ... 167
  articles infected with ... 168–169
  believed to be spread by contact ... 164–169
  droplet infection in ... 167
  fomites infection in, not important ... 169
  infection by kissing ... 168
    non-sexual contact ... 168–169
   latency of ... 116
   not persistent ... 168–169
  sexual act chief mode of infection ... 168
  spirochete of, see Spirochete of syphilis.
  spread solely by contact ... 167–168

Tabanus lineola ... 3
Teacher caused diphtheria ... 97
  contracts diphtheria from pupil ... 98
Telephones, bacillus diphtheriæ not on ... 241
    tuberculosis on ... 195
Tetanus and fomites ... 225–226
  bacillus, see Bacillus tetani.
  decrease of, in Havana ... 226
  from lamp wick used for tying umbilical cord ... 5, 226
  in Red Bank, N. J. ... 5
  on Long Island ... 5
Texas cattle fever, an endemic disease ... 30
   carried by tick ... 112
   first disease proved to be carried by insects ... 381–382
   not due to soil infection ... 30
   persistence in blood ... 112
Thermometer transfers bacillus typhi ... 174
Things not so dangerous as persons ... 225
Ticks and relapsing fever ... 410–411
  Rocky Mountain fever ... 412
  Texas cattle fever ... 112, 122, 381–382
Tidal mud, bacillus typhi in ... 8
Tongue, bacillus tuberculosis on ... 203
Tonsillitis and milk ... 351–352
Tonsils, bacillus tuberculosis in ... 203–204
    typhi in ... 34
  bacteria of suppuration in ... 24
  tuberculosis infection through ... 306
    of ... 204
Tools, diphtheria from ... 215
Towel, see Roller towel.
Toys, bacillus diphtheria on ... 240
Tramcars, bacillus tuberculosis in ... 292
Treasurer of United States, investigation of money as carrier of disease by ... 224
Treponema pallida in gummata ... 116
   life of, short ... 167, 169

PAGE
Trier, typhoid fever in ... 17, 57
Trypanosoma bruccei ... 113
equiperdum ... 113
gambiense ... 115, 399–401
Tsetse flies and sleeping sickness ... 115, 399–401
nagana ... 113
Tuberculosis and flies ... 429
fomites, lack of experiments ... 247
laundries ... 219
meat ... 272–273
bacillus, see Bacillus tuberculosis.
bovine, eradication of ... 364
contact infection in ... 204–205
experiments concerning air-borne infection ... 301–311
feeding experiments ... 354–355
from flies ... 429
house infection ... 220–222
milk ... 354–368
amount of ... 356–362
epidemiological evidence ... 361–362
instances of ... 360
protection against ... 362–363
shuttle ... 192
water ... 332–333
human and bovine reciprocally infective ... 353
infection by air ... 194, 202–203
dust questioned ... 302–303
in the home ... 205
stomach ... 305–308
experiments under natural conditions ... 309–311
in alimentary tract ... 203–204
animals through mouth and pharynx 204, 306
laboratory ... 308–309
unnatural conditions of experiment ... 308
mode of infection, evidence from pathology ... 205
of the nose ... 204
tonsils ... 204
proportion of human and bovine types of bacillus 360–361
spread by animals licking one another ... 204
kissing ... 202–203
through tonsils ... 204, 306
Tuberculous milk consumed by children ... 357–360
Typhoid bacillus, see Bacillus typhi.
carriers ... 18, 38–55, 180
cannot be isolated ... 152
cause disease ... 47–54
infective during incubation stage ... 39–40
number of ... 180
opsonic index in ... 42
percentage of ... 40–44
feces in yard ... 170, 173, 182
fever among nurses ... 173–174
an infection of the blood ... 34–35
and gall stones ... 36, 42

PAGE

Typhoid fever and high temperature....374–375
tonsillitis.... 34
atypical....56–59
believed to be an intestinal disease.... 178
by bathing....324–325
contact....17, 47–51, 169–183
in an almshouse.... 175
civil life....171–173
hospitals....173–174, 436
South Africa....171, 436
Spanish War....170–171, 435–436
the family.... 176
on shipboard.... 176
food infection....169–170
prosedemic infection.... 172
carriers of, among different classes....39–44
duration of infection.... 45
causes of excess in cities.... 321
contact outbreaks in cities....172–173
contracted by laundress from soiled linen.... 175
death rate in Rhode Island.... 18
decreases with removal of privies....181–183
filthy habits cause of....170, 173, 182
from bedbugs.... 418
celery.... 379
clothing.... 219
crawfish.... 378
cream.... 349
dust....275–276
flies....169–171, 182–183, 435–447
correlated decrease....442–444
seasonal distribution....439–442
statistical evidence....439–445
fomites.... 227
handling typhoid cultures.... 175
ice cream....349–350
infected bedding.... 175
milk....51–54, 345–346
mud dumped near intake.... 320
pail closets....181–182
privies....169–170, 179–183
rags.... 222
sewer air....274–275
shellfish....374–378
soil infection.... 29
soiled linen.... 219
springs.... 324
thermometer.... 174
unrecognized cases.... 133
water....317–325
watercress....378–379
wind blowing sewage to water works.... 320
houses, infected flies in....421–422
in barracks due to room infection.... 216

PAGE
Typhoid fever in mines ... 182
soldiers' home due to contact infection from physician ... 175
Spanish War ... 17, 56, 435
Trier ... 17
waitress due to contact infection ... 175
infection stopped by strict cleanliness ... 174
less with water closets ... 181–182, 144
mild cases in Panama ... 57
Spanish War ... 56
Trier ... 57
not an intestinal disease ... 34
dust-borne ... 289–290
outbreaks continued by contact infection ... 172–173
in Providence, R. I. ... 18
prevalent in country ... 173
spread among patients by nurses ... 174
by kitchen help ... 175
waitress ... 175
"Typhoid Mary" ... 47
Typhus fever and flies ... 408
lice ... 405–409
carried in shawl ... 409
considered air-borne ... 408
from clothing ... 216–217
identity of strains ... 409
not air-borne ... 281
of extra-corporal origin ... 29

Uncinaria, see Hookworms, Anchylostoma.
americana ... 186
due chiefly to contact ... 186–187
Urine, bacillus typhi in ... 37
persistence of ... 10
cause of Mediterranean fever ... 22

Vaccine, resistance to drying ... 243–244
transport across ocean ... 242–244
Vaginitis in Babies' Hospital ... 165–166
Vegetables, amebæ dysenteriæ on ... 24
bacillus typhi on ... 8
Venereal diseases, see Gonorrhea; Syphilis.
Vincent's angina ... 117

Wage earners, isolation of ... 152, 162–163
Waitress, typhoid fever spread by ... 175
Warning sign in diphtheria ... 151
Washing soiled linen in running streams cause of cholera ... 325
Water and cholera ... 325–326
diarrhea ... 327–329, 331
dysentery ... 326–329, 331
malaria ... 335, 384
pneumonia ... 333

PAGE
Water and the general death rate ... 331
tuberculosis ... 332–333
typhoid fever ... 317–325
worms ... 336
yellow fever ... 336
bacillus typhi in ... 10–13, 319
recovered from ... 319
bacteria of suppuration in ... 25
closets, typhoid fever less with ... 181–182
filtration of ... 338
infection by ... 316–339
of ... 18
milk by ... 323
micrococcus, melitensis in ... 21
mode of infection with typhoid bacilli ... 320
municipal supplies infected ... 320, 326
outbreaks, characteristics ... 317–319
protection of ... 337–338
purification of ... 338–339
spirillum choleræ in ... 19
sterilization of municipal ... 339
storage of ... 338
Watercress, typhoid fever caused by ... 378–379
Wells, amount of typhoid fever due to ... 322–324
cholera infection from ... 325–326
conditions of safety ... 324
infection from ... 316–317, 321–325
protection of ... 337
White diarrhea of chicks ... 71
Whooping cough, air-borne ... 280
not of extra-corporal origin ... 29
Willard State Hospital, diphtheria in ... 144
Wind blowing sewage to water works cause of typhoid fever ... 320
Wool, anthrax from ... 227
spores in ... 226–227
Worms derived from water ... 336
Wounds, infection of, by air ... 300–301

Yellow fever an endemic disease ... 30
and bagging ... 213
ballast ... 213
cloth ... 213
fomites ... 213–214, 394
experiments in Havana ... 245
grain ... 213
mattress ... 213
merchandise ... 213
mosquitoes ... 293–298
oyster buckets ... 213
quarantine ... 396
discovery of causation ... 392–394
latent period in outbreaks ... 393–394
mild and atypical cases ... 117
mosquito destruction ... 397

PAGE

Yellow fever mosquito, habits of.......... 395
not due to soil infection.......... 30
from water.......... 336
preventive measures.......... 396–397
screening of cases and houses.......... 396–397
success of mosquito destruction.......... 391, 395, 397–398
virus filterable.......... 393–394
in blood.......... 393–394